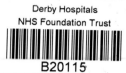
Preventive Dermatology in Infectious Diseases

Robert A. Norman (Ed.)

Preventive Dermatology in Infectious Diseases

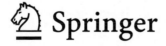 Springer

Editor
Dr. Robert A. Norman
Nova Southeastern University
Ft. Lauderdale, FL, USA and
Private Practice
Tampa
FL, USA

ISBN 978-0-85729-846-1   e-ISBN 978-0-85729-847-8
DOI 10.1007/978-0-85729-847-8
Springer London Dordrecht Heidelberg New York

British Library Cataloguing in Publication Data
A catalogue record for this book is available from the British Library

Library of Congress Control Number: 2011935729

Springer is part of Springer Science+Business Media (www.springer.com)

Foreword

In his latest books, Dr. Rob Norman introduces us to the intriguing concept of preventive dermatology. While dermatologists have long been patient advocates and have stressed vigorously the importance of sun avoidance and protection, there is still much more that we can do to prevent disease.

Dr. Norman and his skilled coterie of collaborators discuss two distinct types of prevention in dermatology: the prevention of skin diseases and the prevention of systemic disorders, some with only very indirect connections to the skin. The first is fairly well known to dermatologists; the second is truly an emerging concept of great importance.

Educational efforts to prevent or at least control skin disease may range from the proper use of sunscreens to weight loss in psoriatic patients, the avoidance of trigger factors in rosacea, proper skin care in atopic dermatitis, or adoption of a low-fat diet to decrease the incidence of actinic keratosis and non-melanoma skin cancer. Another good example is the use of vaccines to protect against diseases such as herpes zoster and genital HPV infection in females.

This book, however, looks beyond the prevention of skin diseases to suggest that dermatologists view their patients through a more holistic lens. This means treating the entire patient not just the skin. Thus Dr. Norman suggests that we be more proactive in addressing health issues such as obesity, smoking, stress management, and nutrition. Consider, for example, the psoriatic patient, whose disease must now be treated as a systemic disorder predisposing to the very serious risks of the metabolic triad.

As dermatologists, we deal with numerous chronic diseases, seeing some patients repeatedly over many years. This longitudinal interaction offers an excellent platform for the practice of preventive dermatology.

Read and enjoy this book. It could make you a better dermatologist.

John E. Wolf Jr., M.D.
Professor and Chairman
Department of Dermatology

Preface

It seems almost counterintuitive to cover dermatology prevention, because so much of what we do in dermatology is based on repair and restructuring of skin maladies. But with the shortage of dermatology providers and the shift to cosmetics and procedures, it is urgent to make sure our patients are given a fair chance to succeed in the fast-changing world of modern healthcare. Although we are specialists in the care of the skin, we are health care providers first, and should treat our patients with a holistic and caring approach that includes prevention.

We live in a world between expectation and reality – and our goal as providers is to help ourselves and our patients anticipate problems and provide solutions. A smoker may have expectations of invincibility. Like many of you, I have succeeded most often in getting the person to quit by appealing to the vanity of the smoker by pointing out the accumulated wrinkles if he or she persists. If that method works, it is a success!

Time's arrow only moves in one direction – forward – and chronological aging takes a toll on all of us, especially visible on the most recognizable features of our facial skin. A rising tide of boomers are arriving daily at the shores of older age and demanding more help, including prevention of skin problems.

Much can be done to prevent the disfiguring effects brought on by the abuse of sun, nicotine and alcohol, excess weight, mobility and exercise difficulties, dysfunctional nutrition, improper hygiene, lack of immunizations, poor reading and comprehension skills, inadequate cosmetic repair, and many other problems. Preventive dermatology focuses on ways we can minimize skin problems, and maximize and enjoy the time we have been given.

We have highly effective sunscreens, a plethora of information about skin care on the internet, and more prevention and treatment modalities than ever before. But even the most informed patients need guidance, and that's why you need the information included in this book. I hope you share this information with your colleagues and patients, and this first book on prevention in dermatology is a springboard for many more books, ideas, and discussions to improve the quality of our lives.

Tampa, FL   Dr. Robert A. Norman

Contents

Contributors

Brian B. Adams Department of Dermatology, University of Cincinnati, Cincinnati, OH, USA

Brian Berman Department of Dermatology and Cutaneous Surgery, University of Miami Miller School of Medicine, Miami, FL, USA

Ivan D. Camacho Department of Dermatology and Cutaneous Surgery, University of Miami Miller School of Medicine, Miami, FL, USA

Gwynn Coatney Department of Family Medicine, University of Medicine and Dentistry of New Jersey, Stratford, NJ, USA

Trisha C. Crisostomo Section of Dermatology, Research Institute for Tropical Medicine, Muntinlupa City, Philippines

Kim K. Dernovsek Departments of Dermatology and Family Medicine, University of Colorado Health Sciences Center, Pueblo, CO, USA

Zoe Diana Draelos Department of Dermatology, Duke University School of Medicine, Durham, NC, USA

Dirk M. Elston Department of Dermatology, Geisinger Medical Center, Danville, PA, USA

Robert Haight Consultant Sarasota, Private Practice Sarasota Florida, Sarasota, FL, USA

Evangeline B. Handog Department of Dermatology, Asian Hospital and Medical Center, Filinvest Corporate City, Muntinlupa, Alabang, Philippines

Camile L. Hexsel Department of Dermatology, Henry Ford Hospital, Detroit, MI, USA

Lisa C. Hutchison Department of Pharmacy Practice, College of Pharmacy, University of Arkansas for Medical Sciences, Little Rock, AR, USA

Oumitana Kajkenova Department of Geriatrics, Thomas and Lyon Longevity Clinic, University of Arkansas for Medical Sciences, Little Rock, AR, USA

Margaret E.M. Kirkup Department of Dermatology, Weston General Hospital, Weston-super-Mare, Avon, UK

Henry W. Lim Department of Dermatology, Henry Ford Hospital, Detroit, MI, USA

Panoglotis Mitropoulos Camp Long Troop Medical Clinic, Suwon-si, Gyeonggi-do, South Korea

Dedee F. Murrell Department of Dermatology, St. George Hospital, University of NSW Medical School, Sydney, NSW, Australia

Robert A. Norman Nova Southeastern University, Ft. Lauderdale, FL, USA and Private Practice, Tampa, FL, USA

Kamaldeep Singh Internal Medicine Resident, Stony Brook University Hospital, Stony Brook, NY, USA

Athena Theodosatos Department of Family Medicine, Florida Hospital, Winter Park, FL, USA

Supriya S. Venugopal Department of Dermatology, St. George Hospital, University of NSW Medical School, Sydney, Australia

Stefan Wöhrl Division of Immunology, Department of Dermatology, Allergy and Infectious Diseases (DIAID), Medical University of Vienna, Vienna, Austria

Lisa C. Hutchison and Oumitana Kajkenova

1.1 Introduction

Adverse drug reactions are defined as noxious or unintended responses to a drug used in standard doses for the purpose of prophylaxis, diagnosis, or treatment.[8] Many side effects to a medication are recognized and accepted as part of the risk/benefit evaluation in determining whether or not it is indicated in a particular patient. For example, diarrhea is a recognized adverse drug reaction associated with the use of erythromycin in 7% of patients.[33] However, it is not an intended response when the drug is used to cure an infection, yet we recognize it as a frequent consequence of oral erythromycin use and are willing to accept this risk in order to achieve the benefit.

Cutaneous drug reactions are one of the most recognized and common types of adverse drug reactions.[35] When asked whether they have allergies or adverse drug reactions, most patients initially report on medications which caused them to have a skin rash with past use. Because most skin rashes develop within 1 week of starting a new medication, this association is reasonable. However, many medications may cause cutaneous reactions after several weeks of therapy and require additional detective work to assess the likelihood of association with a medication. Also, medications cause skin changes that are not immunologic in their mechanism and develop over an extended period of time. Finally, some cutaneous drug reactions may occur in the patient in particular circumstances only

because the patient has an increased risk because of specific time-limited factors. Later use of the same medication may not cause a reaction if the risk factors have resolved.

A focus on prevention of adverse drug reactions has recently gained national prominence. Because treating adverse drug events (which include adverse drug reactions) has been estimated to cost $77 billion in the ambulatory patient population of the United States, prevention of cutaneous drug reactions is not only a preferred patient outcome, it is also a preferred economic outcome.[19] It is imperative for the clinician to be aware of the common cutaneous drug reactions, medications most frequently associated with these reactions and methods to diminish their occurrence and/or severity.

1.1.1 Frequency of Cutaneous Drug Reactions

To identify if one has been successful in reducing the frequency of adverse cutaneous drug reactions, one must first know how often they occur. Several prospective studies have focused upon hospitalized patients and found allergic drug-induced cutaneous reactions to occur in up to 6% of hospitalized patients. A wide variability is seen due to differences in study design, particularly when studies rely upon spontaneous reporting, chart review, or patient recall for information. Table 1.1 provides information from epidemiologic studies on cutaneous drug reactions.

The frequency of cutaneous drug reactions is also related to the relative usage of specific medications that are more likely to cause allergic or other types of skin reactions. In particular, the use of antibiotics in the penicillin family is associated with a higher rate of

L.C. Hutchison (✉)
Department of Pharmacy Practice, College of Pharmacy,
University of Arkansas for Medical Sciences,
Little Rock, AR, USA
e-mail: hutchisonlisac@uams.edu

R.A. Norman (ed.), *Preventive Dermatology in Infectious Diseases*,
DOI 10.1007/978-0-85729-847-8_1, © Springer-Verlag London Limited 2012

Table 1.1 Epidemiologic studies of cutaneous drug reactions

Study	Rate (%)	Comment
Bigby[7]	2.2	Seven-year prospective study in Boston
Hunziker et al.[18]	2.7	Twenty-year prospective study in Switzerland
Naldi et al.[24]	0.01	Spontaneous reporting over 2 years in Italy
Van der Linden et al.[38]	0.36	Retrospective evaluation of medical records over 18 months in The Netherlands
Rademaker et al.[26]	6	Prospective 6 month survey in the hospital setting in New Zealand

cutaneous drug reactions. One study compared the rate of drugs received by at least 1,000 patients reported in nine studies and reported amoxicillin and ampicillin to cause cutaneous drug reactions at a rate of 1.2–8%. Sulfonamides, including co-trimoxazole had a rate of 2.5–3.7% and the rate for cefaclor was 4.8%.[5] Amiodarone will cause a slate blue skin discoloration in 4–9% of patients treated with the drug.[39]

Risk factors have been identified for some allergic cutaneous drug reactions. Infection with human immunodeficiency virus or infectious mononucleosis increases the risk for cutaneous drug reactions. Therefore, an individual who received amoxicillin while infected with mononucleosis may develop a rash; but given the same antibiotic years later, this individual has no reaction. Female sex and either very young age or very old age are inconsistently reported as risk factors.

1.1.2 Serious and Life-Threatening Cutaneous Drug Reactions

Considering that cutaneous drug reactions are the most common type of adverse drug reaction, it is fortunate that they cause serious or life-threatening reactions at a much lower rate. Depending upon the definition of "serious," most reviews place the incidence of serious cutaneous drug reactions in the range of 1/1,000–1/100,000 patients treated whether studied in adults or children.[20,32] Cutaneous skin reactions considered serious are those which cause skin damage or affect multiple organs. In a 6 month prospective

study of hospitalized patients with cutaneous drug reactions, 34% were considered serious because they prompted hospitalization, prolonged hospitalization, or were life-threatening. Only 2% were considered life-threatening, but no deaths were reported.[13]

1.1.3 Preventability of Cutaneous Drug Reactions

For adverse drug reactions in general, studies indicate that 28–57% of those that occur in hospitalized patients are preventable or avoidable.[4,9] However, the preventability rate for cutaneous drug reactions is likely much lower. Many occur upon first exposure to a medication or provide no warning when they occur with a subsequent exposure. Only one study reports assessment of preventability based upon consensus between a dermatologist and a pharmacologist upon retrospective review of the patient records. In this study they determined that 15% of serious cutaneous drug reactions were preventable but did not elucidate beyond providing this rate.[13] This study was limited to allergic cutaneous drug reactions. When one considers the full spectrum of cutaneous drug reactions that includes pharmacologic reactions and cumulative reactions, preventability rates are probably much higher.

1.2 Classification of Adverse Cutaneous Drug Reactions

Adverse drug events, including cutaneous drug reactions, are classified into one of four types.[2] Type A reactions are those that can be anticipated from the pharmacologic properties of the medication. These are expected exaggerations of known pharmacologic effects, may occur at normal doses, and display a dose-dependency. They are nonimmunologic in nature. Few cutaneous drug reactions fall into this category. Type B reactions are usually unexpected reactions, most of which are immune-mediated. Many cutaneous drug reactions fall into this category including urticaria, petechiae, morbilliform reactions, Stevens–Johnson syndrome, and toxic epidermal necrolysis. Type C reactions are associated with cumulative doses of medications over extended periods of time. These are rare for cutaneous drug reactions but include skin discolorations from extended doses of carotenoids or amiodarone. Finally, Type D reactions are delayed effects such as teratogenesis or carcinogenesis and are also rare for cutaneous drug reactions.

1.2.1 Gell-Coombs Classification of Hypersensitivity Reactions

Because the majority of cutaneous drug reactions fall into Type B reactions, it is helpful to further subdivide this category. The Gell-Coombs classification divides immunologically mediated reactions according to pathogenesis.[25,27] This is helpful for investigating the cause of a cutaneous drug reaction or for researchers to find common links. However, one must realize that the Gell-Coombs classification tries to pigeon-hole reactions which may have several mechanisms underlying their development. Nevertheless, the Gell-Coombs classification system remains widely accepted.

Type 1 reactions are immediate reactions that are mediated through IgE immunoglobulins. IgE binds to mast cells causing them to release histamine and other inflammatory mediators. Urticaria, angioedema, pruritis, and anaphylaxis are examples of this type of immune reaction. These reactions occur within minutes to hours after exposure to a medication. Gell-Coombs Type 2 reactions result from the drug combining with cytotoxic antibodies to cause cell lysis. Examples include drug-induced pemphigus and petechia resulting from drug-induced thrombocytopenic purpura.

Gell-Coombs Type 3 reactions are medicated by IgG or IgM immunoglobulins which form immune complexes. These immune complexes are deposited in the basement membrane of small blood vessels and activate complement causing vasculitis or serum sickness. Finally, Gell-Coombs Type 4 reactions are cell-mediated immune reactions causing morbilliform exanthematous rashes, fixed drug eruptions, lichenoid eruptions, Stevens–Johnson syndrome, and toxic epidermal necrolysis.

1.2.2 Clinical Classification

Cutaneous drug reactions may or may not be immunologic in origin and even if they are immunologic in origin, the immunologic classifications do not always clearly follow the clinical picture. For these reasons, a separate classification system based upon the clinical presentation is useful in the discussion of prevention and management.[28]

1.2.2.1 Exanthematous Reactions

Exanthematous reactions are the most common type of cutaneous drug reaction and can be morbilliform or maculopapular. Eruptions usually start on the trunk, spread peripherally, and may be pruritic. With the first exposure to the culprit drug, the patient will produce the reaction in 7–14 days, but with rechallenge the rash occurs more rapidly. Any medication may cause this type of cutaneous drug reaction, but it is most closely associated with the penicillins, sulfonamides, antiepileptic drugs, and nonnucleoside transcriptase inhibitors. Patients with infectious mononucleosis or human immunodeficiency virus have an increased risk of developing exanthematous reactions when treated with a penicillin or sulfonamide.

1.2.2.2 Urticaria and Angioedema

Urticaria is the second most frequent cutaneous drug reaction.[34] Pruritic red wheals of various sizes develop within minutes to hours after exposure to the medication, and occur rapidly upon rechallenge, although intentional rechallenges are rarely attempted. Angioedema may affect only limited parts of the face or neck and is nonpruritic. It may last from 2 h to 5 days. Penicillins and cephalosporins are most commonly associated with urticarial reactions but also consider nonsteroidal anti-inflammatory drugs, phenytoin and carbamazepine as culprits. Angioedema is seen with angiotensin converting enzyme inhibitors.

1.2.2.3 Fixed Drug Eruptions

Fixed drug eruptions are well-delineated lesions dusky red to violet in color that may appear anywhere on the body, primarily the torso, limbs, lips or genitalia. One peculiar feature of fixed drug eruptions is that they will recur in exactly the same location on the body when a patient is rechallenged with the same medication.

Fixed drug eruptions may be confused with macular–papular eruptions, so their reported frequency is likely underestimated. Many drugs can cause fixed drug eruptions including sulfonamides, ciprofloxacin, non-steroidal anti-inflammatory drugs, phenytoin and pseudoephedrine.

1.2.2.4 Drug-Induced Erythema Multiforme, Stevens–Johnson Syndrome, and Toxic Epidermal Necrolysis

Erythema multiforme, Stevens–Johnson syndrome, and toxic epidermal necrolysis are considered severe and life-threatening drug reactions.[20] As such, they require early recognition and discontinuation of all possible offending agents without delay to avoid serious outcomes. Systemic symptoms such as fever, lymphadenopathy, eosinophilia, sore throat, and cough may accompany the skin lesions. Some believe these entities to fit into a continuum with erythema multiforme being self-limited and benign with lesions occurring symmetrically on the extremities and sometimes on the oral mucosa; Stevens-Johnson syndrome always involves at least two mucosal lesions but also includes lesions on multiple organs (eyes, mouth, genitalia, and skin). Detachment of skin occurs over less than 10% of the body surface area in Stevens-Johnson syndrome as compared to toxic epidermal necrolysis, where over 30% of the body surface area may slough off. Patients with toxic epidermal necrolysis must be treated similarly to burn victims with so much skin surface affected.

Causative agents most often identified are phenytoin, carbamazepine, sulfonamides, barbiturates, allopurinol, minocycline, aminopenicillins, and non-steroidal anti-inflammatory agents.[20] The importance of discontinuing all potentially responsible medications cannot be overemphasized. Mortality in one study was 11% for patients who had prompt discontinuation of causative agents compared to 27% when drug withdrawal occurred later.[15]

1.2.3 Associated Nondermatologic Symptoms

Cutaneous reactions must include assessment of associated systemic symptoms along with any skin eruptions.

When systemic symptoms occur, the cutaneous drug reaction is considered to be more serious than when symptoms are limited to the skin and skin structure. Systemic symptoms may be minor or major. Minor symptoms include fever, malaise, and arthralgias. Major symptoms include pharyngitis and lymphadenopathy. Laboratory evidence of a major reaction may be seen such as lymphocytosis, eosinophilia, elevated liver function tests, proteinuria, and renal impairment.[20]

1.3 General Prevention Principles

Luckily most cutaneous drug reactions are self-limiting once the offending agent is discontinued. However, the most basic prevention principle is to avoid using a medication if it is not indicated. Elderly patients in particular seem to be at risk for overprescribing of medication and with each additional drug, the risk of an adverse drug event rises, including the risk for cutaneous drug reactions.[2]

Specific medications have associated recommendations for prevention of cutaneous reactions when the drug is required for therapeutic benefit. These recommendations involve the choice of agent, choice of patient dose, duration of therapy, administration techniques, and monitoring requirements.

1.4 Specific Medications Associated with Cutaneous Reactions

The following discussion provides examples of each type of adverse drug reaction. Type A or pharmacologic adverse reactions are seen with corticosteroids. These are dose-related reactions and can be predicted with long-term use of high dose and high potency corticosteroids. Type B or immunologic adverse cutaneous reactions are seen with anticonvulsants and with tumor necrosis factor alpha inhibitors. However, as our understanding of the mechanisms of reactions increase, our ability to predict who is at greater risk for these reactions to anticonvulsant agents has also grown. Type C or cumulative toxicity is seen with amiodarone skin discoloration. Finally, Type D or delayed effect toxicity is a theoretical risk with topical calcineurin inhibitors which are currently under scrutiny to determine what risk of carcinogenesis they may carry.

1.4.1 Corticosteroids

Both systemic and topical corticosteroids are linked with cutaneous adverse reactions. Long-term use of oral corticosteroids has been implicated in development of localized or disseminated infection caused by grampositive bacteria of the genus *Nocardia*. Cutaneous involvement can manifest as ulceration, cellulitis or subcutaneous abscess.[3] Lipodystrophy was the most frequent adverse event reported during the 3 months use of high dose of prednisone. It has also been considered the most distressing by the patients and was most frequent in women and younger patients. Other skin disorders including hirsutism, spontaneous bruising, and altered wound healing were noted by 46% of patients and were more frequent among women.[12]

Topical corticosteroids cause a multitude of cutaneous adverse effects which were first noted after introduction of higher-potency topical steroids like fludrocortisone.[16] Topical steroids have been classified into very potent, potent, moderately potent, and mild categories. The most common skin change is atrophy. Atrophic skin is described as increased in transparency with increased bruising, tearing, and fragility; the term "cigarette paper consistency" has been used. Telangectasias, striae, and ulcerations may also occur.[31] Topical corticosteroids suppress cell proliferation, reduce collagen synthesis, reduce the thickness of the epidermis and stratum corneum, decrease keratinocyte size, and reduce the number of fibroblasts. Figure 1.1 depicts marked thinning of the skin due to steroid-induced atrophy.

Topical steroids have also been associated with causing acne, rosacea, altered pigmentation, and photosensitization. These reactions occur more commonly with higher potency steroids. Contact sensitization has been reported with a prevalence of 0.2–6%; however, it is more often associated with lower potency nonfluorinated corticosteroids such as hydrocortisone and budesonide.[16]

Cutaneous adverse effects, particularly skin atrophy, from topical corticosteroids can be prevented by following several measures.[6] First, use the least-potent corticosteroid possible for the least amount of time to

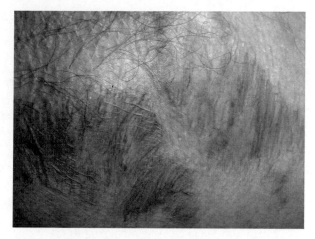

Fig. 1.1 Steroid-induced skin atrophy (Photo courtesy of Charles Goldberg)

obtain therapeutic benefit. If very high potency topical corticosteroids are necessary, consider application only once daily or alternate treatment with nonsteroid therapies. Avoidance of occlusive dressings over the topical corticosteroid will reduce absorption. Use of creams instead of ointments over face, groin, axillae, genital, and perineal areas is recommended because absorption is higher over these sensitive areas. In addition, increased absorption is anticipated over ulcerated or atrophic skin.

1.4.2 Topical Calcineurin Inhibitors

Pimecrolimus cream and tacrolimus ointment have provided a welcome addition to the pharmacological armamentarium against atopic dermatitis. These agents reduce the proliferation of T cells and resultant levels of inflammatory cytokines. The United States Food and Drug Administration has required manufacturers to add a black-box warning and medication guide for patients which communicate that the long-term safety of these agents has not been established and malignancy is a creditable risk with their long-term use.[36] Development of T-cell lymphoma is the primary concern. However, adverse event surveillance in clinical trials and postmarketing has not found a higher rate of malignancies in users of pimecrolimus or tacrolimus. Pharmacokinetic studies indicate that topical application of calcineurin inhibitors results in negligible amounts of systemic absorption. This holds true for children with large percentage of body surface area treated with the medications.[23] It is unlikely that topical calcineurin inhibitors will found to increase the risk for lymphoma, although continued surveillance is warranted.

1.4.3   Anticonvulsants

For many years the anticonvulsants have been tagged with a high frequency of cutaneous reactions, ranging from simple rashes to toxic epidermal necrolysis. Over the decades our understanding of the mechanism by which these reactions occur has grown. Better understanding of the mechanism of cutaneous reactions has led to recommendations for therapy which help to prevent these reactions from occurring. The rash which occurs secondary to anticonvulsant medications is tied to a generalized hypersensitivity reaction that includes fever, lymph node enlargement, and often hepatitis along with mucosal blisters and erythematous skin eruptions.[21] Some investigators have called this syndrome DRESS (drug reactions with eosinophilia and systemic signs).[14] Anticonvulsants are particularly associated with this reaction as it is attributed to an arene oxide metabolite from the aromatic structure of many anticonvulsants. In particular phenobarbital, phenytoin, carbamazepine, and lamotrigine are frequently identified as causative agents.[21,29]

The risk for anticonvulsant cutaneous drug reactions ranges from 1 to 10/10,000.[22,30] These aromatic lipid-soluble drugs are usually oxidized through the cytochrome P450 system into active and inactive metabolites. However, a percentage of the metabolism is routed to form reactive arene oxide metabolites. The percentage which undergoes this pathway of metabolism is generally small, however, if other pathways are inhibited or defective, a higher percentage of the reactive metabolite will be produced, increasing the risk for cutaneous skin reactions.[21,29]

Recently, the United States Food and Drug Administration informed healthcare professionals that dangerous or fatal skin reactions (i.e., Stevens–Johnson syndrome and toxic epidermal necrolysis), can be caused by carbamazepine therapy and are significantly more common in patients with a particular human leukocyte antigen (HLA) allele, HLA-B1502.[37] This allele occurs almost exclusively in patients with ancestry across broad areas of Asia, including South Asian Indians. Patients from these areas should be screened for the HLA-B1502 allele before starting treatment with carbamazepine. If these individuals test positive, carbamazepine should not be started unless the expected benefit clearly outweighs the increased risk of serious skin reactions. However, the reactions generally occur within 2–6 weeks of beginning therapy.[22,30] Patients who have been taking carbamazepine for more than few months without developing skin reactions are at low risk of these events ever developing from carbamazepine. This same mechanism and risk is seen with phenytoin and phenobarbital and cross-reactivity is between 40% and 70%.[21] Therefore, other anticonvulsants such as topiramate, levetiracetam, or gabapentin should be used rather than anticonvulsants with aromatic structures.

Lamotrigine has also been associated with severe cutaneous reactions, and it is metabolized in the same manner as carbamazepine.[17] Therefore, it likely has the same increased incidence in Asian populations. Recommendations to reduce the risk for rash with lamotrigine are to initiate therapy at 25 mg daily for 2 weeks, then increase to 50 mg daily for 2 weeks. Thereafter, doses may be increased by 50–100 mg every week. Other anticonvulsant medications may affect these recommendations because they are potent inducers and inhibitors of the cytochrome P450 system. Lamotrigine increases the levels of the epoxide metabolite of carbamazepine, increasing the risk for toxicity. Other anticonvulsants reduce plasma levels of lamotrigine, requiring higher doses to achieve therapeutic effects.

1.4.4   Tumor Necrosis Factor Alpha Inhibitors

Tumor necrosis factor-alpha inhibitors, such as etanercept (Enbrel), adalimunab (Humira), infliximab (Remicade), and thalidomide have been used in the treatment of autoimmune and lymphoproliferative diseases. Injection site reactions are common but usually minor problems. Incidence in a 6 month study of etanercept was 37%. Urticaria can develop as a part of acute infusion reactions. Current strategies for prevention of acute infusion reactions include premedication with diphenhydramine and acetaminophen 90 min prior to infusion, or use of loratadine for 5 days prior to the infusion. Reactions can also be managed by reducing the rate of infusion. Other adverse cutaneous effects were reported:

- Interstitial granulomatous dermatitis which developed within 1–3 months and in some patients a year later after drug initiation[10]
- Leucoclastic vasculitis, lichenoid eruption, discoid lupus erythematous-like eruption, acute folliculitis, and necrotizing fasciitis,[7,11]

1.4.5 Amiodarone

Amiodarone is an antiarrhythmic agent used for atrial fibrillation, ventricular tachycardia, and several other electrical cardiac disturbances. It has a unique profile of adverse events, causing corneal micro deposits, photosensitivity, thyroid disorders, hepatotoxicity, and pulmonary fibrosis.[39] Unique to amiodarone is the risk for a blue-gray skin discoloration reported to occur in 4–9% of patients treated with the medication. One hypothesis attributed this hyperpigmentation to dermal lipofuscinosis. Macrophages were thought to accumulate lipofuscin in granular sacs and this activity was thought to be related to sunlight because hyper-pigmentation occurs primarily on light-exposed areas of skin. Other researchers note that amiodarone and metabolite concentrations in skin with the blue-gray discoloration have been reported to be 10 times higher than concentrations in nonpigmented skin. One case report of amiodarone associated blue-gray hyperpigmentation showed no lipofuscin pigments leaving the authors to conclude that drug and metabolite deposits in the photo-exposed skin was the primary mechanism of the reaction.[1]

Prevention of the blue-gray hyperpigmentation is related to reducing exposure to the medication. The lowest effective dose should be used for the shortest possible time. Case reports of this cutaneous adverse effect occur after an average of 20 months of treatment. Reversal occurs years after discontinuation of the drug. A cumulative dose of at least 160 g of amiodarone is required for the reaction to occur which is commonly achieved within 3 years of initiation of therapy at an average dose of 200 mg daily.

1.5 Conclusion

Adverse cutaneous drug reactions are common, but most are not severe or life-threatening. The most effective means for prevention of these reactions is to reduce medication exposure by discontinuing medications that are not indicated, using the lowest effective dose and limiting the duration of therapy.

References

1. Ammoury A, Michaud S, et al Photodistribution of blue-gray hyperpigmentation after amiodarone treatment: molecular characterization of amiodarone in the skin. Arch Dermatol. 2008;144(1):92–96
2. Atkin PA, Veitch PC, et al The epidemiology of serious adverse drug reactions among the elderly. Drugs Aging. 1999;14(2):141–152
3. Baldi BG, Santana AN, et al Pulmonary and cutaneous nocardiosis in a patient treated with corticosteroids. J Bras Pneumol. 2006;32(6):592–595
4. Bates DW, Leape LL, et al Incidence and preventability of adverse drug events in hospitalized adults. J Gen Intern Med. 1993;8(6):289–294
5. Bigby M. Rates of cutaneous reactions to drugs. Arch Dermatol. 2001;137(6):765–770
6. Brazzini B, Pimpinelli N. New and established topical corticosteroids in dermatology: clinical pharmacology and therapeutic use. Am J Clin Dermatol. 2002;3(1):47–58
7. Chan AT, Cleeve V, et al Necrotising fasciitis in a patient receiving infliximab for rheumatoid arthritis. Postgrad Med J. 2002;78(915):47–48
8. Cousins DD. Medication Use: A Systems Approach to Reducing Errors. Oakbrook Terrace, IL: Joint Commission on Accreditation of Healthcare Organizations; 1998
9. Cullen DJ, Bates DW, et al The incident reporting system does not detect adverse drug events: a problem for quality improvement. Jt Comm J Qual Improv. 1995;21(10):541–548
10. Deng A, Harvey V, et al Interstitial granulomatous dermatitis associated with the use of tumor necrosis factor alpha inhibitors. Arch Dermatol. 2006;142(2):198–202
11. Devos SA, Van Den Bossche N, et al Adverse skin reactions to anti-TNF-alpha monoclonal antibody therapy. Dermatology. 2003;206(4):388–390
12. Fardet L, Flahault A, et al Corticosteroid-induced clinical adverse events: frequency, risk factors and patient's opinion. Br J Dermatol. 2007;157(1):142–148
13. Fiszenson-Albala F, Auzerie V, et al A 6-month prospective survey of cutaneous drug reactions in a hospital setting. Br J Dermatol. 2003;149(5):1018–1022
14. Gaig P, Garcia-Ortega P, et al Drug neosensitization during anticonvulsant hypersensitivity syndrome. J Investig Allergol Clin Immunol. 2006;16(5):321–326
15. Garcia-Doval I, LeCleach L, et al Toxic epidermal necrolysis and Stevens-Johnson syndrome: does early withdrawal of

causative drugs decrease the risk of death? *Arch Dermatol.* 2000;136(3):323–327

16. Hengge UR, Ruzicka T, et al Adverse effects of topical glucocorticosteroids. *J Am Acad Dermatol.* 2006;54(1):1–15; quiz 16–18

17. Hilas O, Charneski L. Lamotrigine-induced Stevens-Johnson syndrome. *Am J Health Syst Pharm.* 2007;64(3): 273–275

18. Hunziker T, Kunzi UP, et al Comprehensive hospital drug monitoring (CHDM): adverse skin reactions, a 20-year survey. *Allergy.* 1997;52(4):388–393

19. Johnson JA, Bootman JL. Drug-related morbidity and mortality. A cost-of-illness model. *Arch Intern Med.* 1995; 155(18):1949–1956

20. Knowles SR, Shear NH. Recognition and management of severe cutaneous drug reactions. *Dermatol Clin.* 2007; 25(2):245–253, viii

21. Krauss G. Current understanding of delayed anticonvulsant hypersensitivity reactions. *Epilepsy Curr.* 2006;6(2):33–37

22. Mockenhaupt M, Messenheimer J, et al Risk of Stevens-Johnson syndrome and toxic epidermal necrolysis in new users of antiepileptics. *Neurology.* 2005;64(7):1134–1138

23. Munzenberger PJ, Montejo JM. Safety of topical calcineurin inhibitors for the treatment of atopic dermatitis. *Pharmacotherapy.* 2007;27(7):1020–1028

24. Naldi L, Conforti A, et al Cutaneous reactions to drugs. An analysis of spontaneous reports in four Italian regions. *Br J Clin Pharmacol.* 1999;48(6):839–846

25. Posadas SJ, Pichler WJ. Delayed drug hypersensitivity reactions – new concepts. *Clin Exp Allergy.* 2007;37(7): 989–999

26. Rademaker M, Oakley A, Duffill MB. Cutaneous adverse drug reactions in a hospital setting. *N Z Med J.* 1995; 108(999):165–166

27. Rajan TV. The Gell-Coombs classification of hypersensitivity reactions: a re-interpretation. *Trends Immunol.* 2003; 24(7):376–379

28. Riedl MA, Casillas AM. Adverse drug reactions: types and treatment options. *Am Fam Physician.* 2003;68(9):1781–1790

29. Roychowdhury S, Svensson CK. Mechanisms of drug-induced delayed-type hypersensitivity reactions in the skin. *Aaps J.* 2005;7(4):E834–E846

30. Rzany B, Correia O, et al Risk of Stevens-Johnson syndrome and toxic epidermal necrolysis during first weeks of antiepileptic therapy: a case-control study. Study Group of the International Case Control Study on Severe Cutaneous Adverse Reactions. *Lancet.* 1999;353(9171):2190–2194

31. Schoepe S, Schacke H, et al Glucocorticoid therapy-induced skin atrophy. *Exp Dermatol.* 2006;15(6):406–420

32. Segal A, Doherty K, et al Cutaneous reactions to drugs in children. *Pediatrics.* 2007;120(4):e1082–e1096

33. Semla TP, Beizer JL, et al *Geriatric Dosage Handbook.* Hudson, OH: Lexi-Comp; 2006.

34. Shipley D, Ormerod AD. Drug-induced urticaria. Recognition and treatment. *Am J Clin Dermatol.* 2001;2(3): 151–158

35. Svensson C, EW C, et al Cutaneous drug reactions. *Pharmacol Rev.* 2000;53(3):357–379

36. U.S. Food and Drug Administration, (March 10, 2005). FDA Public Health Advisory Elidel (Pimecrolimus) Cream and Protopic (Tacrolimus) Ointment. Retrieved 21 December 2009, from http://www.fda.gov/Drugs/DrugSafety/PublicHealthAdvisories/ucm051760.htm

37. U.S. Food and Drug Administration, (December 12, 2007). Information for Healthcare Professionals: Dangerous or Even Fatal Skin Reactions - Carbamazepine (marketed as Carbatrol, Equetro, Tegretol, and generics). Retrieved 21 December 2009, from http://www.fda.gov/Drugs/DrugSafety/PostmarketDrugSafetyInformationforPatientsandProviders/ucm124718.htm

38. van der Linden PD, van der Lei J, et al Skin reactions to antibacterial agents in general practice. *J Clin Epidemiol.* 1998;51(8):703–708

39. Vassallo P, Trohman RG. Prescribing amiodarone: an evidence-based review of clinical indications. *JAMA.* 2007; 298(11):1312–1322

Xerosis and Stasis Dermatitis

2

Margaret E.M. Kirkup

2.1 Introduction

Dry skin and stasis dermatitis are common conditions of senescence although they can occur at any age given the predisposing constitutional or environmental factors.

In this chapter, I will attempt to describe the differences between dry and normal skin and the influences which can contribute to dryness with emphasis on those which are reversible before a clinical problem develops. In addition, I shall discuss the nature of and preventative measures possible in stasis dermatitis.

Knowledge of the microstructure of the epidermis, particularly the stratum corneum, is important in understanding how dry skin occurs and the efficacy of the preventative measures which are available. Stasis dermatitis, a common condition of the lower limb, is due to failure of the tissue drainage mechanisms. The result is abnormality of appearance of the skin including discoloration, followed by inflammation. Ultimately fibrosis and ulceration can occur.

Prevention of dry skin requires avoiding contact with irritant substances, attention to the environment of the skin, and regular application of moisturizing and emollient agents. Prevention of stasis dermatitis requires avoidance of pooling of blood and tissue fluids in the lower limbs by exercise, weight control, and prompt and continuous treatment of vein and lymphatic disease. Also required is prevention of localized xerosis with its loss of skin-barrier function that leaves the limbs vulnerable to dermatitis.

M.E.M. Kirkup
Department of Dermatology, Weston General Hospital,
Weston-super-Mare, Avon, UK
e-mail: maggie@kirkup.plus.com

The fact that there is no universally accepted definition of dry skin has hampered research in this area. It may be perceived as cosmetic rather than pathological by some physicians. Indeed there is a spectrum of severity from a few dry patches on the face to a generalized pruritic condition. Dry skin can be severe and symptomatic, involving a detrimental effect on quality of life. Left untreated, it may be major reason for itching, especially in the elderly. Dry skin can be constitutional or hereditary. It can be acquired by poor skin care or contact with irritants, including friction and exposure. It can also be a component sign of skin disease such as atopic eczema or associated with systemic diseases, including renal failure, thyroid disease, and malignancies. The term xerosis (Greek *xeros* > dry) is frequently used interchangeably with "dry skin." Dry skin is considered here to mean skin which is free of dermatological disease but which feels dry and rough to the touch. The surface appears to lack the normal, smooth, slightly oily feel and can appear to be covered in white powdery flakes. In established cases, the skin has a mosaic-like appearance sometimes described as "crazy paving" or eczema *craquelé* (Fig. 2.1). Such skin will often be described as feeling "tight" and will lack elasticity. It can and often does itch. It has a tendency to worsen in winter but can also be exacerbated by sun exposure. Dry skin is vulnerable to damage from friction, shearing forces, and trauma. This can lead to development of fissures, which heal poorly. Dry skin shows increased penetration by substances, rendering it more susceptible to development of irritant contact dermatitis.[1]

Chronic stasis dermatitis has several synonyms, including gravitational eczema, venous stasis eczema, and varicose eczema. The onset is gradual after many months or years of venous hypertension or lymphedema, signs of which may be relatively subtle

R.A. Norman (ed.), *Preventive Dermatology in Infectious Diseases*,
DOI 10.1007/978-0-85729-847-8_2, © Springer-Verlag London Limited 2012

clinically when the skin changes begin to appear. Failure of drainage of the skin and subcutaneous tissue of the leg due to inadequacy of the venous or lymphatic systems leads to malnourishment of those tissues and poor oxygenation of the cells. However, the mechanism of development of dermatitis is unclear. The epidermal changes are speculated to be secondary to alterations in the function of the dermal blood vessels.[2] Signs of chronic venous stasis disease include edema, varicosities of the veins due to failure of the valves in the superficial venous system or perforating veins and variable skin changes. There is extravasation of blood into the skin which is clinically seen as hemosiderin staining (Fig. 2.2). Dryness and erythema are common features.

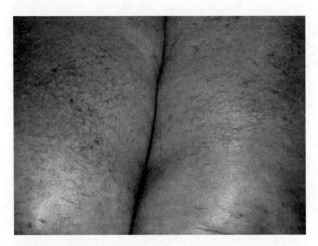

Fig. 2.1 Eczema Craquelé on the thighs

2.2 Xerosis

2.2.1 Pathogenesis of Xerosis

The major component of the skin which is altered when dryness occurs is the epidermis, principally the stratum corneum. Stratum corneum consists of the terminally differentiated keratinocytes known as corneocytes. Corneocytes are fl attened in shape compared to the keratinocytes in the deeper layers of the epidermis. They have no nucleus and consist of a cell envelope surrounding a compacted mass of keratin and amorphous matrix. Part of this intracellular matrix is a complex mixture of compounds described as the natural moisturizing factor, the function of which seems to be to retain water in the stratum corneum. The corneocytes are arranged rather like a brick wall, the mortar of which consists mainly of a bilayer of lipid. The effect of this layer is to waterproof the skin, preventing evaporation and waterlogging, yet allow diffusion of hydrophilic materials.

The cells of the epidermis are held together by desmosomes. In the stratum corneum the corresponding structures, the corneodesmosomes, break down naturally allowing the spent cells to be shed imperceptibly. Water is necessary for the activity of the enzymes involved in this process. In xerotic skin there is failure of the corneocytes to be shed in the normal way. The corneodesmosomes do not break down at the normal rate and the cells are shed in clumps, perceived macroscopically as scale and roughness (Fig. 2.3). The rough,

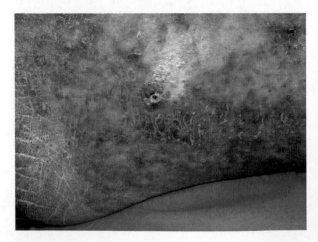

Fig. 2.2 Venous stasis disease showing early ulceration, xerosis, and hemosiderin staining

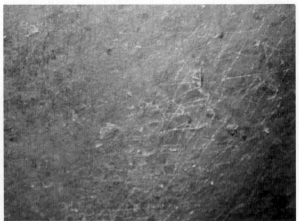

Fig. 2.3 Very dry skin in an elderly lady

dry appearance and feeling is due to this dysfunctional desquamation but also due to increased evaporation of water and reduction in intercellular lipid.

Dry skin cannot perform all of its functions. Being in direct contact with the external environment, the epidermis is particularly vulnerable to physical and chemical influences. Dry skin has reduced barrier function, which renders it more vulnerable to these environmental influences. This loss of function is in part due to the reduced levels of lipid and in part due to the dehydration of the cellular component, allowing the skin to fissure and permitting entry of chemical substances and microbiological invaders.

In most cases, it is likely that a combination of genetic predisposition and environmental influences are involved. Individual thresholds for barrier function breakdown are very variable. Contributing environmental factors are

- Cold
- Heat
- Wind
- Low humidity
- Ultraviolet radiation
- Soaps, detergents, and other cleaning products
- Friction

Systemic medication may contribute to dry skin. For example, diuretics which are very widely used may have a dehydrating effect on the skin and retinoids have an effect on keratinization with a dose-related drying effect.

Measuring skin dryness is essential in experimental work but is of no practical use in a clinical setting. Among the measures commonly used are electrical impedance, which is an indicator of the water content by its ability to conduct electricity, and transepidermal water loss (TEWL), an indicator of the protective skin barrier function.

2.2.2 Epidemiology of Xerosis

Studies reveal that xerosis is one of the most common abnormalities of older skin.[3,4] Some evidence suggests that females are more likely to describe their skin as dry at all ages[5] and dry skin was found to be more common in females than males in study of non-institutionalized older individuals.[3] Clinically

recognizable xerosis is most common on the face and lower legs and is of increased prevalence with increasing age. Institutionalized elderly people are at particular risk due to the conditions of low humidity and high environmental temperatures often to be found in care homes and hospitals. Prevalence rates of 29–58% are reported in nursing home patients.[6,7] It is more diffi-cult to perform epidemiological studies in non-institutionalized people and studies in unselected populations are sparse. Epidemiological studies of skin do not always include xerosis as a pathological condition. However, there is a high prevalence of xerosis reported in several studies of patients attending dermatology facilities.[8,9]

While women are more likely than men to complain of dry skin, inflamed dry skin known as asteatotic eczema is more common in men.[10,11] Outdoor workers are at risk because of exposure to the effect of temperature extremes, UV radiation, and wind. Definition of dry skin and cultural values make it difficult to compare populations. There is some evidence that immigrant men from East Asia, the Middle East, and North Africa are more aware of dry skin than other groups following migration to a Western community.[12]

2.2.3 Prevention of Xerosis

Prevention of dry skin and treatment of established cases follow the same principles. These are avoidance of aggravating factors, manipulation of the micro-environment of the skin surface, and application of topical agents to enhance or support the functions of the stratum corneum. There is limited evidence of benefit from systemic pharmaceutical agents.

2.2.3.1 Manipulation of the External Environment of the Skin

The environment needs to be manipulated to avoid the skin being exposed to extremes of temperature. Suitable clothing should be worn to protection against wind, rain, and sunlight. Use of sun-protective topical agents may help in two ways, both by preventing UV radiation damage to the DNA of the skin cells and by having a moisturizing effect. Clothing is being developed which is made from very fine, smooth fibers which may have a place in primary prevention of xerosis. Measures should be taken to increase the humidity of the local environment. This may require reduction in ambient temperature or adjustment of the time exposed to air conditioning or central heating. Some additional increase in moisture in the air may be gained by placing open containers of water around the home or workplace. Indoor plants may also help.

2.2.3.2 Personal Care

Since indoor bathrooms became commonplace in the twentieth century, there has been a tendency toward frequent showering and bathing. Millions are spent every year on advertising soaps, shower and bath gels, and shampoos. We are encouraged to believe that we should be sweet-smelling at all times and over-washing may be a factor in development of xerosis. Water, soap, and detergent skin-washing liquids are generally the most common irritants applied to the skin. In my experience, many people with dry, itchy skin find the application of water gives temporary relief and reduces the feeling of dryness. They may need considerable persuasion to convince them to reduce excess contact with water that, in the long term, is damaging their skin.

There is a huge industry involved in developing and marketing skin cleansing products. A study of commonly used soaps and cleansers in Mexico showed that the majority of washing agents were irritants as assessed by a 5 day patch test technique.[13] Soaps, soap-free cleansers, shampoos, shower and bath gels and creams may be described as "moisturizing" but as a general rule contain surfactants which strip the natural lipid from the stratum corneum, contributing to dryness. Reducing washing frequency and use of soap-substitutes goes a long way toward preventing xerosis.

2.2.3.3 Topical Agents

Almost any moisturizer or emollient can be used as a soap-substitute or applied directly to the skin. Emollients are skin softeners, reducing the feeling of roughness; moisturizers also add water to the epidermis, improving its function. In practice, they can be used interchangeably in most cases and the terms are often used as synonyms. Instruction needs to be given in how to use these products. While they can be added to very hot water and whipped into a suspension or emulsion, allowing use as a liquid skin cleanser, it is equally effective to use these products by applying them directly to the skin. Gentle removal with sponge or flannel in the bath or shower is cleansing and leaves a pleasant layer of the product on the skin. The water must not be very hot or cold. Moisturizers and emollient preparations containing antimicrobial agents may be helpful on a short-term basis where scratching or other skin trauma increases the risk of infection. Bath oils and liquid emollients added to the bath water, form a film on the surface of the water. Some of this will cling to the skin on leaving the bath giving additional benefit. Emollients and moisturizers can cause the surface of the bath to be slippery and extra care is required to avoid falls, particularly in children and the elderly.

After bathing, the skin should be gently patted dry with a soft towel to avoid frictional trauma and a further layer of emollient or moisturizer applied. Ideally this should be done before the skin is quite dry. Emollient or moisturizer should be reapplied throughout the day to protect from the environment and prevent development of signs of dryness. The frequency of application will depend partly on the severity of the xerosis or tendency to dryness but should be at least twice daily. Social circumstances and clothing may well have an influence on what is practical.

2.2.3.4 Moisturizing

As well as spending vast sums of money on production and advertising of skin cleansers, the cosmetics and toiletries industries are investing heavily in developing and advertising moisturizers. While those at risk from genetic and environmental factors are well-advised to be liberal with applications of moisturizing agents, what is the evidence that regular moisturizing actually prevents dryness in those at low risk? There is good evidence that regular moisturizing reduces the incidence of irritant dermatitis in those at risk and prevents recurrence of the dry skin, suggesting that primary prevention would also be effective.[14] Moisturizing has been shown to have a significantly protective effect against detergents in healthy volunteers.[15]

2.2.4 *Choice of Moisturizer and Soap-Substitute*

The range of moisturizers available is vast and includes lotions (solutions, suspensions or emulsions of lipid and water) creams (emulsions of water in oil or oil in water), ointments (with hydrophilic or hydrophobic bases), pastes (solids suspended in a base), and gels.[16] The ideal emollient might be a simple preparation, such as soft white paraffin, which softens the skin and provides a waterproof film, preventing contact with irritants and preventing evaporation of water from the stratum corneum. However, it is not always cosmetically acceptable to use and can stain clothing and make skin surface slippery, reducing grip. A balance has to be struck between cosmesis and effectiveness. The best topical agent is the one which the individual will actually use and it may take some time to find the best one for each individual. Compromise between effectiveness and cosmetic acceptability may be necessary.

When xerosis is established, it can take many weeks of persistence with a good moisturizing regimen before normal skin barrier function is restored. Secondary prevention in the form of continued moisturizing and avoidance of irritants is wise.

Moisturizers and emollient ingredients vary. While the best combination for any given patient may be found by trial and error, it can be useful for healthcare professionals to have some knowledge of the constituents of these products. Ideally, the chosen preparation should include a humectant, which retains or attracts water, and a grease or lipid to act as a waterproof barrier, preventing evaporation of water and protecting the skin from the influences of an adverse environment. Examples of humectants are lactic acid, glycerol, and urea. Some products also contain physiological lipids, which may improve the differentiation of the epidermis and may help reform the lipid bilayer.[17] Additional ingredients such as ammonium lactate may improve the efficacy by keratolysis, thus normalizing desquamation. The risk of skin irritation and development of contact allergy is reduced by careful selection of products to avoid irritant and allergenic ingredients. It may also be necessary to select different products for different areas of the body and for different times of day; a heavier, greasier product may be more acceptable at night than before dressing for the day. A compromise product is better than none.

Ingredients used in emollient and moisturizer manufacture are shown in Table 2.1. Most commercial products will also contain preservatives, perfumes, and emulsifying agents and some contain coloring materials.

2.2.5 *Adverse Effects of Moisturizing*

Serious reactions are rare but allergic contact dermatitis to contents of these products can occur. Irritant dermatitis

Table 2.1 Ingredients commonly used in emollients and moisturizers

Ingredient	Example	Primary function
Water	–	Adds moisture
Fats and oils	Liquid paraffin, petrolatum	Prevents evaporation
Physiological lipid	Cholesterol, ceramides	Prevent evaporation and may play a role in restoration of function of the stratum corneum
Humectant	Glycerol, lactic acid, urea	Restore water content of stratum corneum
Antioxidants	Tocopherols, gallates	Inhibit oxidation
Keratolytics	Ammonium lactate	Enhancelysis of corneodesmosomes
Preservative (antimicrobial)	Parabens, alcohol	Reduce microbial growth in opened container
Emulsifying agent	Stearic acid, palmitic acid, sodium lauryl sulfate	Collect at interface of two phases to promote emulsification
Perfumes		Increase acceptability of the product
Color	–	Increase acceptability of the product

is more common with frequent and prolonged use of preparations containing potential irritants such as sodium lauryl sulfate. Humectants such as urea and lactic acid are associated with causing a subjective sensation in some individuals.[16]

2.2.6 Specific Body Areas

Some areas of the body may require special attention. Among these are hands, feet, and flexures.

2.2.6.1 Hands

Those in occupations which involve frequent unavoidable exposure to water, such as domestic cleaners, catering workers, healthcare workers, hairdressers, and bar staff will need additional advice on protection of the hands. Dry skin is the precursor to irritant hand eczema. It is always best to place a barrier between the skin and the water where possible. Gloves form a better barrier than topical agents. Gloves need to be appropriate to the task and may not be easily accepted. Powdered latex must be avoided to reduce the risk of latex allergy. Hand washing with an emollient is acceptable in most settings but liberal and frequent application of emollients or moisturizers after washing or other exposure to water is also vital. Wearing gloves in cold and wet weather will also help prevent drying of the skin. Cotton gloves can be useful to wear after liberal application of topical agents.

2.2.6.2 Feet

The skin on the soles of the feet is thick, mainly due to hyperkeratosis of the stratum corneum, maximal on weight-bearing areas. While this is likely to be a physiological response it is more pronounced with advancing age and with obesity and is exacerbated by frictional stresses including ill-fitting footwear. This thick epidermal layer tends to desiccate and crack especially in middle age and beyond, leading to fissures which can be deep, painful, and slow to heal. The thick layer itself can cause difficulty with walking and shoe-fitting. Paring away the build-up of thick skin may give temporary relief but the skin responds by rebuilding the thick stratum corneum unless measures are taken to alter the local environment of the feet. Application of emollients will soften the hyperkeratotic skin and improve comfort while helping reduce further build-up. Particular care is needed in those with diabetes and peripheral ischemia.

2.2.6.3 Flexures

Body flexures are vulnerable areas because the epidermis tends to be thin with a thin stratum corneum and because the skin folds can trap topical agents and irritants if not adequately cleansed. Build-up of sweat, retained cleaning agents and other applications such as talcum powder can contribute to the development of irritation.

2.2.7 Occupational Factors

In the workplace and in domestic cleaning, it is essential to avoid direct contact of the skin and irritants. Water is an irritant, especially if contact is prolonged. Protective gloves are widely available. The gloves chosen need to be appropriate for the task. Nonpowdered latex should be avoided as it increases the risk of sensitization to latex. It is the duty of the employer to ensure that appropriate gloves and other protective clothing are available but it is the duty of the employee to make sure that they use them. Training may be required.

Regulations exist to protect the workforce against extremes of temperature. Control of humidity is less well-regulated.

2.3 Stasis Dermatitis

2.3.1 Introduction

Stasis dermatitis affects the lower legs bilaterally, often beginning insidiously on the shin or "gaiter" area above the ankles. It is believed to be due to stasis of tissue fluids but is an under-researched condition. The stasis may not be clinically overt when the skin changes present. Reduced efficacy of the activity of the drainage mechanisms of the lower limbs results in inflammation and gross changes of appearance of the skin. Etiology can be multifactorial; lymphatic or venous obstruction or insufficiency may be implicated. Lymphatic drainage can be overwhelmed and impaired by systemic disease of the cardiovascular, renal or hepatic systems and by obstruction to the drainage by lymphatic involvement in malignancy or obesity. Local damage to the lymphatics can occur after deep venous thrombosis (DVT), repeated attacks of cellulitis, or as a result of trauma. Congenital lymphatic insufficiency can be symptomless until adult life. Venous disease may be overt as in DVT or varicose veins but can occur insidiously in immobility and advancing age when lymphatic insufficiency is likely to be worsened by venous stasis. Obesity compounds the problem whatever primary cause is involved due to increased hydrostatic pressure, which can overcome the capacity to drain the interstitial tissues. Flow may also become retrograde when the limbs are dependent and immobile.

2.3.2 Pathogenesis of Stasis Dermatitis

The pathogenesis of stasis dermatitis has not been fully elucidated. Poorly drained skin demonstrates changes microscopically before clinical problems present. The lymphatics are dilated, dermal blood vessel walls thicken and passage of fluid and cells in either direction becomes impaired. The inflammatory process leading to stasis dermatitis seems to involve white blood cells sequestration in postcapillary venules which increases cell adhesion leading to leucocyte activation in the superficial dermal microvasculature.[2] This process becomes self-perpetuating. Left untreated the process leads to fibrosis and ultimately ulceration. Extravasated blood cells cannot reenter the circulation and are broken down slowly in situ leading to hemo-siderin staining (Fig. 2.2). The skin becomes xerotic and inflammation ensues. Dry skin may itch and scratching may be the final straw in developing signs of dermatitis. However, itch is not a prominent clinical feature in many cases. The "gaiter" area just above the ankles seems to be the most vulnerable site and this is the most common site for development of ulceration if stasis problems are not addressed.

2.3.3 Epidemiology of Stasis Dermatitis

There is a slight female preponderance in this condition. Females have increased risk factors for the conditions which predispose to the development of the underlying stasis. Frequency increases with advancing age. It is estimated that 2–5% of the adult population of the United States shows changes associated with venous insufficiency.

2.3.4 Predisposing Factors to Stasis Dermatitis

Factors predisposing to stasis dermatitis are:

- Obesity
- Cardiac failure
- Immobility
- Renal failure
- Advancing age
- Hepatic failure
- Xerosis
- Hypothyroidism
- Venous disease
- Hypoalbuminemia
- Lymphatic obstruction
- Malignancy
- Smoking

2.3.5 Prevention of Stasis Dermatitis

Primary prevention of stasis dermatitis requires correction of the condition of tissue fluid stasis, reducing pressure on the venous or lymphatic return. This restores the physiological state of tissues toward normal. Depending on the underlying predisposition, it may not be possible to completely correct the problem.

Leg elevation, exercise of the lower leg musculature, compression hosiery, and prevention of xerosis, as outlined above, all have a part to play.

2.3.5.1 Leg Elevation

Dependency of the lower limb causes the drainage systems to be under conditions of increased hydrostatic pressure. Simple elevation of the legs when at rest will relieve this pressure. This can be achieved by recumbence with raising of the foot end of the bed. There are many comfortable chairs available which include the facility to raise the feet at least level with the hips.

2.3.5.2 Exercise

The calf muscles act as a pump, aiding venous and lymphatic return. Simple exercises to increase the activity of these muscles are a useful adjunct to management and help prevent the condition. Exercises can be performed while sitting or recumbent.[18,19]

2.3.5.3 Compression

Where it is not possible to restore the drainage to normal, external support in the form of compression hosiery or bandaging will encourage fluid into the deep venous or lymphatic system and reduce the tissue fluid pressure in the skin. Compression must not be introduced if it will compromise the arterial supply of the limb or if there is any infection present. It is essential to palpate the limb pulses and observe for signs of ischemia. If there is doubt, Doppler studies of the pressure in the peripheral arteries give an indication of suitability for compression but it may be necessary to formally investigate for arterial disease surgeon before proceeding. A useful rule of thumb is not to introduce compression if the ankle bra-chial pressure index (ABPI) is greater than 0.8. The method of measuring ABPI is shown in Table 2.2.

There are many suppliers of compression hosiery and many different methods of classification of the degree of support provided by the products. Compression hosiery classifications vary from country to country. Examples of the systems in use are shown in Table 2.3.

The higher the class of garment, the lower is the likelihood of compliance. There is some evidence that there is little difference in reduction of edema between classes I and II in preulcer states.[20] Therefore, to optimize compliance, class I compression may be sufficient for prevention. As few as 21% of those prescribed compression for venous disease use the compression on a daily basis.[21] The more compressive the garment, the more difficult it is to put on, the higher grades requiring considerable dexterity and strength. The

Table 2.2 Ankle brachial pressure index (ABPI)

Measure blood pressure in brachial artery as normal
Apply blood pressure cuff to lower limb and inflate
Use handheld Doppler probe over the posterior tibial artery and dorsalis pedis artery in turn to measure systolic

ABPI = systolic pressure at ankle divided by the systolic pressure at brachial artery. For example, with blood pressure of 170/80 and post tibial pressure of 150, the ABPI = 0.88

Table 2.3 Classification of compression hosiery in various countries

	UK (mmHg)	France (mmHg)	Germany (mmHg)	USA (mmHg)
Class 1	14–17	10–15	18–21	15–30
Class 2	18–24	15–20	23–32	30–40
Class 3	25–35	20–36	34–46	40+

physical act of putting on compression hosiery can be extremely difficult or impossible for those who have impaired joint mobility, flexibility, weakness, or cognitive dysfunction. Many suppliers can provide aids to assist but there is no substitute for having someone to help.

2.3.5.4 Emollients

Emollient therapy as outlined above is the most appropriate topical therapy for reducing the appearance of stasis dermatitis. Xerosis is an important part of the pathophysiology of the condition. Application is easier if there is someone to help as the lower legs can be out of reach of many obese, elderly, ill people. Application is best done by smoothing the agent on in the direction of hair growth to avoid occlusion of follicles.

2.3.5.5 Pharmaceutical Interventions

There is unconfirmed evidence that oral flavonoids, which are botanical antioxidants, are venotropic and can help reverse venous stasis disease.[22] Other pharmaceutical agents such as the angiogenesis inhibitor calcium dobesilate and xanthine derivative pentoxy-fyline may have a role in management of established stasis dermatitis but their place in prevention is untested.[23,24]

References

1. Smith HR, Rowson M, Basketter DA, McFadden JP. Intra-individual variation of irritant threshold and relationship to transepidermal water loss measurement of skin irritation. *Contact Derm.* 2004;51:26–29

2. Cheatle TR, Scott HJ, Scurr JH, et al White cells, venous blood flow and venous ulcers. *Br J Dermatol.* 1991;125:288–290

3. Beauregard S, Gilchrest BA. A survey of skin problem and skin care regimens in the elderly. *Arch Dermatol.* 1987;123:1638–1643

4. Weisman K, Krakauer R, Wanscher B. Prevalence of skin disease in old age. *Acta Derm Venereol.* 1980;60:352–353

5. Jemec GBE, Serup J. Scaling, dry skin and gender. *Acta Derm Venereol.* 1992;177:26–28

6. Norman RA. Xerosis and pruritus in elderly patients, part 1. *Ostomy Wound Manage.* 2006;52:12–14

7. Smith DR, Atkinson R, Tang S, Yamagata Z. A survey of skin disease among patients in an Australian nursing home. *J Epidemiol.* 2002;12:336–340

8. Thaiisuttikul Y. Pruritic skin diseases in the elderly. *J Dermatol* 1998;25:153–157

9. McFadden N, Hande KO. A survey of elderly new patients at a dermatology outpatient clinic. *Acta Derm Venereol.* 1989;69:260–262

10. Anderson C. Asteatotic eczema. E medicine, emedicine. com; 2006

11. Fritsch PO, Reider N. Other eczematous disorders. In: Bolognia JL, Jorizzo JL, Rapini R, eds. *Dermatology.* Philadelphia: Mosby; 2003:218

12. Dalgard F, Holm JO, Svensson A, et al Self reported skin morbidity and ethnicity: a population based study in a Western community. *BMC Dermatol.* 2006;7:4

13. Baranda L, Gonzalez-Amaro R, Torres-Alvarez B, et al Correlation between pH and irritant effect of cleansers marketed for dry skin. *Int J Dermatol.* 2002;41:494–499

14. Simion FA, Abrutyn ES, Draelos Z. Ability of moisturisers to reduce dry skin and irritation and to prevent their return. *J Cosmet Sci.* 2005;56:427–444

15. Ramsing DW, Agner T. Preventive and therapeutic effects of a moisturizer. *Acta Derm Venereol.* 1997;77:335–337

16. Loden M. Role of topical emollients and moisturizers in the treatment of dry skin barrier disorders. *Am J Clin Dermatol.* 2003;4:771–788

17. Proksch E, Lachapelle J-M. The management of dry skin with topical emollients – recent perspectives. *J Dtsch Dermatol Ges.* 2005;3:768–774

18. Hansson C. Optimal treatment of venous (stasis) ulcers in elderly patients. *Drugs Aging.* 1994;5:323–334

19. Padberg FT Jr, Johnston MV, Sisto SA. Structured exercise improves calf muscle pump function in chronic venous insufficiency: a randomized trial. *J Vasc Surg.* 2004;39:79–87

20. Gniadecka M, Karlsmark T, Bertram A. Removal of dermal oedema with class I and II compression stockings in patients with lipodermatosclerosis. *J Am Acad Dermatol.* 1998;39:966–970

21. Raju S, Hollis K, Neglen P. Use of compression stockings in chronic venous disease: patient compliance and efficacy. *Ann Vasc Surg.* 2007;21:790–795

22. Katsenis K. Micronized purified flavonoid fraction (MPFF): a review of its pharmacological effects, therapeutic efficacy and benefits in the management of chronic venous insufficiency. *Curr Vasc Pharmacol.* 2005;3:1–9

23. Ciapponi A, Laffaire E, Roque M. Calcium dobesilate for chronic venous insufficiency: a systematic review. *Angiology.* 2004;55:147–154

24. Pascarella L, Schoenbein GW, Bergan JJ. Microcirculation and venous ulceration: a review. *Ann Vasc Surg.* 2005, 19:921–927

Photoprotection

3

Camile L. Hexsel and Henry W. Lim

Author contributions: Dr. Lim and Dr. Hexsel have participated in the conception and design, drafting and critical revision of the chapter for important intellectual content.

Conflict of interest: Dr. Lim is a consultant for La Roche-Posay, Orfagen, Johnson and Johnson, and Dow Pharmaceuticals; and he has received research grant support from Johnson and Johnson. Dr. Hexsel has no conflicts of interest to declare.

3.1 Cutaneous Effects of Ultraviolet Radiation

Ultraviolet (UV) radiation consists of UVC (270–290 nm [nm]), ultraviolet B (UVB) (290–320 nm) and ultraviolet A (UVA), which is further classified into UVA1 (340–400 nm) and UVA2 (320–340 nm). UVC radiation does not reach the surface of the earth as it is filtered by the ozone layer. On the surface of the earth, there is 20 times more UVA than UVB.

Cutaneous effects of UV radiation can be divided into acute and chronic. Acute effects include erythema, edema, blisters, and immediate and delayed pigment darkening followed by tanning or neomelanogenesis, acanthosis, and dermal thickening. Exposure to UV can also induce immunosuppression, vitamin D synthesis, and development of photodermatoses.

Erythema and edema are primarily induced by UVB, start at 3–4 h after UVB exposure, and peak at 8–24 h. They last 24–48 h or longer in light-skinned individuals. Delayed tanning or neomelanogenesis peaks at 72 h after UV radiation. UVB-induced delayed tanning requires a preceding erythemal response and has a sun protection factor (SPF) of 3.

In contrast to UVB, UVA-induced erythema peaks at 1–2 h after exposure and subsides gradually over 24–72 h. Because of the longer wavelength of UVA, it takes 1,000-fold more fluence (dose) to induce erythema by UVA compared to UVB. UVA also induces immediate and delayed pigment darkening followed by tanning. Immediate pigment darkening (IPD) occurs within seconds after UVA and visible light irradiation, and resolves in 2 h; it is due to photo-oxidation of preexisting melanin.[1] Persistent pigment darkening (PPD) is also a result of a photo-oxidation and redistribution of preexisting melanin; PPD persists from 2 to 24 h after irradiation.[1,2] UVA-induced delayed tanning, which is secondary to neomelanogenesis, appears usually 3 days after exposure.[1]

Chronic effects of UV radiation include photoaging and the development of actinic keratosis, basal cell carcinoma, and squamous cell carcinoma.[1,3,4] Melanoma has been associated with intermittent intense acute sun exposure and history of sunburns. The specific wavelengths associated with melanoma have not completely been identified; therefore, although sunburns are associated with an increased risk of melanoma, the specific wavelengths of UV responsible for sunburn may not be the same wavelengths responsible for the development of melanoma.[3]

Although solar radiation comprises a broad range of wavelengths, several eye disorders are related to UV, visible and infra-red radiation. Examples of acute opthalmological effects include photokeratitis (welder's flash or snow blindness) from UVC and UVB radiation; solar retinitis (blue light retinitis or eclipse blindness) from unprotected exposure to intense

C.L. Hexsel (✉)
Department of Dermatology, Henry Ford Hospital,
Detroit, MI, USA
e-mail: chexsel1@hfhs.org

sunlight; retinal photochemical burn from short-wavelength visible light (blue–violet light); retinal thermal damage from longer wavelengths and short pulses of intense visible light. Long-term effects of UV radiation associated with long-term exposure to sunlight include age-related macular degeneration, cataracts, pterygium, and pinguecula.[5]

3.2 General Photoprotection Recommendations and Their Rationales

Cutaneous effects of UV radiation can be effectively prevented with the use of multiple photoprotection measures.

UV radiation is more intense between 10 AM and 4 PM.[1] Approximately 20–30% of total UV radiation reaches the earth between 11 AM and 1 PM, and 75% between 9 AM and 3 PM. Maximal irradiance occurs in the summer months, although seasonal variation in UV radiation decreases with latitude. Furthermore, there is an increase of about 3% in UV reaching the surface per degree decrease in latitude. Because of the wide range of geographical, latitude, and time zone distribution,[6] the "shadow rule" has been proposed as a simple way to determine the peak hours of UV radiation. During peak hours of UV radiation, a person's shadow is shorter than their height, while during off-peak hours, it is longer. [4,6] Therefore, *the first recommendation in photoprotection is:* seek shade during peak hours of UV radiation (between 10 AM and 4 PM)[1] or when one's shadow is shorter than one's height (Table 3.1).[4,6]

An effective and widely used photoprotection method is sunscreen. Discussion of the sunscreen actives available will be discussed in detail in this chapter. Correct use, appropriate amounts, and reapplication frequency are important factors for the effectiveness of sunscreens. Studies have shown that most of those who use sunscreens apply them inadequately. Concentrations of sunscreen used by consumers (0.5–1 mg/cm^2), compared to that used in testing (2 mg/cm^2) is the reason that in-use SPF frequently is only 20–50% of the labeled SPF value.[1,6] To achieve a 2 mg/cm^2 concentration, the average adult should apply approximately 35 mL evenly, which is the equivalent of a full 1-ounce shot glass. Sunscreen should be

Table 3.1 Recommendations for photoprotection

Seek shade during peak hours of UV radiation (between 10 AM and 4 PM or when a person's shadow is shorter than their height)
Use sunscreens with broad spectrum UVB and UVA coverage with minimum sun protection factor (SPF) 15, preferably 30
First apply sunscreen 15–30 min before sun exposure followed by another application 15–30 min later
Reapply sunscreen at least every 2 h and after swimming, perspiring, and towel drying
In addition to sunscreen, use other physical barriers such as shade, a wide-brimmed hat, tightly woven or specifically designed protective clothing
In children younger than 6 months of age, use physical measures for photoprotection (shade, clothing, hat). If absolutely necessary, use sunscreen limited only on exposed areas and infrequently
If you are at risk for vitamin D deficiency, take a minimum of 800–1,000 IU of vitamin D supplementation
If planning multiday sun exposure, use higher SPFs

applied 15–30 min before going out in the sun, followed by a second application 15–30 min after sun exposure.[1] The second application can provide up to three times increase in photoprotection, thus compensating for improper first application. Sweating, swimming, and towel drying can considerably decrease the efficacy of sunscreens[1]; towel drying can remove up to 85% of a product.[4] With swimming and sweating, even the most water-resistant product requires a more frequent application than every 2 h. Therefore, *the second recommendation in photoprotection is:* use sunscreens with broad-spectrum UVB and UVA coverage and a minimum SPF 15, preferably 30. Sunscreen should be reapplied at least every 2 h and after swimming, perspiring, and towel drying. Sunscreen should be first applied 15–30 min before sun exposure followed by another application 15–30 min later (Table 3.1).

As will be outlined in more detail below, sunscreens do not provide complete protection to the whole spectrum of UV radiation. Therefore, in addition to sunscreens, other physical barriers, such as shade, a wide-brimmed hat, tightly woven or specifically designed protective clothing, and sunglasses are an integral part of photoprotection strategy.

Because of the higher skin-surface-to-body-weight ratio, and because the metabolism and excretion of absorbed substances are not completely developed in children under 6 months of age, it is *recommended* that for children younger than 6 months of age, photoprotection be achieved by physical measures (shade, clothing, hat). If absolutely necessary, limited and infrequent use of sunscreen on exposed areas may be done.[1] The 1999 sunscreen monograph recommends that physicians be consulted for the use of sunscreen in this age group.[7]

Vitamin D oral supplementation is practical and inexpensive. Therefore, oral vitamin D supplementation is *recommended* for individuals at risk for vitamin D deficiency. These individuals at risk of vitamin D deficiency include those living in northern latitudes (above 35°), elderly, housebound, and darker-skinned individuals. Intake of vitamin D should be 400–800 IU/day depending on the age, for individuals at low risk for vitamin D deficiency; the recommended intake of vitamin D for high-risk individuals is 800–1,000 IU/day or up to 50,000 IU of vitamin D per month (Table 3.1).[4]

Other factors should be considered for effective photoprotection. Multiday exposure affects the sensitivity to the sun since erythema peaks at 8–24 h of sun exposure. Therefore, higher SPFs are *recommended* for multiday sun exposure.[1] Various surfaces cause significant reflection of UV radiation. Snow reflects 30–80% of absorbed radiation, sand 15–30%, water less than 5%, and most ground surfaces less than 10%. UV radiation can penetrate through water to a depth of 60 cm. Although complete cloud cover reduces surface UV radiation by approximately 50%, light scattered cloud cover has minimal impact on surface UV radiation.[8]

3.2.1 Sunscreens

Organic sunscreens, previously called chemical sunscreens, act by absorbing UV radiation in the UVB and/or UVA spectra. Inorganic filters, previously called physical sunscreens, act by either reflecting or absorbing UV radiation, depending on the particle size.[1] Sunscreens have been shown to prevent both acute and most chronic effects of UV radiation.[3,9,10]

In the United States, the Food and Drug Administration (FDA) regulates sunscreens as over-the-counter drugs. The most recent version of the final FDA sunscreen monograph was issued in 1999 with a list of 16 approved sunscreen drugs (Table 3.2), approved

Table 3.2 Sunscreen drugs listed in the 1999 FDA sunscreen monograph

Inorganic sunscreen drugs
Titanium dioxide
Zinc oxide
Organic sunscreen drugs
UVB
Para-aminobenzoic acid (PABA)
Padimate O
Octinoxate
Cinoxate
Octisalate
Homosalate
Trolamine salicylate
Octocrylene
Ensulizole
UVA
Oxybenzone
Sulisobenzone
Dioxybenzone
Avobenzone
Meradimate

All listed as United States adapted name (USAN)
FDA Food and Drug Administration, *UVB* ultraviolet B, *UVA* ultraviolet A

maximum concentration, testing procedures, and labeling requirements.[1,7] A proposed amendment to the 1999 monograph was published in August, 2007.[2]

There are two different methods available for application of FDA approval for sunscreen drugs: the new drug application (NDA), and the time and extent application (TEA). To be considered for TEA approval, the FDA requires submission of the data acquired from at least 5 years of over-the-counter marketing of the product in the same country outside the United States.[11]

Various broad-spectrum sunscreen products containing ecamsule (terephtalydene dicamphor sulfonic acid, Mexoryl SX™) were recently approved by the FDA, the first one in July 2006.[12] Ecamsule is not listed among the approved sunscreen drugs since ecamsule-containing products were approved as final products rather than individual UV sunscreen drugs by the NDA process.

3.2.2 Organic UVB Filters

SPF is the ratio of the dose of UV radiation (290–400 nm) needed to produce one minimal erythema dose (MED) on sunscreen-protected skin (2 mg/cm² of product) over the dose needed to produce one MED on unprotected skin.[1,3] Therefore, SPF is a reflection of predominantly the erythemogenic effect of UVB, and to a lesser extend, UVA2.

A proposed amendment to the 1999 monograph was published by the FDA on 27 Aug 2007.[2] Key propositions comprise a new grading system for UVB and UVA protection, a cap of the SPF at 50+, and several recommendations in directions of use and labeling, including the requisite of a sun alert statement warning.

In the 2007 amendment, the FDA suggests modifying the acronym "SPF" from "SPF" to "UVB *sunburn* protection factor" to better differentiate the biologic effects of UVB and UVA. Furthermore, a grading system for UVB sunburn protection factor was proposed based on the following four categories: low UVB sunburn protection (SPF 2 £ 15), medium UVB sunburn protection (SPF 15 £ 30), high UVB sunburn protection (SPF 30–50), highest UVB sunburn protection (SPF over 50).

The FDA is of the opinion that there are no current data reporting the accuracy and reproducibility of SPF values over 50. Thus, the FDA proposes that manufacturers label their products with the specific SPF values up to, but no greater than 50; those products with SPF>50 would be labeled as 50+. Products would need to have SPF of 60 to obtain a SPF50+.[2]

FDA-approved UVB sunscreen drugs are listed in Table 3.2. Several important points regarding UVB filters listed in Table 3.2 need to be made.

Octinoxate (ethylhexyl methoxicinnamate, Parsol MCX™) is the most widely used UVB sunscreen drug in the United States. Octinoxate has maximum peak absorption at 311 nm but it is less potent and photostable than Padimate O, and hence, requires additional photostable UVB drugs, or stabilizers, to achieve a high SPF value. *Octisalate (ethyl hexyl salicylate), homosalate (homomenthyl salicilate)*, and o *ctocrylene (2-ethylhexyl-2-cyano-3, 3-diphenylacrylate)* are photostable; they are often combined with other sunscreen drugs to enhance the photostability of the final product.

3.2.3 Organic UVA Filters

The 2007 proposed amendment to the FDA sunscreen monograph presents a new grading system of the level of UVA protection, comprising a four-star rating system that ranges from low, medium, high, to highest UVA protection (Table 3.3). The rating system is based on both in vivo and in vitro testing procedures.

The PPD test is proposed by the FDA as the standard method of in vivo UVA testing. UVA protection factor is subsequently determined by the ratio of the minimal pigmentation dose in sunscreen-protected skin to the minimal pigmentation dose in unprotected skin, evaluated between 3 and 24 h after the irradiation.[2]

Since UVA2 is the portion of UVA mostly represented in the PPD testing,[13] the FDA proposed an in vitro testing that provides a measure of UVA1 protection, specifically, the ratio of UVA1 absorbance to total UV (290–400 nm) absorbance.

When discordances between in vitro and in vivo test results occur, the final rating will be the lowest rating determined by either of these two methods. For example, a product with an in vivo UVA-PF of 15 and an in vitro UVA1/UV ratio of 8 would be rated as a three-star product.

FDA-approved organic UVA sunscreen drugs are listed in Table 3.2. The FDA recently approved sunscreen products containing ecamsule (terephtalydene dicamphor sulfonic acid, Mexoryl SX™). There are at least five ecamsule-containing sunscreen products in the US market.

Oxybenzone (benzophenone-3, Bp-3), is a photostable UVB and UVA2 filter; it is the most common cause of photoallergic contact dermatitis from UV

Table 3.3 Grading system of the level of UVA protection recommended by the FDA in the 2007 proposed amendment of the 1999 sunscreen monograph

Star	UVA-PF	UVA1/UV	Rating
None	<2	<0.2	No UVA protection
*	2 to <4	0.2–0.39	Low
**	4 to <8	0.4–0.69	Medium
***	8 to <12	0.7–0.95	High
****	>12	>0.95	Highest

UVA ultraviolet A, *FDA* Food and Drug Administration, *UV* ultraviolet, *UVA-PF* ultraviolet A protection factor filters.[1] *Avobenzone (butyl methoxydibenzoylmethane, Parsol 1789™)* is the best UVA1 sunscreen drug available in the United States; however, it is photolabile and must be combined with photostable UVB sunscreen drugs; in some products, nonultraviolet-filter stabilizers, such as diethylhexyl 2,6-naphtalate, are also used.[1]

Other broad-spectrum and intrinsically photostable UVB and UVA sunscreen actives, currently unavailable in the United States, include silatriazole (drometriazole trisiloxane, Mexoryl XL™), bisoctrizole (methylene-bis-benzotriazoyl tetramethylbutylphenol, Tinosorb M™), and bemotrizinol (anizotriazine, bis-ethylhexyloxyphenol methoxyphenol triazine, Tinosorb S™)[11]; the last two are undergoing the FDA TEA approval process.[1,11]

3.2.4 Inorganic Filters

Inorganic sunscreen drugs are photostable; they photoprotect by reflecting or absorbing UV radiation, depending on the particle size. They are less efficient UV absorbers than organic UV filters. Thick coating is required to achieve satisfactory degree of reflection. Reducing the particle size considerably improves cosmetic acceptability, but also results in less scattering of visible light and shifts the protection toward shorter wavelengths and toward absorbency function. Opaque inorganic sunscreen actives may protect against visible light-induced photosensitivity.

Microfine zinc oxide is a photostable sunscreen drug that protects from the UVB to the UVA1 range. *Microfine titanium dioxide* is a photostable sunscreen drug that is conversely more protective in the UVB and UVA2 range. *Titanium dioxide* has a higher refractive index and is therefore whiter, despite a smaller particle size.[1,3]

3.2.5 Contact, Photocontact, and Phototoxic Reactions to Sunscreen

Considering the widespread use of sunscreens, irritant and allergic contact, photocontact allergic and phototoxic reactions to sunscreen are rare. Currently oxybenzone is the most common contact photoallergen, replacing para-aminobenzoic acid (PABA), which is not as frequently used anymore. The UVB filters methylbenziledene camphor, octinoxate and ensulizole, padimate O, and UVA filters avobenzone and sulizobenzone may only rarely induce contact allergic and photoallergic reactions.[1,3]

3.2.6 Controversies on Sunscreens

3.2.6.1 Compensation Hypothesis

The compensation hypothesis postulates that the use of high SPF sunscreen may encourage longer exposure to UV radiation, resulting in higher exposure to UVA radiation. Therefore, sunscreens could theoretically increase skin cancer susceptibility, especially melanoma.[6] However, a systematic review by Dennis et al.[14] that examined 18 heterogeneous case control studies published from 1966 to 2003 found no association between melanoma and sunscreen use.[3,14]

3.2.6.2 Hormonal Effects

In vitro, Schlumpf et al.[15] demonstrated an increased MCF-7 breast cancer cell proliferation after exposure to five different UVB filters. In vivo, they also demonstrated a dose dependent increase in uterine weight of immature Long-Evans rats after oral administration of two UVB filters, enzacamene and octinoxate. In addition, a dose-dependent increase in uterine weight in immature hairless rats after dermal administration of enzacamene was reported.[15] Another study from the same group by Ma et al. reported the in vitro antiandrogenic activity of the sunscreen drugs oxybenzone and homosalate in the human breast carcinoma cell line MDA-kb2.[16] Nakagawa and Suzuki reported the estrogenic effect of some hydroxylated intermediates of sulizobenzone in human breast cancer cells in vitro.[17] It should be noted that the doses of sunscreen drug products used were unrealistically high compared to human exposure scenarios.[1] Furthermore, a study by Janjua et al.[18] reported no effects on reproductive hormone levels in 32 volunteers after topical application of oxybenzone, octinoxate, and enzacamene, daily for 5 days.[18] The scientific committee of cosmetic products and nonfood products, a European Committee based in Belgium, stated that the relative estrogenic potencies of UV sunscreen products were about one million less than estradiol, the positive control substance used in these studies.[1]

Therefore, while the reported estrogenic effect of UV sunscreen actives is still not completely clear, it most likely has no biologic relevance in otherwise healthy human subjects.

3.2.7 Other Topical, Oral, and Dietary Photoprotection Agents

These agents are listed in Table 3.4. Selected ones are discussed below.

UVB can induce immunosuppression by generating damage to DNA, directly via the formation of cyclobutane pyrimidine dimers (CPD), or indirectly, via reactive oxygen species formation. *Photolyase*, a DNA repair enzyme has been shown to decrease the number of UVB-induced dimers by 40–45% in human skin when applied immediately after UVB exposure[1] and therefore, prevents immunosuppression, erythema, and sunburn formation.[19] *T4 endonuclease V* is a bacterial DNA excision repair enzyme that repairs CPD in DNA. Its liposome form used as topical treatment was shown to remove dimers in DNA in the epidermis of animals and human beings, and nearly completely prevented UV-induced upregulation of IL-10 and tumor necrosis factor-alpha messenger RNAs. Application of T4 endonuclease V immediately after UV exposure partially protects against sunburn cell formation, local suppression of contact hypersensitivity, and suppression of delayed-type hypersensitivity and has minimal or no effect on UV-induced skin edema.[1] Topical application of T4 endonuclease V for 1 year lowered the rate of development of actinic keratoses and basal cell carcinomas in patients with xeroderma pigmentosum.[1,19]

UV irradiation generates short DNA fragments during the course of excision repair process. One small single-stranded DNA fragment, *thymidine dinucleotide*, has been extensively studied. Thymidine dinucleotides mimic cellular responses to UV radiation including increased DNA repair, reversible cell growth arrest, tumor necrosis factor-alpha expression and secretion, induction of IL-10 expression, and enhanced melanogenesis. Some of these effects are mediated through activation of p53 and increased messenger RNA levels for the responsible proteins. In human fibroblasts, pretreatment with thymidine dinucleotide enhances activation of p53 and p53-upregulated proteins. Therefore, thymidine dinucletides may play a role in photoprotection.

Antioxidants agents have been administered both orally and topically for photoprotection. Topical antioxidants are inefficient UV filters and have low SPF; therefore, they are commonly used in combination with sunscreens to enhance their efficacy. They are less potent than sunscreens in preventing sunburn. The limitations of topical antioxidants are the requirement of compliance with application, difficulties with diffusion into the epidermis, instability, and dose or concentration-dependent effectiveness. Commonly used antioxidants in sunscreen products include vitamin E and vitamin C.

Topical application of *calcitriol (1,25-dihydroxyvitamin D3, 1,25 hydroxyvitamin D)*, the active form of vitamin D, has been reported to inhibit UVB-induced sunburn cell formation in mice skin by inducing the expression of metallothionein,[1,20] a sulfhydryl-rich protein that acts as a potent radical scavenger.

Green tea, consumed regularly by two-thirds of the world's population, contains four main polyphenolic compounds, (−)-epicatechin (EC), (−)-epicatechin gallate (ECG), (−)-epigallotechin (EGC), and (−)-epigallo-techin-3-gallate (EGCG). EGCG is considered the main polyphenol responsible for the antioxidant effects.[21] Green tea polyphenols have absorption maximum at 273 nm, in the UVC range. These compounds exhibit anti-inflammatory activity, causing inhibition of UV radiation-induced skin erythema, edema, depletion of the epidermal antioxidant defense system, induction of epidermal cycloxygenase and ornithine decarboxylase enzyme activities, immunosuppression, a decrease in the number of sunburn cells, downregulation of UVB-induced production of IL 10, increased production of IL12, suppression of contact hypersensitivity,[21] and inhibition of phosphorylation of MAPKs and NF-kB pathways.[1] Effects on photocarcinogenesis include a decrease tumor burden, inhibition on the formation and size of malignant and nonmalignant tumors and regression of these tumors in mice with established tumors, enhanced UVB-induced increases in epidermal wild type p53, p21 and apoptotic sunburn. EGCG has also been reported to inhibit UV-induced lipid peroxidation, to restore UV-induced decrease

Table 3.4 Photoprotective agents other than sunscreens

Agent	Photoprotective properties	Source
T4 endonuclease V, Photolyase	Repair of cyclobutane pyrimidine dimer	Bacterial DNA excision enzyme
Thymidine dinucleotide	Enhancement of melanogenesis, increase of DNA repair	Synthetic
Alpha tocopherol (vitamin E)	Reduction of erythema, sunburn cell formation, chronic UVB-induced photodamage, photocarcinogenesis. Reduction in epidermal Langerhans cell density and contact hypersensitivity	Plants and vegetables, dietary supplements
L-ascorbic acid (vitamin C)	Reduction of erythema, sunburn cell formation, UVB-induced immunosuppression and contact hypersensitivity	Plants and vegetables, dietary supplements
Carotenoids	Protective against squamous cell carcinoma, visible light-induced retinal damage and aged-related macular degeneration, reduction in photosensitivity in patients with erythropoietic protoporphyria	Plants and vegetables, dietary supplements
Calcitriol (1,25-dihydroxyvi-tamin D3)	Induction of metallothionein (scavenger of free radicals). Induction of p53 protein expression, improved survival of keratinocytes post-UV radiation, reduction in nitric oxide products, sunburn cells, cyclobutane pyrimidine dimers (CPD) formation	Synthesized in kidneys after diet and sun exposure
Zinc	Antioxidant, reduction in sunburn cell formation, UVA1-induced early and delayed apoptosis of fibroblasts	Diet and dietary supplements
2-Furildioxime	Iron chelator, reduction of erythema, sunburn cell formation, acanthosis, infiltration of inflammatory cells	Synthetic
Polyphenolic compounds	Antioxidant	Green tea
Caffeine	Enhancement of apoptosis, reduction in the formation of nonmalignant and malignant tumors and photodamage	Plant
Caffeic acid and ferulic acid	Antioxidant and radial scavenging	Plants and vegetables
Genistein	Protection against UV-induced inflammation and immunosuppression, UV-induced carcinogenesis, photoaging, contact hypersensitivity	Soybean, Greek oregano, Greek sage, ginko biloba extract
Equol	Protection against UV-induced inflammation and immunosuppression, UV-induced carcinogenesis by induction of metallothionein	Red clover
Flavonoid cocoa	Protection against UV-induced inflammation, skin thickening, and epidermal water loss	Diet
Pomegranate extract	Inhibits the phosphorylation of NF- k B and MAPK pathways, reduces UV-induced inflammation, hyperplasia, hydrogen peroxide and CPD formation	Fruit extract
Cistus	Free radical scavenging and inhibition of lipid peroxidation	Mediterranean shrubs
Plant xyloglucans	Prevention of UVB-induced systemic immunosuppression	Tamarind seeds
Aloe plant poly/oligosaccharide	Suppression of delayed-type and contact hypersensitivity	Aloe barbadensis
Polypodium leucotomos	Antioxidant and antiinflammation	Plant extract
Omega-3 polyunsaturated fatty acid	Decrease of sunburn cell formation, inflammation, UVA provocation response	Fish oil
N-acetylcysteine (NAC)	Increase of glutathione level (endogenous antioxidant)	Synthetic

in glutathione levels, to prevent CPD formation, to reduce prostaglandin metabolites, particularly prostaglandin E2, which plays a major role in skin tumor promotion. Effects of green tea polyphenols in photoaging include the inhibition of UVB-induced expression of matrix metalloproteinases and reduction of UVB-induced collagen cross-linking.[1]

The plant extract *Polypodium leucotomos* does not have significant absorption in either UVB or UVA range. In humans and animal models, the plant extract *Polypodium leucotomos* exhibits antioxidant and anti-inflammatory properties.[1] Other proposed effects include prevention of UV-induced photoisomerization of transurocanic acid,[22] suppression of the production of nitric oxide and induction of TNF alpha expression,[23] and prevention of UV-induced apoptosis in human keratinocytes and fibroblasts.[24] After topical and oral administration, *Polypodium leucotomos* was reported to increase the UV dose required for IPD, MED, minimal melanogenic dose and minimal phototoxic dose. In humans, oral and topical administration of *Polypodium leucotomos* was shown to be photoprotective against psoralen-UVA-induced phototoxic reaction and pigmentary and histological changes.

Fish oil, which is rich in *omega-3* polyunsaturated fatty acid, has been shown to decrease UVB-induced sunburn cell formation and inflammation and reduce UVA provocation response. Due to the latter properties, it has been used for patients with polymorphous light eruption; however, relatively large amount of fish oil needs to be ingested for such effect; therefore it is not widely used for the management of this condition.

N-acetylcysteine (NAC) is an agent that increases the levels of the endogenous antioxidant glutathione. Topical application of NAC before UVB exposure can protect against immunosuppression in mice. The mechanism of action is unclear. NAC has also been reported to have antioxidant properties against UVA cytotoxicity in human fibroblasts.[1]

3.2.8 Shade

The sun protection provided by shade varies with diurnal variation of the angle of the sun and the amount of area or density of coverage provided.[1,6] Shade alone reduces solar irradiation by 50–95% and is, therefore, an important adjuvant of other photoprotective measures.[3]

3.2.9 Clothing

Clothing is an essential part of photoprotection not only for the general population, but also and especially for particular groups of the population such as children, employees exposed to artificial sources of UV radiation, and those working outdoors and performing outdoor recreational activities and hobbies[4,25] photosensitive patients,[25] and patients with risk factors for skin cancer.

UV protection factor (UPF) is the measurement of UV photoprotection of fabrics. UPF is measured in vitro with a spectrophotometer that determines the transmission of UVA and UVB through fabrics. This in vitro method was reported to be accurate and reproducible, particularly for samples with UPF below 50,[1] and appears to be the most suitable method for the evaluation of UPF.[3]

Recent advances in clothing photoprotection have included specifically designed clothing with UPF, and the development of regulation standards of photoprotection by clothing, the first one being the Australian/New Zealand standard issued in July 1996. Subsequently, other standards have been developed, such as the United Kingdom, the European and the United States. These standards usually address the minimum UPF and the minimum recommended body coverage for photoprotection (e.g., trunk, upper arms).[25]

Several factors affect the UPF of fabrics, and should be taken into account when using clothing as a photoprotection method. These include the construction and the color of fabrics, hydration, washing and wearing, chemical treatments, stretching, and distance of the fabric from the skin.[1,25]

Clothing with tightly woven fibers (wool and synthetic materials such as polyester) and thick fibers have higher UPF than loosely woven (cotton, linen, acetate, and rayon) and thin fabrics. Typical summer cotton T-shirts provide UPF of five to nine, and when wet, the UPF decreases to only three to four. Denim provides UPF of 1,700.

When wet, changes in the UPF are variable due to scattering and absorption properties of the fabrics. In general, hydration results in a decline in the UPF because the presence of water in the interstices of the fabrics enhances UV transmission. Conversely, the UPF frequently increases when the textile becomes wet in fabrics made of viscose or silk, or those that have been treated with broad-spectrum UV absorbers.[1]

Washing shrinks and reduces the gaps between fibers. UPF is also affected by chemical treatment of the fabrics with optical brightening agents and UV absorbers. Optical brightening agents are compounds which that absorb the energy and fluoresce at the visible light range, leading to reduced UV transmission and the appearance of being bright.[1] White fabrics with an optical whitening agent have slightly higher UPF than other pale-colored fabrics.[25] Dark-colored fabrics have greater UPF and visible light absorption than light-colored fabrics.[1]

The laundry additive containing UV absorber Tinosorb FD has been shown to result in significantly increased UPF than fabrics exposed to regular washing.

The UPF decreases considerably when fabrics are stretched. Unstretched Lycra (DuPont, Wilmington, Del) may block 100% of UV radiation; on the other hand, the UPF may decrease to two when stretched.

Another factor that affects the UPF of fabrics is the distance of the fabric from the skin. The closer to the skin, the lesser the photoprotection the fabric provides because the smaller the distance is between the fabric and the skin, the lesser the diffusion of the UV beam reaching the skin.[1]

3.2.10 Hats

Hats can provide protection not only to the face and neck, but are highly recommended for scalp protection of individuals with alopecia or thin or short hairs.[6] Photoprotection of hats depends on the brim width, material, and weaving. A wide-brimmed hat (>7.5 cm) has SPF 7 for nose, three for cheek, five for neck, and two for chin. Medium-brimmed hats (2.5–7.5 cm) provide SPF 3 for nose, two for cheek and neck, and none for chin, whereas narrow-brimmed hats provide SPF 1.5 for nose, and little protection for chin and neck.[1]

3.2.11 Makeup

Foundations containing UV filters with high SPF are of great value and recommended for daily photoprotection. Foundation makeup without sunscreen provides SPF 3–4 due to its pigment content. This photoprotective property and ability to create an even cosmetic film on the skin surface lasts up to 4 h after application; subsequent decrease in photoprotective property is due to migration into the dermatoglyphs and accumulation in the follicular ostia. The loss in photoprotective property could occur in a shorter period as a result of perspiration, tearing, sebum production, and accidental removal. Thus, reapplication at least every 2 h is recommended for patients who rely on their facial foundation engaging in outdoor activities.[1]

3.2.12 Sunless Tanning Agents

Dihydroxy acetone, the active ingredient of sunless tanning preparations have an SPF of two, and has photoprotective properties against UVA and the low end of visible light for approximately 5–6 days.[1,3] It acts by an oxidative effect that changes skin color to orange–brown; the color binds chemically to the stratum corneum and does not interfere with normal skin function.[1] Dihydroxy acetone may provide some protection against UVA and visible light induced photodermatosis.[26]

3.2.13 Sunglasses

Sunglasses should reduce glare and provide protection against UV radiation. UV radiation is recognized to be potentially hazardous to the structure of the eyes, predominantly the cornea, lens, and retina. The cornea absorbs wavelengths below 295 nm, the crystalline lens between 295 and 400 nm and the retina between 400 and 1,400 nm; thus visible and infrared light are transmitted to the retina.

Sunglasses standards have been developed to ensure quality, performance, and adequate protection to consumers. Australia, Europe, and the United States have all developed standards. While the Australian and European standards are mandatory, the United States standard is voluntary and not followed by all manufacturers.

Sunglasses have been classified in three categories: cosmetic (which provide minimal UV protection), general purpose (which reduce the glare of bright light) and special purpose sunglasses (which are indicated for specific activities such as skiing and going to the beach). Furthermore, polarizing lenses reduce glare but do not add UV-blocking properties. For general purpose sunglasses, the United States standard (ANZI Z80.3) requires less than 1% of the wavelengths below 310 nm to be transmitted.

For ideal photoprotection, sunglasses should wrap around the eyes maximizing eye and eyelid protection, since a significant amount of UV can reach unprotected eyes. For added photoprotection, a wide-brimmed hat is recommended to reduce the level of radiation reaching the eyes.

Extensive and dark-tinted sunglasses can cause pupillary dilatation and increase lid opening, thus resulting in increased UV exposure to the lens of the eye. Clear glasses absorb the vast majority of UVB radiation but no UVA radiation, thus, for UVA protection a plastic film containing zinc, chrome, nickel or other metals with broad spectrum UV coverage is recommended. There is no regulation regarding lens color; in spite of this, the effect of the color should not interfere with the ability to see color-coded signals, especially red and green traffic signals. Neutral gray and amber brown are two popular colors that allow color discrimination. Only visible light, not UV radiation, is required for human vision. Therefore the ideal sunglasses should substantially reduce UV to cornea and lens, including that from lateral directions. Additional retinal protection can be accomplished with lenses that reduce the transmission of short-wavelength violet/blue light since this portion of visible light is considered to be hazardous to the retina.

3.2.14 Window Glass

In daily activity, considerable time is spent indoors and in vehicles. Contemporary residential and commercial architectural design increasingly incorporates more and larger window areas. Nonetheless, exposure to UV radiation through architectural window glass and automobile glass is generally unappreciated. Recent developments in the glass industry have resulted in window glass that provides broad UV protection without the historically associated loss of visible light transmission. Factors affecting the UV protective properties of glass are glass type, glass color, interleave between glass and glass coating. In contrast, thickness of glass has limited effect on the properties of visible light and UV transmission.

Window glasses can have a single pane of glass (monolithic glass); however, this type of glass was largely replaced by insulating glass units, which comprise two or more panes of glass separated by a perimeter spacer to keep the glasses apart and sealed with curable adhesive material to hold the pieces together.

While standard glass filters out UVB but not UVA, visible light, and infrared radiation, several types of glass are now available commercially in which the use of additional filters for UVA and infrared radiation are incorporated.

The interlayer is virtually invisible. It can filter 99% of UV (up to 380 nm). It also reduces the transmission of sound. Laminated glass is widely used in automobiles, airports, museums, schools, sound studios, and large public spaces.

3.2.15 Automobile Glass

For safety reasons, all car windshields are made of laminated glass, which is produced by binding two pieces of glass together with a plastic interlayer; if broken, glass fragments will adhere to the interlayer rather than fall free. Laminated glass blocks the vast portion of UVA radiation. On the other hand, rear and side windows are usually made from nonlaminated glass that transmits a significant amount of UVA. Yet, it is possible to add tints to rear and side windows to reduce the transmission of UVA radiation, visible and infrared light resulting in reduced unwanted heat gain and minimizing the fading of the interior components.

Photosensitive patients are advised to choose vehicles with complete laminated window glass packages or to apply a plastic film to nonlaminated rear and side windows. Nevertheless, this does not substitute general photoprotection measures such as sunscreen and protective clothing use.[5]

3.3 Summary

Effective photoprotection measures should be undertaken by all individuals to prevent transitory and permanent harmful effects of UV radiation. If possible, sun exposure should be avoided during peak hours of UV radiation (between 10 AM and 4 PM[1] or when one's shadow is shorter than one's height).[4,6] Since often sun avoidance during those hours is not possible or practical, other effective photoprotection measures should be undertaken. Sunscreens with broad spectrum UVB and UVA coverage of minimum SPF 15, preferably 30, should be correctly applied at least every 2 h and after swimming, perspiring, and towel drying. To account for frequent inadequacy of application, sunscreen should be first applied 15–30 min before sun exposure followed by another application 15–30 min later. Sunscreens do not completely block all UV radiation, especially UVA. The use of physical barriers in addition to sunscreen, such as shade, a wide-brimmed hat, tightly woven or specifically designed protective clothing, sunglasses and window glass is an essential adjunctive method of photoprotection to sunscreen.

Children younger than 6 months of age should be photoprotected mainly by physical measures. Oral vitamin D supplementation is recommended for individuals at risk for vitamin D deficiency.[1]

References

1. Kullavanijaya P, Lim HW, Photoprotection. J Am Acad Dermatol. 2005;52:937–958; quiz 959–962
2. Food and Drug Administration. 21 CFR Parts 347 and 352. Sunscreen drug products for over-the-counter human use: proposed amendment of final monograph; proposed rule. Federal Register 2007;72:49070–49122
3. Lautenschlager S, Wulf HC, Pittelkow MR. Photoprotection. Lancet. 2007;370:528–537
4. Palm MD, O'Donoghue MN. Update on photoprotection. Dermatol Ther. 2007;20:360–376
5. Tuchinda C, Srivannaboon S, Lim HW. Photoprotection by window glass, automobile glass, and sunglasses. J Am Acad Dermatol. 2006;54:845–854
6. Eide MJ, Weinstock MA. Public health challenges in sun protection. Dermatol Clin. 2006;24:119–124
7. Food and Drug Administration. Sunscreen drug products for over-the-counter human use; final monograph. Food and Drug Administration, HHS. Final rule. Federal Register 1999;64: 27666–27693
8. Rai R, Srinivas CR. Photoprotection. Indian J Dermatol Venereol Leprol. 2007;73:73–79
9. Green A, Williams G, Neale R, et al Daily sunscreen application and betacarotene supplementation in prevention of basal-cell and squamous-cell carcinomas of the skin: a randomised controlled trial. Lancet. 1999;354:723–729
10. van der Pols JC, Williams GM, Pandeya N, et al Prolonged prevention of squamous cell carcinoma of the skin by regular sunscreen use. Cancer Epidemiol Biomark Prev. 2006;15: 2546–2548
11. Tuchinda C, Lim HW, Osterwalder U, Rougier A. Novel emerging sunscreen technologies. Dermatol Clin. 2006;24: 105–117
12. The FDA approves new over-the-counter sunscreen. FDA consumer 2006;40:4
13. Bissonnette R, Allas S, Moyal D, Provost N. Comparison of UVA protection afforded by high sun protection factor sunscreens. J Am Acad Dermatol. 2000;43:1036–1038
14. Dennis LK, Beane Freeman LE, VanBeek MJ. Sunscreen use and the risk for melanoma: a quantitative review. Ann Intern Med. 2003;139:966–978
15. Schlumpf M, Cotton B, Conscience M, et al In vitro and in vivo estrogenicity of UV screens. Environ Health Perspect. 2001;109:239–244
16. Ma R, Cotton B, Lichtensteiger W, Schlumpf M. UV filters with antagonistic action at androgen receptors in the MDA-kb2 cell transcriptional-activation assay. Toxicol Sci. 2003;74:43–50
17. Nakagawa Y, Suzuki T. Metabolism of 2-hydroxy-4-methoxybenzophenone in isolated rat hepatocytes and xenoestrogenic effects of its metabolites on MCF-7 human breast cancer cells. Chem Biol Interact. 2002;139:115–128
18. Janjua NR, Mogensen B, Andersson AM, et al Systemic absorption of the sunscreens benzophenone-3, octyl-methoxycinnamate, and 3-(4-methyl-benzylidene) camphor after whole-body topical application and reproductive hormone levels in humans. J Invest Dermatol. 2004;123:57–61
19. Verschooten L, Claerhout S, Van Laethem A, et al New strategies of photoprotection. Photochem Photobiol. 2006;82: 1016–1023
20. Lee J, Youn JI. The photoprotective effect of 1, 25-dihydroxyvitamin D3 on ultraviolet light B-induced damage in keratinocyte and its mechanism of action. J Dermatol Sci. 1998;18:11–18
21. Afaq F, Mukhtar H. Botanical antioxidants in the prevention of photocarcinogenesis and photoaging. Exp Dermatol. 2006;15:678–684
22. Capote R, Alonso-Lebrero JL, Garcia F, et al Polypodium leucotomos extract inhibits trans-urocanic acid photoisomerization and photodecomposition. J Photochem Photobiol. 2006;82:173–179
23. Janczyk A, Garcia-Lopez MA, Fernandez-Penas P, et al A Polypodium leucotomos extract inhibits solar-simulated radiation-induced TNF-alpha and iNOS expression, transcriptional activation and apoptosis. Exp Dermatol. 2007; 16:823–829
24. Alonso-Lebrero JL, Dominguez-Jimenez C, Tejedor R, et al Photoprotective properties of a hydrophilic extract of the fern Polypodium leucotomos on human skin cells. J Photochem Photobiol. 2003;70:31–37
25. Gies P. Photoprotection by clothing. Photodermatol Photoimmunol Photomed. 2007;23:264–274
26. Deleo V. Sunscreen use in photodermatoses. Dermatol Clin. 2006;24:27–33

Biologics

4

Panoglotis Mitropoulos and Robert A. Norman

Modern advances in our understanding of immuno-logic processes, along with discoveries in disease pathophysiology, have led to the development of inno-vative therapeutic tools. In several fields of medicine, *biologic response modifiers, selective immunoregula-tory drugs*, or simply *biologics* are now being used in the treatment of conditions for which either no other effective therapies exist or the existing therapies pro-vide substandard therapeutic results.

Biologic agents comprise a variety of medicinal products already in use, such as vaccines, human cells and tissues, recombinant therapeutic proteins, allergenic products, blood components, and human gene therapy products. The term *biologics*, however, is more com-monly used to describe a class of medications produced by means of biological processes involving recombinant DNA technology. These are immunoregulators and bio-engineered proteins, such as fusion proteins, chimeric or fully humanized monoclonal antibodies, or recombinant cytokines that directly interfere with the pathological effects of T cells.

4.1 Indications

Currently, the only US Food and Drug Administration-approved indication of biologics in dermatology is for the treatment of psoriasis (Table 4.1).[1-5]

Nonetheless, the treatment potential of these medi-cations has led to their off-label use for several other conditions in dermatology. Some of these include

pemphigus vulgaris, paraneoplastic pemphigus, epi-dermolysis bullosa acquisita, primary cutaneous B-cell lymphoma, dermatomyositis, atopic dermatitis, chronic urticaria, sarcoidosis, granuloma annulare, Sweet's syndrome, lupus erythematosus, and several other granulomatous, autoimmune, inflammatory, and neu-trophilic dermatoses.[1]

For psoriasis, biologics do not constitute first-line treatment. Biologic therapy should be reserved for moderate-to-severe plaque psoriasis, and in cases where traditional treatments do not appear to be ade-quate or are contraindicated. Current initial therapies for psoriasis include topical agents (corticosteroids, coal tar, anthralins, vitamin A and D derivatives) and systemic agents (methotrexate, cyclosporine, retin-oids) as well as phototherapy.

Biologic therapy may be reasonable for patients who fall in two or more of the following categories:

- Age ≥ 18 year old
- Chronic (≥6 months) moderate/severe plaque psoriasis
- Psoriasis-area severity index (PASI) score of ten or more (or body surface area (BSA) of 10% or greater if PASI score not applicable), and a dermatology quality life index (DQLI) of less than ten
- Inadequate response or intolerance to standard therapy
- Higher than average risk of developing clinically important drug-related toxicity with the standard treatments
- Significant coexistent unrelated morbidity (i.e., unstable congestive heart failure [CHF], liver dis-ease) which precludes the use of systemic agents like cyclosporine or methotrexate
- Disease requiring repeated inpatient management for control

P. Mitropoulos (✉)
Camp Long Troop Medical Clinic,
Suwon-si, Gyeonggi-do, South Korea
e-mail: panagiotis.mitropoulos@amedd.army.mil

R.A. Norman (ed.), *Preventive Dermatology in Infectious Diseases*,
DOI 10.1007/978-0-85729-847-8_4, © Springer-Verlag London Limited 2012

Table 4.1 Currently FDA approved biologics for treatment of psoriasis and psoriatic arthritsis[1-5]

Name	Type	Principal mechanism of action	FDA approval
Alefacept (*Amevive®*)	Fusion protein/immunoglobulin G1 (IgG1)	T-cell depletory	Psoriasis
Etanercept (*Enbrel®*)	Fusion protein/soluble tumor necrosis factor-alpha (TNF-α) receptor	TNF-α antagonist	Psoriasis, psoriatic arthritis
Infliximab (*Remicade®*)	Chimeric monoclonal antibody	TNF-α antagonist	Psoriasis, psoriatic arthritis
Adalimumab (*Humira®*)	Fully humanized monoclonal antibody	TNF-α antagonist	Psoriasis, psoriatic arthritis
Ustekinumab (*Stelara*)	Chimeric monoclonal antibody	Human monoclonal antibody targets the activity of cytokines interleukin-12 (IL-12) and interleukin-23 (IL-23)	Psoriasis, psoriatic arthritis

- Patient not receiving any immunosuppressive medications except those used for the treatment of psoriasis
- Presence of psoriatic arthritis

4.2 Dosage and Administration

There are two methods of administration for the biologic agents currently used in dermatology (Table 4.2), subcutaneous (SC) or intravenous (IV). Since these medications are composed of relatively large molecules, parenteral administration, rather than oral, ensures better absorption and bioavailability.

Following appropriate education and demonstration from their physician, patients may choose to self-inject themselves at home subcutaneously according to their recommended dosing regimen. Intravenous administration should be completed at a clinic or other medical environment under the supervision of a physician.

4.3 Side Effects

The side effects of biologic medications vary. The most frequently reported event with all biologics is skin irritation at the site of injection. Other common adverse reactions may include flu-like symptoms, headache, dizziness, chills, low-grade fever, nausea, asthenia, myalgia, or arthralgia. Typically, these

Table 4.2 Administration and dosing of biologics for the treatment of psoriasis

Drug	Route of administration	Recommended dosage
Alefacept (*Amevive®*)	Intramuscular or intravenous	IM: 15 mg injection once a week for 12 weeks IV: 7.5 mg bolus once a week for 12 weeks
Etanercept (*Enbrel®*)	Subcutaneous (SC)	Twice a week 50 mg injection for 3 months; then once a week for maintenance
Infliximab (*Remicade®*)	Intravenous	Initially: infusion (over 2–3 h) 5 mg/kg on weeks 0, 2, and 6; then one infusion every 8 weeks for maintenance
Adalimumab (*Humira®*)	SC	Initial dose of 80 mg; then 40 mg once bi-weekly starting a week after initial dose
Ustekinumab (*Stelara*)	SC	45 mg (for pts < 200 lbs) at week 0, 4 & q 12 weeks 90 mg (for pts > 200) at week 0, 4 & q 12 weeks

symptoms are mild and transient. They are most likely to occur after the first two initial treatments and generally do not recur with subsequent doses.

Overall, biologics are well-tolerated and contrary to the conventional systemic antipsoriatic agents (methotrexate, cyclosporine) they have a limited organ-toxicity profile. Biologics are being used successfully in patients with renal insufficiency or hepatic dysfunction; when indicated they may be preferable to the aforementioned traditional systemic psoriasis treatments. The most serious side effects of biologic therapy are related to their immunosuppressive and immunoregulatory properties.

4.3.1 Infections

There is an increased risk of reactivation of latent infections or emergence of new infections associated with tumor necrosing factor (TNF)-α (alpha) inhibition. All the biologics currently used in dermatology contribute to immunosuppression via their depleting or modulation effect on B cells, T-cells, cytokines, or other molecules of the body's immune mechanism. Upon infection, TNF-α (alpha) plays a key role in the recruitment of defense cells to the site of infection, and in the formation and maintenance of granulomas. Tuberculosis (TB) and other serious opportunistic infections, including histoplasmosis, listeriosis, aspergillosis, toxoplasmosis, coccidioidomycosis, candidiasis, cutaneous Nocardia, and pneumocystosis, have been reported in both clinical research and postmarking surveillance settings.[6-8] Physicians must be cautious when prescribing biologics to patients who reside in geographical areas where the aforementioned diseases may be endemic. Additionally, the risk for opportunistic infections increases further more in patients who are receiving one or more immunosuppressant agents, or are HIV positive.

4.3.2 Neurological Disease

Development or worsening of nervous system disorders, including demyelinating diseases such as multiple sclerosis, transverse myelitis, seizures, Parkinson's disease, and optic neuritis, has been documented in patients who were receiving treatment with biologics.[8,9] It is suggested that biologic agents be withheld

from patients who have a history of, or a first degree relative with, a demyelinating disease.

4.3.3 Cardiovascular Disease

Higher incidence of mortality and hospitalization for worsening heart failure has been documented in patients with moderate-to-severe CHF (New York Heart Association classes III or IV) who were being treated with TNF-α (alpha) antagonists and, specifically, infliximab, and etarnecept.[3,8] Caution should be used when using TNF inhibitors in patients with unstable cardiac dysfunction.

4.3.4 Hepatitis/Hepatic Dysfunction

Several clinical studies have demonstrated evidence of hepatic enzymes elevation with use of all of the biologic medications.[6,10] These abnormalities are thought to be confounded by comorbid conditions and concomitant use of medications, as nonsteroidal anti-inflammatory drugs (NSAIDs), methotrexate, or cyclosporine have also been associated with hepatic dysfunction.

Autoimmune hepatitis and liver damage is a rare but increasingly recognized serious complication of treatment with the TNF-α (alpha) blocking agent, infliximab. It is noteworthy that a number of cases of liver failure resulting in liver transplantation or death have been reported in patients receiving infliximab.[11-13] Signs of severe hepatic reaction may include jaundice, cholestasis, and marked elevation (more than five times the upper limit of normal) in liver enzymes. The rest of the biologic medications used in the treatment of psoriasis have more favorable hepatic dysfunction profile which mainly involves a mild increase in liver enzymes.

Some reports are emerging regarding fulminant hepatic failure in patients with chronic hepatitis B virus (HBV) infection. HBV reactivation has been reported very rarely in patients with chronic hepatitis B infection receiving a biologic medication.[3,8,14] This is why serologic screening for viral hepatitis (HBV and hepatitis C virus) is recommended prior to initiation of therapy with biologics. For patients who are hepatitis B surface antigen (HBsAg)-positive, prophylaxis with lamivudine or other antiviral agent should be considered. Roux and colleagues evaluated the safety of TNF inhibitors in patients with concurrent chronic viral hepatitis.[15] Their retrospective study demonstrated that TNF inhibitors can be given safely in patients with chronic hepatitis B who were receiving lamivudine, and no changes were seen in their serum aminotransferase levels.

4.3.5 Occurrence of Autoantibodies and Autoimmunity

The development of antibodies (human antichimeric antibodies, antinuclear antibodies, antidouble stranded DNA antibodies, anticardiolipin, antiphospholipid antibodies) and autoimmune disorders has been associated with TNF-α (alpha) antagonism treatment.[7]

TNF-α (alpha) instigates its immunosuppressive effect by regulating antigen-presenting cell functions and apoptosis of potentially autoreactive T cells. Therefore, antagonizing TNF and its suppressive effects may lead to the development or unmasking of autoimmune diseases. There are reports of lupus-associated antibodies occurring after administration of biologics.[7] Patients may develop positivity for antinuclear antibodies (ANAs), antihistone, and anti-DNA. However, no evidence exists that patients who develop new autoantibodies are at significantly increased risk of developing lupus-like syndrome or lupus erythematosus.[6,7,16] Although progressive reduction in ANA titers takes place after discontinuation of treatment the majority of patients will remain ANA-positive.[17] Furthermore, formation of antibodies against the biologic drug itself is an emerging issue. Autoantibodies formation and autoimmunity appears to be more commonly associated with infliximab therapy, than treatment with etanercept, and only limited reports exist for adalimumab.[7,11,13] Whether these antibodies attenuate the efficacy of the treatment or whether they have no measurable effect on the activity of the agent has yet to be determined.

4.3.6 Blood Disorders

Rare reports of patients developing pancytopenia and aplastic anemia on infliximab and etanercept have been described. Leucopenia and thrombocytopenia, although not common, are recognized side effects of TNF-blocking therapy.[3,18] The exact mechanism of cytopenias as a result of TNF-block therapy is still unclear.

4.3.7 Malignancy

The risk for developing malignancies (non-Hodgkin lymphoma, melanoma, and nonmelanoma skin cancer) while under therapy with biologic medications has been investigated. However, no compelling evidence exists that biologics are directly related to an increase in the rate of malignancies.[3,19] Specifically, in patients with psoriasis, no clear findings identify whether lymphoma risk is associated with disease severity, treatment, other unidentified factors, or a combination of factors.[20]

Patients who have been exposed to more than 1,000 J cumulative dosage of psoralen and UVA (PUVA) (more than 200 treatments) may be at increased risk for cutaneous malignancies.[21] The risk is greatest for squamous cell carcinomas, but melanoma is not excluded. Nonmelanoma skin cancer is not an absolute contraindication to biologic therapy. Nevertheless, because these patients represent a particular, high-risk group, caution is warranted when considering biologics.

The known excess of malignancies in immunosuppressed populations, and the known immunosuppressive effects of the biologic agents do, however, provide a biologic basis for concern and justification for the initiation of additional epidemiologic studies to confirm a clear association. Meanwhile, current practice recommendation should probably not go any further than awareness that certain malignancies have been associated with biologics, and alertness for any suspicious symptoms should be maintained.

4.3.8 Anaphylaxis/Allergic Reactions

Formation of antibodies against the biologic drug itself has been reported. More specifically, antibodies against infliximab have been associated with immediate as well as delayed hypersensitivity reactions.[7,8,22] Symptoms may range from mild urticaria and pruritus to more severe anaphylaxis, hypotension, and shock. A reaction may develop during or within 2 h of infliximab infusion, and it is most likely to occur during the first and second infusion. Reinstitution of infliximab after a prolonged period without treatment (more than 16 weeks) can cause a delayed hypersensitivity or serum-like sickness reaction. Symptoms of delayed reaction may include muscle or joint pain with fever or rash, itching, swelling of the hands, lips or face, difficulty swallowing, nettle-type rash, sore throat, and headache. There has been promising success in decreasing the risk of infusion reactions with daily low dose of corticosteroids.[22,23] In addition, diphenhydramine 25–50 mg IV 1.5 h prior to infusion is commonly practiced. All patients receiving infliximab infusions must be medically observed for 1–2 h following the infusion in case a reaction develops.

Individuals who are sensitive to latex should be careful not to handle the rubber cover in the single prefilled autoinjectors of adalimumab (*Humira*) and etanercept (*Enbrel*).[4,24]

4.3.9 Pregnancy/Breast-Feeding

All the biologic medications currently in use in dermatology are pregnancy category B (no human studies conducted, but no adverse effects have been noted in animal studies). An exception to this is efalizumab which has been labeled category C (animal reproduction studies have shown an adverse effect on the fetus and there are no adequate and well-controlled studies in humans). Since no human data is available, initiation of biologic therapy should be avoided in women who are pregnant, planning for pregnancy, or currently breast-feeding. For women of reproductive age, efficient contraception methods should be suggested and implemented prior to therapy.

4.4 Treatment Risk Reduction Strategies

Not all patients are suitable candidates for treatment with a biologic agent. Appropriate patient selection is key in order to achieve treatment success and avert potential unfavorable outcomes. A thorough physical examination and detailed personal and family medical history should be an essential part of all patient encounters. Even for a patient with a "clean bill of health," the physician should offer the option of treatment with biologics to those patients who they feel will be compliant with the dosing schedule and with follow-up visits, and will comprehend how to self-assess and report the onset of signs or symptoms that may signal the onset of an adverse event.

4.4.1 Treatment Exclusion Criteria

Biologics are generally *not indicated* for patients who meet one or more of the following criteria:

- Active TB
- Moderate to severe CHF
- History of demyelinating disease or optic neuritis
- Hepatitis B or C positivity
- HIV positivity
- Active infections (i.e., chronic leg ulcers, persistent or recurring chest infections, indwelling urinary catheter)
- Septic arthritis or sepsis of prosthetic joint within last 12 months
- Pregnancy, planning to become pregnant, or currently breast-feeding
- Premalignant states
- Patients who have had extensive immunosuppressant therapy or prolonged PUVA treatment

4.4.2 Baseline Screening Tests

Specific, guidelines regarding objective screening and monitoring prior to and during treatment with biologics have not been established. In accordance with good clinical practice, baseline and follow-up laboratory tests and imaging studies ought to be offered to all patients when considering therapy with a biologic agent. Initial laboratory testing and subsequent monitoring should be determined on an individual basis according to patient, region of practice, and medication to be utilized.

The United States FDA only mandates TB testing prior to initiating treatment with adalimumab and infliximab. However, because of the increased risk of granulomatous disease with all immunoregulatory medications it is prudent to offer TB screening (tuberculin purified protein derivative [PPD] and/or a chest X-ray) to all patients who are being considered for treatment. Table 4.3 lists the current FDA-mandated laboratory and imaging testing according to biologic agent.

A number of patients may already be receiving medications for the same or different medical condition. A psoriasis patient may already be on an immunosuppressant medication, such as methotrexate. In this case, if biologic therapy is considered, a stricter monitoring strategy may be implemented. The recommended baseline studies shown in Table 4.3 may be used as a guideline. Ultimately, it should be each patient's medical history, family history, social history, physical examination, and individualized risk assessment that directs the appropriate screening and monitoring.

4.4.3 Periodic Monitoring

Close, routine follow-up physical examination and laboratory testing, although not FDA-mandated, are reasonable in order to evaluate the safety of the biologic drug the patient is receiving along with its therapeutic efficacy.

4.4.3.1 Physical Examination

Patient health status should be monitored regularly and any changes or pertinent positives in the review of systems need to be identified and addressed promptly, with special attention to:

- Symptoms and signs of infection
- Symptoms and signs of CHF
- Symptoms and signs of demyelinating disease

4.4.3.2 Laboratory Tests

Many patients do well and feel fine while on biologics and may not see the need for frequent follow-up visits and tests. Regular reevaluation, however, is strongly recommended as biologics are not benign medications. Monthly evaluations are prudent during the initial months of treatment. If the progression of treatment is satisfactory then patient and physician may agree to decrease frequency of follow-up to every 3 months and, subsequently, to every 6 months. At a minimum, monitoring tests should include:

- Complete blood count (CBC)
- Liver function tests (LFT)
- Renal function tests (RFT)

Table 4.3 Guidelines for screening and monitoring studies according to biologic agent

Drug	FDA required	Recommended (non-FDA-mandated) baseline screening	Recommended (non-FDA-mandated) periodic monitoring
Alefacept (*Amevive®*)	Baseline CD4 level; monitor biweekly. Withhold treatment for at least 1 month if CD4 < 250 cells/mL	PPD/Chest X-ray, complete blood count (CBC) with differential, liver function tests (LFT), renal function tests (RFT), β-hcg, HIV	CBC, LFT, RFT, and clinical evaluation every 6 months
Etanercept (*Enbrel®*)	None mandated	PPD/Chest X-ray, RFT, LFT, Hepatitis B and C serology, β-hcg, HIV	
Infliximab (*Remicade®*)	PPD and/or Chest X-ray for latent TB screening	CBC, RFT, LFT, Hepatitis B and C serology, β-hcg, HIV	
Adalimumab (*Humira®*)	PPD and/or Chest X-ray for latent TB screening	CBC, RFT, LFT, Hepatitis B and C serology, β-hcg, HIV	
Ustekinumab (*Stelara*)	PPD and/or Chest X-ray for latent TB screening	CBC, RFT, LFT, Hepatitis B and C serology, β-hcg, HIV	CBC, LFT, RFT, and clinical evaluation every 6 months

4.4.4 Tuberculosis Risk

Before initiating biologic therapy, all patients must have their TB risk assessed.[25] This should include a history of any prior TB infection and treatment, BCG (bacillus Calmette Guérin) vaccination, a thorough clinical examination, and a chest X-ray. The chest X-ray needs to be taken as close as possible to the planned start date of the biologic therapy.[25] A PPD test is advised. However, one should keep in mind that the accuracy and reliability of the tuberculin skin test is significantly affected by immunosuppressive therapy. If the patient is currently on immunosuppressive medications, such as methotrexate or cyclosporine, the PPD test should be regarded as unreliable. The same holds true for patients who have stopped immunosuppressive therapy for a period of less than 3 months from the test.

Referral to a pulmonologist or TB specialist is warranted for individuals with a positive PPD, abnormal chest X-ray, or history of TB infection.[25] If the patient is found to have active TB infection or have had inadequate treatment of past infection, then appropriate TB treatment should be commenced. Initiating biologic therapy in this case is contraindicated.

If the patient is found to have had adequate treatment of a previous TB infection, then biologic therapy may be initiated. However, a repeat chest X-ray 3 month after the initiation of therapy should be acquired to help rule out TB reoccurrence.[25]

For patients with normal chest X-ray, negative PPD (less than 5 mm induration), and no history of TB, therapy with biologic medications may be initiated.

4.4.5 Vaccinations

Seasonal influenza vaccine is not mandated but recommended and commonly administered to patients who are being treated with biologics. The exception to this is the intranasal *FluMist* vaccine which is a live, attenuated influenza virus vaccination product and its administration to patients who are on immunosuppressants, including biologics, is contraindicated.[5]

Several other live, attenuated vaccines currently licensed for use and distribution in several countries, including the United States are also *contraindicated* in patients who are receiving biologic therapy. These include:

- Measles, mumps, and rubella (MMR)
- BCG
- Poliomyelitis (oral Sabin vaccine)
- Yellow fever
- Typhoid (oral)
- Varicella (*Varivax*)
- Zoster (*Zostavax*)
- Smallpox (Vaccinia)

If for any reason a patient requires a live vaccination while on therapy with a biologic agent, it would be prudent that therapy be stopped at least 2 weeks prior to immunization and, ideally, not be resumed until at least 4 weeks after.

4.4.6 Withdrawal of Therapy

As with any medication, treatment should be promptly withdrawn in the event of an adverse event. According to the circumstances, withdrawal may be temporary or permanent. Table 4.4 lists some of the reasons therapy with a biologic medication should be interrupted:

- If a patient develops lupus-like symptoms, blood tests for antinuclear antibodies and antidoublestranded DNA antibodies should be repeated before considering any further treatment.
- If disease response is unsatisfactory after 3–6 months of treatment, switching to a different biologic agent may be appropriate. Failure of one agent to produce results does not equate failure of the medication class as a whole.[26]

Table 4.4 Indications for withdrawal of biologic therapy

Permanent withdrawal of treatment	Temporary withdrawal of treatment
Malignancy	
Severe drug-related toxicity	
Drug-associated allergic reaction	Pregnancy
Neurological symptoms	Need for surgical procedure
Congestive heart failure (CHF)	Severe intercurrent infection
Lupus-like symptoms	

- A high index of suspicion for infection should be kept at all times and appropriate screening should be undertaken if required.
- Patient should be educated to promptly report any neurologic events including visual changes.
- Therapy should be discontinued 2–4 weeks prior to any major surgical procedure and not resume until at least 4 weeks after.
- Effective contraception in women of reproductive age and avoidance of breast-feeding while on biologics is warranted.

4.5 Combination Therapy/Concomitant Medications

Hepatotoxicity and nephrotoxicity have been associated with the most commonly used systemic psoriasis treatment agents, methotrexate and cyclosporine. Combining these traditional agents with biologic therapy may achieve not only improved therapeutic efficacy but also a decrease in the risk of end organ toxicity. The concern of combination therapy leading to increased immunosuppression and its consequences has been addressed. However, there are a number of case reports in literature of successful use of biologic agents concurrently with methotrexate. Additionally, phototherapy is generally considered safe to implement concomitantly with biologic agents.

To date, no long-term clinical studies on quantifying risks and benefits of combination therapy exist, and therefore combination therapy should only be cautiously recommended. As our knowledge and experience with this class of medication increases, the intricacies and potential of combination therapy will continue to be refined.

4.6 Pediatrics

Treatment of psoriasis in children is challenging. Trials of biologic agents for managing psoriasis in children are being conducted but information is currently limited and the long-term safety profile still being evaluated. To date, none of the biologics in use in dermatology are FDA-approved for treating psoriasis in individuals less than 18 years of age.

Etanercept has been approved for treatment of juvenile rheumatoid arthritis (JRA) for children as young as 4 years of age. Both psoriasis and rheumatoid arthritis share similarities in their pathogenesis at the molecular level. The fact that a biologic agent has succeeded in studies and gained approval for use in children with JRA foreshadows potential future approval for the use of these agents in children with psoriasis and/or psoriatic arthritis.

4.7 Elderly

The elderly (65 years of age or older) take more medications (prescription and nonprescription) than any other age group. The risk of side effects and drug–drug interaction increases proportionally with the number of medications. Additionally, the more medications a patient is asked to take the higher the risk of nonadherence. One should also keep in mind that as the body ages the pharmacokinetics and pharmacodynamics of drugs are also altered. However, there are no studies to date that indicate any differences in the safety or efficacy of biologic agents between older and younger patients.

Certain additional practical considerations should be implemented prior to initiating biologic therapy to treat psoriasis in an older individual:

- Obtain complete medication history that includes prescription, nonprescription, and herbs. Patient should be instructed to bring medications in at every visit.
- Discontinue any medications if the benefit is marginal or if a nonpharmacologic alternative exists.
- Be sure the patient understands how to take the medication. If necessary write and provide clear instructions for the patient and anyone who is assisting in treatment.
- Be sure the patient understands the potential risks and side effects of each drug taken.
- In-home support and supervision should be encouraged.
- Because of the increased risk of infections in the elderly a higher suspicion index should be maintained.
- Consider the cost of the drug.

Safe medication use in the elderly requires vigilance and awareness from everyone involved in the patient's treatment. Everyone should be alert for any subtle changes that may signal a potential adverse event. It is especially important to keep track of all maintenance drugs and ensure they are taken properly. The patient must understand and feel comfortable in directing all medical questions and concerns promptly to their physician.

References

1. Alexis AF, Strober BE. Off-label dermatologic uses of anti-TNF- a therapies. *J Cutan Med Surg*. 2005;9:296–302
2. Biogen Inc. Amevive (alefacept), package insert. 2008
3. Desai SB, Furst DE. Problems encountered during antitumour necrosis factor therapy. *Best Pract Res Clin Rheumatol*. 2006;20(4):757–790
4. Immunex Corporation. Enbrel (etanercept), package insert. 2008
5. National Psoriasis Foundation. Flu vaccines warranted for psoriasis patients. 2004. At: www.psoriasis.org; 2008 Accessed 15.01.08
6. Jackson Mark J. TNF-α inhibitors. *Dermatol Ther*. 2007; 20(4):251–264
7. Rott S, Mrowietz U. Recent developments in the use of biologics in psoriasis and autoimmune disorders. The role of antibodies. *BMJ*. 2005;330:716–720
8. Tandon VR, Mahajan A, Khajuria V, Kapoor V. Biologics and challenges ahead for the physician *Indian Acad Clin Med*. 2006;7(4):334–343
9. Robinson WH, Genovese MC, Moreland LW. Demyelinating and neurological events reported in association with tumor necrosis factor alpha antagonism: by what mechanisms could tumor necrosis alpha antagonists improve rheumatoid arthritis but exacerbate multiple sclerosis. *Arthritis Rheum*. 2001;44:1977–1983
10. Suissa S, Ernst P, Hudson M, et al Newer disease modifying antirheumatic drugs and the risk of serious hepatic adverse events in patients with rheumatoid arthritis. *Am J Med*. 2004;117(2):87–92
11. Centocor. Remicade (infliximab), package insert. 2007
12. Tobon GJ, Cañas C, Jaller JJ, et al Serious liver disease induced by infliximab. *Clin Rheumatol*. 2007;26(4):578–581
13. United States Food and Drug Administration. Safety alerts for drugs, biologics medical devices, and dietary supplements.
14. Thiele DL. Is anti-TNF therapy safe in patients with rheumatic disease who also have concurrent B or C chronic hepatitis? *Nat Clin Pract Rheumatol*. 2007;3:130–131
15. Roux CH, Brocq O, Breuil V, et al Safety of anti-TNF- a therapy in rheumatoid arthritis and spondylarthropathies with concurrent B or C chronic hepatitis. *Rheumatology*. 2006;45(10):1294–1297
16. Eriksson C, Engstrand S, Sunddqvist KG, Rantapaa-Dahlqvist S. Autoantibody formation in patients with rheumatoid arthritis treated with anti-TNF alpha. *Ann Rheum Dis*. 2005;64:403–407
17. Vermeire S, Noman M, Van Assche G, et al Autoimmunity associated with anti-tumor necrosis factor alpha treatment in Crohn's disease: a prospective cohort study. *Gastroenterology*. 2003;125(1):32–39
18. Pathare SK, Heycock C, Hamilton J. TNFα blocker-induced thrombocytopenia. *Rheumatology*. 2006;45(10):1313–1314
19. Wolfe F, Michaud K. The effect of methotrexate and anti-tumor necrosis factor therapy on the risk of lymphoma in rheumatoid arthritis in 19, 562 patients during 89, 710 person-years of observation. *Arthritis Rheum*. 2007;56: 1433–1439
20. Gelfand JM, Berlin J, Van Voorhees A, Margolis DJ. Lymphoma rates are low but increased in patients with psoriasis: results from a population-based cohort study in the United Kingdom. *Arch Dermatol*. 2003;139(11):1425–1429
21. Lindelöf B, Sigurgeirsson B, Tegner E, et al. PUVA and cancer: a large-scale epidemiological study. *Lancet*. 1991;338 (8759):91–93
22. Baert F, De Vos M, Louis M, et al. Immunogenicity of infliximab: how to handle the problem? *Acta Gastroenterol Belg*. 2007;70(2):163–170
23. Augustsson J, Eksborg S, Ernestam S, et al Low-dose glucocorticoid therapy decreases risk for treatment-limiting infusion reaction to infliximab in patients with rheumatoid arthritis. *Ann Rheum Dis*. 2007;66:1462–1466
24. Abbot Laboratories. Humira (adalimumab), package insert. 2008
25. Ledingham J, Wilkinson C, Deighton C. British thoracic society (BTS) recommendations for assessing risk and managing tuberculosis in patients due to start anti-TNF- a treatments. *Rheumatology*. 2005;44(10):1205–1206
26. Menter A, Hamilton TK, Toth DP, et al Transitioning patients from efalizumab to alternate psoriasis therapies: findings from an open-label, multicenter, Phase IIIb study. *Int J Dermatol*. 2007;46(6):637–648

Remicade (infliximab). Washington, DC: FDA, 2004. At: http://www.fda.gov/medwatch/SAFETY/2004/safety04. htm#Remicade2; 2008 Accessed 2.02.08

Occupational Dermatology

5

Athena Theodosatos and Robert Haight

5.1 Introduction

Occupational medicine specializes in treating patients with injuries and illnesses from exposures in the workplace. People often encounter very harsh environments in the workplace. Although today's workplace in general is considerably tamer than that of the past, skin problems remain a serious issue.[1]

The bureau of labor statistics (BLS) calculates the frequency of work-related injuries and illnesses for private industry. According to BLS, skin diseases accounted for 15.6% of the nonfatal illnesses in private industry in 2004.[2] This is hardly insignificant. Many occupational medicine physicians rarely see skin disorders. This might be because occupational skin problems are from specific exposures which are associated with specific industries. These industries do not have a uniform geographic distribution.[2]

5.2 Diagnosis

Occupational dermatology includes a broad spectrum of disorders but the majority are acute and chronic contact dermatitis. The most commonly cited are irritant contact dermatitis and allergic contact dermatitis. Since sunlight can be an occupational exposure, skin disorders caused by the sun can therefore be considered work-related for some jobs. Likewise, skin injuries from other physical agents like hot, cold, pressure, friction, electricity, and ionizing radiation can, under some circumstances, be occupational. Water can even cause skin lesions under the right conditions. Toxins and infectious agents are found in some workplaces. The classic occupational skin diseases were chloracne and chrome ulcers. Those diseases are rare in the developed world today. Less acute skin lesions such as hyperpigmentation, leukoderma, alopecia, and lichenification can be occupational.[1-3] Other dermatoses are the major differential to consider when evaluating occupational skin disorders. Any nondermatologist who deals with occupational skin lesions must be able to differentiate them from dermatitis and the other common nonwork-related diagnoses. This means that the physician needs to be able recognize and understand them.

5.2.1 Relevant History

Occupational skin disorders require a detailed history of the skin findings and a work history. The basic questions to consider when evaluating an occupational skin disorder include:

- What does the patient do for a living?
- How long has the patient been doing this job? (the position)
- What is the patient exposed to at work? (Chemicals? Physical agents?)
- What personal protective equipment does the patient use at work?
- Has there been any change to any of the processes at work?
- Do other people at work have similar skin conditions?
- What is the patient exposed to outside of work?

A. Theodosatos (✉)
Department of Family Medicine, Florida Hospital,
Winter Park, FL, USA
e-mail: athenatheo@hotmail.com

R.A. Norman (ed.), *Preventive Dermatology in Infectious Diseases*,
DOI 10.1007/978-0-85729-847-8_5, © Springer-Verlag London Limited 2012

- Has the patient had a work-related skin disorder in the past?
- Has the patient had any exposure-related skin disorders?
- Does the patient have any nonwork-related skin disorders?
- Does the patient have any chronic medical conditions?
- Does the patient have any allergies or a history of atopy?
- Does the patient take any medications?

Material safety data sheet (MSDS) is a brief description of a chemicals physical properties and health effects.[1,2] Data that should be included are: chemical identity; hazardous ingredients; physical and chemical characteristics; fire and exposure hazard data; reactivity data; health hazards; precautions for safe handling and use; and control measures. Although the Hazardous Communication Standard (29 CFR 1910.1200) requires employers to have an MSDS on all of the chemicals to which workers might be exposed, they may be little help to the medical professional except for providing the names of the chemicals to which an employee was exposed.[1,3]

5.3 Worker's Compensation

Each state has a different worker's compensation system. Each of these systems has so many idiosyncrasies that dealing with them has become a major part of the practice of occupational medicine. Not surprisingly, the willingness of other specialists to deal with these systems is related to how the reimbursement compares to that of other payers and how difficult the rules are to deal with.[4]

Part of the extra awkwardness of a worker's compensation system comes from the extra dimension of work-relatedness. Causation is a topic that is unique to occupational medicine. To thrive in the realm of occupational medicine, specialists need to have some understanding of causation.[4]

5.3.1 Assessing Causation

Causation is often a matter of major contention. The worker's compensation system is a compromise. As with most compromises, neither party is satisfied.

The employers and the insurance companies would prefer that an injury not be labeled as work-related. The injured worker has an interest in an occupational etiology. Often, not only is payment for the injury on the line but disability compensation is at stake. This is many times more than enough money to inspire litigation. Highly contested cases might require an independent medical examination (IME). In IMEs, the physician is approached as a consultant to answer specific questions. Causation is a very common question. If a dermatologist or another specialist wants to get some of IME business, the ability to discuss causation intelligently becomes important.[4] In particular, hand dermatitis and nail disorders require careful evaluation since many of them may be work-related or nonwork-related.[5]

Contact dermatitis is the most common occupational skin disorder.[3] Mathias suggested that the presence of four of seven criteria favor an occupational dermatitis[4]:

1. Is the clinical appearance consistent with contact dermatitis?
2. Are there workplace exposures to potential cutaneous irritants or allergens?
3. Is the anatomic distribution of dermatitis consistent with cutaneous exposure in relation to job task?
4. Is the temporal relationship between exposure and onset consistent with contact dermatitis?
5. Are nonoccupational exposures excluded as probable causes?
6. Does dermatitis improve away from work exposure to the suspected irritant or allergen?
7. Do patch or provocation test identify a probable causal agent?

Mathias also suggested that a preexisting dermatitis can probably be said to be aggravated if new dermatitis has occurred on a skin surface that was not previously affected or the dermatitis has become more severe in an area that was already affected by the preexisting dermatitis. If an aggravation has developed, the above seven criteria can be used to determine if the aggravation is due to a superimposed occupational dermatitis.[4]

5.3.2 Determination of Impairment

When a worker's compensation patient reaches the point of maximum medical improvement, the physician determines the degree of permanent impairment. The level of impairment is a frequent point of contention because it affects the amount of compensation. The American Medical Association publishes the Guides to the Evaluation of Permanent Impairment to help to standardize the determination of impairment ratings. A number of states have developed their own guides to calculating impairment ratings.[1,4]

There is a chapter that provides criteria for rating permanent impairment due to skin disorders. There are five classes of impairment due to skin disease with impairment ratings ranging from 0% to 95%. The class of impairment is determined by whether the signs and symptoms are present intermittently or constantly, if there is limitation of the activities of daily living, and if they require intermittent or constant treatment.[6]

5.4 Phototoxic Reactions and Photoallergic Reactions

A phototoxic reaction occurs when a chemical forms free radicals by reacting with ultraviolet light. Classically, phototoxic reactions occur in workers that are exposed to tars. Photoallergic reactions occur when an allergen is produced from an interaction of a chemical with light. Photosensitivity can refer to phototoxic or photoallergic responses. Either form of photosensitivity requires that both the chemical and the proper wavelength of light are present. These reactions can occur following topical exposure or an internal dose.[7]

5.5 Occupational Acne

Folliculitis is an inflammation of the hair follicles. It may be caused by irritants or infections. The folliculitis is seen in the areas that are exposed to the irritant chemical. Acne is most commonly seen with exposures to oils and tars.[1,3]

Chloracne is a specific folliculitis caused by halogenated aromatic hydrocarbons,[1] most often polychlorinated biphenyls (PCBs). Small, straw-colored cysts typically occur on the sides of the forehead, around the lateral aspects of the eyelids, and behind the ears. The neck, groin, chest, back, and buttocks may also be involved. The nose is rarely involved. While an ordinary folliculitis normally resolves in a week or less, chloracne may persist for decades.[1] This is not surprising because the serum half-life of highly chlorinated PCBs is 15 years.[1]

5.6 Pigment Changes

Some authors differentiate occupational vitiligo from leukoderma. Both are acquired depigmentation disorders with selective destruction of melanocytes. A number of chemicals are implicated in occupational vitiligo from leukoderma. The major difference is that contact vitiligo may spread beyond the areas of contact while leukoderma remains confined to the areas of contact.[8] Hypopigmentation can be a nonspecific consequence of contact dermatitis or burns.

Hyperpigmentation is caused by an increase in melanin production. This most often occurs with coal tar pitch, psoralens, heavy metals, and ionizing and non-ionizing radiation.[8]

5.7 Occupational Skin Cancers

Occupational exposures are seldom considered for skin cancers. It is estimated that occupational exposures account for 2% or less of cancers.[9] Cancer may be caused by occupational exposure to chemical carcinogens such as polycyclic aromatic hydrocarbons or radiation from exposure to the sun or X-rays. Skin cancers can also arise from scarring of burns acquired in the workplace.[10] Carcinogens to be considered in the indoor air include: tobacco smoke, radon, and pollutants from cooking and heating.[9]

5.8 Occupational Skin Infections

Worker can be exposed to a number of organisms that can result in a skin infection. The organisms can often be predicted based on the occupation and the exposure (Table 5.1).[1,3]

Table 5.1 Occupational exposures and infectious agents

Exposure	Infectious agent
Any skin trauma	*Staphylococcus*, *Streptococcus*
Fresh- or saltwater fish, crustacea, poultry	*Erysipelothrix rhusiopathiae* (gram-positive rod)
Wet work	Candida
Soil, foliage	Sporotrichosis
Fish tanks	*Mycobacterium marinum*
Healthcare	Scabies
Healthcare (puncture)	*Herpes simplex*
Sheep, goats	Orf

5.9 Skin Notations

The absorption of chemicals through the skin depends on a number of factors. These include: solute concentration, exposure time, the amount of skin surface exposed, the anatomical site of the exposed skin, and the hydrophobicity of the chemical.[1]

5.10 Specific Industries and Exposures

Since solar radiation can be an occupational exposure, photoaging, skin cancer, phototoxic, and photoallergic reactions can be attributed to occupational skin disease.[7] Segmental vibration can result in Raynaud's phenomenon.

Chromium (VI) is a powerful skin irritant. Although rarely seen today in the developed world, exposure can cause painful ulcers known as chrome holes.[1,3,7]

5.11 Occupational Dermatitis

About 15% of all workplace injuries are due to dermatoses.[11] It is therefore an important area of medicine for physicians and healthcare workers. Morbidity associated with these occupational exposures is significantly high in the working population and the cost of care is continually rising. The ultimate goal should be to enable healthcare workers to be able to assess risk factors and develop interventions that will reduce job-related skin injury and disease.[11]

Occupational contact dermatitis is an inflammatory skin condition that can develop with exposure to various agents in the workplace. The two most common forms are irritant and allergic contact dermatitis.[12] It is important to differentiate between the two forms because, although treatment may be the same, diagnosis and prevention strategies differ. Irritant dermatitis is a cutaneous inflammatory reaction that results from a direct cytotoxic effect of a chemical or physical agent. Allergic contact dermatitis is an acquired sensitivity to different substances that produce inflammatory reactions in those who have been previously sensitized to the allergen.[12,13] Approximately 80% of the cases of contact dermatitis have been shown to be due to chemical irritants and about 20% have been shown to be due to allergic reactions.[11] Some new data suggest that allergic contact dermatitis may actually be more prevalent than irritant dermatitis.[13] The 5-year study indicated an under-diagnosis of allergic dermatitis based on the under-utilization of patch testing. Comparison studies in other countries showed higher rates of diagnosis of allergic contact dermatitis in multiple studies. Results suggest the need for a wider array of allergens to be used in patch testing and also encourage a stronger emphasis on performing patch testing.[13] The importance of proper patch testing and patience needed by the physician and patient in order to diagnosis the correct condition is also underscored.[13]

5.11.1 Causes

The skin initially becomes red and may burn or itch when it comes in contact with an irritating or sensitizing substance. After the initial contact cutaneous erythema sets in, small vesicles and papules can develop. Later scales and crusts form. The most commonly affected areas are the hands and forearms. Although the most commonly affected areas are the exposed regions of the body, if the offending agent is a chemical, it has the ability to soak through the clothing and affect the normally unexposed areas such as the chest, back, and upper thighs. If the causative agent does not remain in contact with the skin, the rash will disappear. Sometimes it may take a few weeks or longer for complete resolution of the skin reaction. One factor that significantly increases the time it takes for the dermatitis to resolve is prolonged length of exposure. Prolonged or chronic exposure leads to hyperpigmentation, fissure formation, and often, secondary infections. Other factors that increase resolution time include increased age, due to the altered skin response that occurs as our skin ages, and pigmentation; darker skin burning more easily than lighter. Genetic predisposition and environmental factors such as extremes in temperature may also lead to lengthy recovery times.[11-13]

Women have been noted to be more likely to develop occupational hand dermatitis than men. This may be due to occupations that many women have that increase their risk for exposure to irritating chemicals and other substances. An example may be kitchen work and other household cleaning jobs that women tend to do more than men.[14,15] The presence of atopic dermatitis or allergic contact dermatitis has been associated with more severe outcomes. Lower socioeconomic status has been postulated as a possible risk factor for development of occupational contact dermatitis.[15] Prolonged sick leave and frequent change of jobs are common in individuals with a chronic job-related skin dermatosis.[16]

Almost any substance has the ability to cause a skin reaction; the most frequently encountered ones will be mentioned here. Irritant dermatitis is most often encountered with use of scented soaps and detergents, other cleaning agents, and many food varieties. Allergic contact dermatitis is often caused by plants, dyes, rubber additives, nickel, and plastic resins. Certain occupations may increase risk of exposure and development of contact dermatitis. Agriculture and manufacturing jobs have been shown by the BLS to be the highest affected occupations.[2] Construction workers have a substantial risk of developing irritant or allergic dermatitis. Within construction, tile workers and terrazzo workers have a strikingly high incidence of occupational skin disease.[11,12] Hairdressers also have a high-risk of developing hand dermatitis; 50% have been shown to develop it within the first 3 years of beginning work.[17] Massage therapists are at increased risk of developing hand dermatitis, mainly due to the use of aromatherapy products in massage oils. Their patients are also at increased risk for occupational dermatitis from the sensitizing effects of massage oils.[18]

An uncommon but interesting cause of occupational dermatosis has been documented in some hairdressers and dog groomers.[19] In these cases, the affected individuals developed an inflammatory response to penetration of hair fragments into the interdigital spaces of the hands. The affected individuals had a recurrence of erythema, papules, and draining pustules in the interdigital web spaces and went on to require foreign body removal of the hairs. Eventually, they were diagnosed with trichogranuloma, also known as a pilonidal sinus. Antibiotics are generally resistant in this condition, therefore prevention is key. The use of gloves and prompt removal of any embedded hairs is encouraged. This condition, although rare, is important to be aware of because multiple sinuses can form leading to fistula formation and further morbidity.[19]

The food industry is a known source of exposure to various agents responsible for dermatological problems. The seafood processing centers have been reported to be a cause of dermatitis in up to 78% of workers in a study done in South Africa. The study reveals a major cause for contact dermatitis development to be unprotected skin exposure, due to the lack of protective equipment.[20] The majority of seafood industry related skin conditions were found to be due to particular irritants such as spices, onions, garlic, and vinegar.[20]

Antimicrobial allergy from plastic gloves is a rare cause of allergic contact dermatitis. It has been reported that some people have had hand dermatitis developing after using gloves that were manufactured with benzisothiazolinone, which is a biocide used in the manufacture of disposable polyvinyl chloride (PVC) gloves. It may benefit patients to have patch testing done with benzisothiazolinone if they experience a skin reaction after using PVC gloves.[21]

Latex allergies have been increasing drastically in the United States. Latex is a known contributor to morbidity and mortality in the hospital and the only way to improve the adverse reactions associated with latex is education of the causes, signs and symptoms, and prevention measures. Avoidance is the only way to prevent allergic reactivation but proper diagnosis via patch testing and serological assays are also very important in making sure the proper diagnosis was made.[22] Latex gloves are the primary barrier used in healthcare settings for protection against infection. Natural latex is produced from the *Hevea brasiliensis* tree.[23] A coagulation process occurs after the liquid is collected from the tree and mixed with other chemicals. The demand for latex gloves has been growing, resulting in less refined production procedures. Latex allergies may occur from a delayed hypersensitivity or an immediate hypersensitivity reaction. If symptoms develop within

30 min, the reaction is immediate and skin findings such as erythema and vesicle formation develop. This reaction is due to the proteins in the latex. Experts believe that the change in the manufacturing process that increased the natural rubber latex proteins has been a huge factor in the development of allergic reactions.[22,23] Other contributing factors include better awareness and universal precautions leading to increased glove use.

The most severe, immediate allergic reaction to natural rubber latex proteins is an IgE-mediated (type 1) hypersensitivity.[24,25] Once sensitization occurs the next exposure will lead to a more serious reaction. Despite the increased recognition of latex rubber allergies, powder-free gloves and patient education has led to a decrease in the number of latex allergies overall.[26]

5.11.2 Patch Testing

The patch test can help to identify the offending agent in a patient with contact dermatitis. The role of a suspected material as an inciting agent can be supported by the observation of an inflammatory response after it is applied to an unaffected area of skin.

The patch test is performed by applying solids, liquids, or powders to the back under metallic disks or in a hydrogel suspension.[27] The procedures are standardized in respect to the concentration of antigen, type of vehicle, character of the vehicle, and the testing and interpretation procedure. The Finn chamber test uses aluminum cups, which are affixed with polyacrylate adhesive tape.[28] The True test uses strips of tape with measured amounts of antigen in hydrophilic gel film on 9×9 mm patches.[29] Standardized concentrations of chemicals are applied to the back in vertical rows and covered with hypoallergenic tape. The patch test remains in place for 48 h.

In occupational medicine it is important to determine what materials will be informative based on the history and physical examination. The patch test should never be performed with unknown exposure chemicals that the employee might bring with him. Simply using a standard panel may not provide the necessary information. For instance, in a study where the number of antigens was increased to 49, an additional 12.4% of the patients were defined as allergic.[1,27-29] In occupational medicine, the potential for a fruitless result is increased by the fact that there are more exposures that may not be recognized by the primary care physician.

If done correctly, the patch test can distinguish an irritant from an allergen. This is an issue because many allergens are also irritants. To do this it is important to use a concentration of the agent that will usually only cause a reaction in sensitized patients. The assumption is that patients who are allergic will react against the agent at a concentration below that at which an irritant reaction will be observed. Using the proper dilution and understanding the mechanisms of the reactions is the key.[27]

The exposed area is examined at the time that the test is removed and again 24–72 h later. The reactions are quantified: a weak positive reaction (+) is defined by erythema, infiltration, and discrete papules. A strong positive reaction (++) is defined by erythema, infiltration, papules, and discrete vesicles. An extreme positive reaction (+++) is defined by coalescing vesicles or bullae. A patient that has an extreme reaction will be capable of reacting to a lower concentration of antigen than a patient with a 1+ reaction. Interpreting the skin reactions is a skill which must be developed through experience. If the intensity of the reaction increases between 24 and 48 h, this supports an allergic reaction; a decrease of intensity favors an irritant reaction.[27-29]

5.11.2.1 TRUE Test

The 24 antigen patches used in the TRUE test are listed in Table 5.2.[27] Wood alcohol is found in cosmetics, soaps, and topical medications. Potassium dichromate may cause a reaction in patients who are allergic to cement, tanned leather, welding fumes, cutting oils, antirust paints, or other industrial chemicals. Colophony is a resin that is found in cosmetics, adhesives, and industrial and household products. Parabens are used as preservatives in a number of topical preparations. Balsam of Peru is found in cosmetics, topical medications, and foods. Ethylenediamine dihydrochloride may cause a reaction in patients who are allergic to topical medications, eye drops, anticorrosive agents, or industrial solvents. Cobalt is found in cement, metal plated objects, and paints. The p-tert-butylphenol formaldehyde resin reacts in patients who are allergic to waterproof glues, bonded leather, construction materials, paper, or fabrics. Epoxy resins are found in two-part adhesives, surface coatings, and paints. The carba

Table 5.2 Antigen patches used in the true test

Nickel sulphate
Wood alcohol
Neomycin sulphate
Potassium dichromate
Caine mix
Fragrance mix
Colophony
Paraben mix
Negative control
Balsam of Peru
Ethylenediamine dihyrochloride
Cobalt dichloride
p-tert-Butylphenol formaldehyde resin
Epoxy resin mix
Carba mix
Black rubber mix
Cl+Me- Isothiazolinone
Quaternium-15
Mercaptobenzothiazole
p-Phenylenediamine
Formaldehyde
Mercapto mix
Thimerosol
Thiuram

Table 5.3 Rule of nines

Body area	Total body surface area (%)
Each upper limb	9
Each lower limb	18
Anterior and posterior trunk	18 anterior, 18 posterior
Head and neck	9
Perineum and genitalia	1

Dehydrated forms of these standardized antigens are incorporated into hydrophilic gels and attached to waterproof backings. There is no allergen preparation required on the part of the physician. The patches are simply placed on the patient's back where perspiration will dehydrate the antigen. The antigens are supplied in two panels. The panels are applied to healthy hairless skin that is free of any dermatological lesions on each side of the patient's upper back approximately 5 cm from the midline. Cleaning with potential irritants is unnecessary and may interfere with the test. The test is removed 48 h later. The reactions are interpreted at 72–96 h after the application of the test. The reactions arc interpreted as shown in Table 5.3. The more positive the test the more likely is that it represents a true allergic reaction. The patient should be instructed to return if a late reaction occurs 4–5 days after the application. This is most often seen with p-phenylenediamine.[1,27-29]

Application of the test during an extensive ongoing dermatitis may intensify the reaction. The application to a previously affected site may result in a false positive. A false positive may also result from hyperirritable skin. False negatives may result from inadequate contact between the allergen and the skin or corticosteroid use.[27]

mix may react in individuals who are allergic to rubber products, leather glues, pesticides, vinyl soaps, or disinfectants. Patients that are allergic to preservatives in cosmetics, skin products, polishes, or cleaners may react to quaterium-15. Patients that are allergic to rubber products, adhesives, fl ea sprays or powders, or film emulsion may react to mercaptobenzothiazole.

Workers that are allergic to dyed textiles, printing ink, or photo developer may react to p-phenylenediamine. Formaldehyde is found in fabric finishes, plastics, synthetic resins, glues, textiles, and a number of construction materials.

The negative control is an uncoated polyester patch. The manufacturer claims that this panel accounts for 80% of the cases of allergic contact dermatitis.[1,27]

5.11.2.2 Finn Chamber

The Finn chamber test uses (8 or 12 mm) aluminum or polypropylene (8, 12, or 18) coated chambers. The chambers must be filled by the clinician. Like the TRUE test the Finn test is applied to the upper back and utilizes an occlusive method. The makers of the Finn test recommend cleaning the skin with alcohol if necessary. The test is removed in 1–2 days. A ring-shaped depression at the time of removal verifies that there was adequate occlusion. The test is read 20 min after the chambers are removed and 3–7 days after application. The patient should avoid vigorous activity or shower while the test is in place.[28]

The Finn chamber offers a choice in antigens but requires more work from the physician. Since the antigen concentration (depending on the selection of the examiner) may be less standardized, there is more of an opportunity for an irritant reaction to cause confusion. Drying of the filter paper may result in a false negative. Using the causative agent in an insufficient strength will also result in a false negative test. False positives may be observed due to the aluminum.[28]

Patch testing will not be helpful if the causative agent is omitted. An allergic reaction pattern along with the right indicates an allergic contact dermatitis. In contrast, an irritant reaction does not add significant support to an irritant contact reaction. The patch test is the only technique available to demonstrate that an allergen causes an allergic contact dermatitis. As with any test the patch test must be considered in the context of the patient's history and physical examination.[27-29]

5.11.3 Prevention and Treatment of Occupational Dermatitis

The use of gloves has been a significant factor in the reduction of hand dermatitis, but improper glove use has led to more severe dermatitis due to the repeated exposure to chemicals and or irritating substances.[30] These findings show a need to make sure that proper glove use is taught and encouraged in the workplace. There are a variety of mechanisms that can lead to glove failure. When gloves are used more than once the chance to be exposed to the contaminated exterior of the glove is increased.[31] Permeation of small amounts of certain chemicals through the glove occurs if the glove is worn longer than the breakthrough time, which is the minimum time needed for a particular chemical to diffuse through the glove. Penetration through a glove occurs when an opening or hole develops in the glove.[30,31] Altered skin pH has also been shown to play a role in the development of dermatitis.[32] Gloves have the ability to maintain skin pH and therefore reduce dermatitis. Gloves should be changed frequently and examined for defects often to minimize the chance of contamination and development of hand dermatitis.[30-33]

There are many ways to intervene and treat patients with occupational dermatitis. Some of the most common treatments are barrier creams and moisturizers.[33] Other treatments are more effective for moderate-to-severe dermatitis, including topical steroid creams. Eventually, nonsteroidal creams should be used because they do not cause thinning of the skin.[31-33]

5.12 Burns

Although we have improved strategies to decrease morbidity and mortality in burn patients, skin care is often neglected. Reports show that there are over two million burn injuries each year in the United States. They result from direct or indirect transfer of heat to the body and they are encountered in a variety of workplaces. Prompt treatment is important to avoid infections and long-term sequlae.[34] The location, type, and classification of a burn help determine the aggressiveness needed in its treatment. Acute treatment with wound debridement helps decrease the risk for hypertrophic scar formation and allows donor sites to be found if a skin graft is needed.[35] Burned skin is fragile and very susceptible to sunburn. Without appropriate postburn care, skin breakdown occurs. Pruritus, caused by the destruction of the sebaceous glands, is a symptom of healing burns. These glands are destroyed most commonly in full-thickness burns but can be seen in some partial-thickness burns. Treatment of pruritus is generally accomplished with emollient creams and short-term antihistamine use.[34-36] Scar formation is hastened and cosmetic outcomes improved when tretinoin creams, topical steroids and hydroquinones are used. The treatment time varies but usually lasts for several months. Proper patient education and involvement of multiple healthcare professionals in treatment and follow-up yield the best results.[35]

5.12.1 Chemical Burns in the Workplace

Industrial exposures are a frequent cause of chemical burns. Cleaning products and agricultural products are also common offending agents resulting in many chemical burns. These burns account for 2.1–6.5% of admissions to burn units. The cutaneous manifestations of chemical burns include necrosis at the site of injury with surrounding erythema and blistering. The greater the depth of the chemical burn, the more persistent the necrosis is. Chemical agents that can lead to systemic complications include various acids, oxidizing agents, protoplasmic poisons, and vesicants.[37-39]

Acids and alkalis cause injury to the body by different mechanisms. Most acids denature proteins when they come in contact with the skin and produce a coagulative necrosis. Hydrofluoric (HF) acids are different in that they produce a liquefactive type of necrosis, like alkalis. Chemicals that cause liquefactive necrosis may result in more extensive burns because they are able to extend further and deeper into the skin. The process leading to liquefactive necrosis starts with denaturation of proteins and saponification of fats.[35-39]

History and physical exam should not only focus on the history obtained by the affected person. The physician examining the patient should try and obtain the container that the substance was in and also contact poison control. The mode of exposure is also very important, in addition to the duration of exposure. Once airway, breathing, and circulation are maintained, special attention must be made to keep burned patients from becoming hypothermic. Further injury prevention is also important; therefore removal of contaminated clothing and attention to the area of affected skin is necessary.[40,41]

Oral burns may lead to contractures of the oropharynx. These burns typically result from caustic lye ingestion. Initial oral and gastrointestinal symptoms are erythema, swelling, and pain. Later progression to drooling, stridor, and airway obstruction may develop. Ocular exposures need immediate decontamination followed by a thorough ophthalmologic evaluation. Decontamination with irrigation should be continued until the pH of the eye is returned to normal (pH 7–8). Ophthalmologic evaluation should also include fluorescein staining to check for corneal abrasions. Slit lamp examination can be helpful in evaluating the anterior chamber of the eye, following the ocular irrigation and examination.[34,39]

Cutaneous burn depth and size should be carefully documented. First degree burns are superficial and present as erythematous areas with intact sensation. Second degree burns are deeper involving varying levels of the dermis. They can form blisters although sensation is still intact. Third degree burns are known as full-thickness burns, as they involve all layers of the dermis. They appear swollen, dry, mottled, and white and they do not elicit any sensation. Fourth degree burns go deeper into the muscle or bone.[34,36]

Burn severity is determined by the depth and total body surface area involved. Total body surface area is estimated using the rule of nines (Table 5.3). This rule estimates a percentage of the body involved by each body part.

HF acid has many applications and is a common cause for severe chemical injury. It can be found in plastics, pesticides, fertilizers, high octane fuels, and heavy duty household cleaners. There are two forms: anhydrous HF and aqueous HF. The anhydrous form is stronger and more deadly than the aqueous form, but the majority of HF burns are due to the aqueous form. These burns manifest as pain, erythema, blister formation, and finally tissue destruction. Since this acid is mostly found in household cleaners the affected site is usually the fingertips. HF causes injury by first penetrating the epidermis and then lipophilic fluoride ions. Finally, it goes into the cells where it binds calcium and magnesium. When this occurs, necrosis of soft tissue begins and pain develops from the immobilization of calcium.[39]

Phenol is a weak organic acid with a variety of uses in medicine. It is used frequently for facial peels and topical and injectable anesthetics. It damages the skin through corrosive effects, which cause the skin the slough. Skin exams may reveal partial-thickness burns, although full-thickness burns are also common. Phenol is rapidly absorbed and systemic symptoms are a major concern. Systemic findings include: premature ventricular contractions, tachycardia, hypotension, central nervous system (CNS) depression, and finally respiratory failure.[41]

Chromic acid burns produce localized coagulative necrosis and sometimes gastrointestinal, renal, and CNS complications. When chromium is absorbed it produces a hexavalent form that can be absorbed by red blood cells and bind hemoglobin, impairing its oxygen-carrying capacity. Formic acid is also used in industry and it produces a localized chemical burn similar to one caused by chromic acid. One major systemic effect is acidosis, which develops when formic acid interferes with cellular respiration. Complex acidosis increases proximal tubule reabsorption, decreasing formic acid excretion. Other systemic findings are hypotension, hematuria, hemoglobinuria, renal failure, and end organ damage.[34-38]

Alkali agents are also common causes of chemical burns. Some frequently encountered alkali agents include: anhydrous ammonia, cement burns and airbag injuries.[42] Anhydrous ammonia is a colorless gas found in cleaning products used in the home. These burns may appear grayish-yellow in appearance in partial-thickness burns and leathery and white in full-thickness burns. Cement burns are encountered in the lower extremities of some construction workers.[37] These burns develop from calcium oxide penetration, causing a liquefactive type of necrosis. The skin is damaged from abrasions due to the coarse consistency of cement. Airbag injuries are associated with the release of sodium azide and sodium hydroxide.[42] It has been estimated that skin injuries account for approximately 8% of all injuries from airbag deployment. White phosphorus can cause corrosive damage to the skin by a chemical and thermal combined burn. This oxidizing agent is used in weaponry, some fertilizers, and fireworks. Immediate removal of this chemical from the skin is important to prevent the progression to systemic effects, such as liver and kidney damage.[38] Sulfur mustard is a blistering agent, used in the past in warfare. This chemical has the ability to cause the skin to blister after an asymptomatic period. This blistering effect mostly involves the intertriginous areas, although it does spread easily. They may coalesce and form larger bulla. Systemic effects are also observed, therefore prompt treatment is important. Betadine is an antiseptic containing water, iodine, and polyvinyl pyrrolidine. It has the ability to cause burns especially on areas of the skin that are not dried properly. Dependent areas of the body are most commonly affected. Other skin cleansing agents must be used with caution, especially in babies and the elderly.[43] Table 5.4 lists some common burn-causing chemical agents, their uses, and medical treatment.

Laboratory studies can be useful in burns that are known to cause systemic effects and in burns involving mild-to-moderate amounts of skin. The common systemic effects that occur vary by the type of chemical involved. Fluid and electrolyte monitoring may be necessary to identify patients needing closer monitoring in the hospital. Initial management of any burn patient requires removal of the offending agent. Next, contaminated clothes should be removed and affected areas of the skin should be irrigated. Earlier irrigation has been shown to limit burn depth and also decrease the duration of time spent in the hospital. Fluid resuscitation is important in chemical burns because these burns tend to be deeper in the tissue than other types of burns. Irrigation dilutes the chemical and removes unreacted chemicals from the skin. Burn treatment also includes pain management, physical therapy, and occupational therapy. Sometimes skin grafting may be needed along with cosmetic reconstruction. Some studies have shown that certain biological dressings can be used effectively in second degree burns. For example, xenoderm can lead to a reduction in dressing times, reduce hospital stay, and decrease the formation of scars.[34,44]

Burn patients who receive the earliest care have been shown to have the best clinical outcomes. In order to be able to treat a burn patient appropriately early on, healthcare providers need to be have a clear clinical picture of the different types and causes of burns, especially in the workplace. This can be accomplished by setting up burn education and prevention measures, especially in high-risk jobs.[34,44]

Table 5.4 Chemical agents, their uses, and medical management

Chemical agent	Uses	Medical management
Hydrofluoric (HF) acid	Fertilizers, pesticides, dyes, plastics, and household cleaners	Irrigation, ammonium compounds (to inactivate free fluoride ions), calcium gluconate gels (neutralization), and sometimes debridement
Phenol, carbolic acid, hydoxybenzene	Sewage treatment, topical and systemic anesthetics, chemical face peels	Irrigation, polyethylene glycol (PEG)
Chromic acid	Dye production	Irrigation, phosphate buffers, thiosulfate soaks, EDTA
Formic acid	Descaling agent, rubber processor	Irrigation, IVF hydration, bicarbonate therapy, folic acid, dialysis (severe)
Cement	Construction products	Irrigation, dry lime, soap and water
White phosphorus	Weaponry, manufacture of insecticides and fertilizers, fireworks	Irrigation, wet compresses, and surgical debridement

References

1. Rom WM. *Environmental and Occupational Medicine.* 3 rd ed. Philadelphia: Lippincott-Raven; 1998
2. US Department of Labor, US Bureau of Labor Statistics. Occupational Injuries and Illnesses: counts, rates, and characteristics, 2004. *Bulletin 2584.* 2006
3. Emmett EA. Occupational dermatitosis. In: Fitzpatrick TB, Eisen AZ, Wolf K, et al eds. *Dermatology in General Medicine.* 3rd ed. New York: McGraw-Hill; 1987
4. Mathias CGT. Contact dermatitis and workers' compensation: criteria for establishing occupational causation and aggravation. *J Am Acad Derm.* 1989;20(5):842–848
5. Dhir H. Hand dermatitis and nail disorders of the workplace. *Clin Occup Environ Med.* 2006;5(2):381–396
6. Cocchiarella L, Anderson GBJ. *Guides to the Evaluation of Permanent Impairment.* 5th ed. Chicago: American Medical Association; 2000
7. Pharda V, Gruber F, Kastelan M, et al Occupational skin diseases caused by solar radiation. *Coll Antropol.* 2007;31(1): 87–90
8. Boissy RE, Manga P. On the etiology of contact/occupational vitiligo. *Pigment Cell Res.* 2004;17(3):208–214
9. Boffetta P. Epidemiology of environmental and occupational cancer. *Oncogene.* 2004;23(38):6392–6403
10. Gawkrodger DJ. Occupational skin cancer. *Occup Med.* 2004;54(7):458–463
11. McCall BP, Horwitz IB, Feldman SR, Balkrishnan R. Incidence rates, costs, severity, and work-related factors of occupational dermatitis-A workers compensation analysis of Oregon 1990–1997. *Arch Dermatol.* 2005;141:713–718
12. Rietschel RL. Occupational contact dermatitis. *Lancet.* 1997;349:1093–1095
13. Kucenic MJ, Belsito DV. Occupational allergic contact dermatitis is more prevalent than irritant contact dermatitis: a 5 year study. *J Am Acad Dermatol.* 2002;46:695–699
14. Robinson JK, Ramos-e-Silva M. Women's dermatologic diseases, health care delivery, and socioeconomic barriers. *Arch Dermatol.* 2006;142:362–364
15. Cvetkovski RS, Zachariae R, et al Prognosis of occupational hand eczema. *Arch Dermatol.* 2006;142:305–311
16. Olsen J, Mathiesen L, et al Relation between diagnoses on severity, sick leave and loss of job among patients with occupational hand eczema. *Br J Dermatol.* 2004;152:93–98
17. Worth A, Arshad SH, Sheikh A. Occupational dermatitis in a hairdresser. *Br Med J.* 2007;335:399
18. Crawford GH, Katz KA, Ellis E, James WD. Use of aromatherapy products and increased risk of hand dermatitis in massage therapists. *Arch Dermatol.* 2004;140:991–996
19. Vaccaro M, Guarneri F, Barbuzza O, et al A prickly pair. *Am J Med.* 2007;120:1026–1027
20. Jeebhay MF, Lopata AL, Robins TG. Seafood processing in South Africa: a study of working practices, occupational health services and allergic problems in the industry. *Occup Med.* 2000;50:406–413
21. Aalton-Korte K, Alanko K, et al Antimicrobial allergy from polyvinyl chloride gloves. *Arch Dermatol Oct.* 2006;142: 1326–1330
22. Wilkinson SM, Beck MH. Allergic contact dermatitis from latex rubber. *Br J Dermatol.* 1996;134:910–914
23. Sinha A, Harrison P V. Latex glove allergy among hospital employees: a study in the north-west of England. *Occup Med.* 1998;48:405–410
24. Woods JA, Lambert S, Thomas AE, et al Natural rubber latex allergy: spectrum, diagnostic approach, and therapy. *J Emerg Med.* 1997;15:71–85
25. Bock M, Schmidt A, et al Occupational skin disease in the construction industry. *Br J Derm.* 2003;149:1165–1171
26. Henning A, et al Primary prevention of natural rubber latex allergy in the German health care system through education and intervention. *J Allergy Clin Immunol.* 2002;110: 318–323
27. True Test Physician's Reference Manual. At: www.truetest. com; 2009 Accessed 17.02.09
28. Finn Chamber on Scanpor. At: www.epitest.fi; 2009 Accessed 17.02.09
29. Marks JG, Belsito DV, DeLeo VA, et al Clinical and laboratory studies: North American contact dermatitis group patch test for the determination of delayed- type hypersensitivity to topical allergens. *J Am Ac Derm.* 1998;38(6):911–918
30. Saary J, et al A systematic review of contact dermatitis treatment and prevention. *J Am Acad Dermatol.* 2005;53: 843–855
31. Soonyou K, Lauren S, et al Role of protective gloves in the causation and treatment of occupational irritant contact dermatitis. *J Am Acad Dermatol.* 2006;55:891–896
32. Mirza R, et al A randomized, controlled, double blind study of the effect of wearing coated pH 5.5 latex gloves compared with standard powder free latex gloves on skin pH, transepidermal water loss and skin irritation. *Contact Derm.* 2006; 55:20–25
33. Wigger-Alberti W, Elsner P. Prevention of irritant contact dermatitis-new aspects. *Immunol Allergy Clin N Am.* 1997; 17:443–450
34. Monafo WW. Initial management of burns. *N Engl J Med.* 1996;335(21):1581–1586
35. Ho WS, Chan HH, Ying S Y, et al Skin care in burn patients: a team approach. *Burns.* 2001;27:489–491
36. Kales SN, Christiani DC. Acute chemical emergencies. *N Engl J Med.* 2004;350(8):800–808
37. Spoo J, Elsner P. Cement burns: a review 1960–2000. *Contact Derm.* 2001;45(2):68–71
38. Chou TD, Lee TW, Chen SL, et al The management of white phosphorus burns. *Burns.* 2001;27(5):492–497
39. Hatzifotis M, Williams A, Muller M, et al Hydrofluoric acid burns. *Burns.* 2004;30(2):156–159
40. Browne TD. The treatment of hydrofluoric acid burns. *Occup Med.* 1974;24:80–89
41. Horch R, Spilker G, Stark GB. Phenol burns and intoxications. *Burns.* 1994;20(1):45–50
42. Corazza M, Bacilieri S, Morandi P. Airbag dermatitis. *Contact Derm.* 2000;42(6):367–368
43. Maenthaisong R, Chaiyakunapruk N, et al The efficacy of aloe vera used for burn wound healing: A systematic review. *Burns.* 2007;33:713–718
44. Cox RD. Burns, Chemical. At www.emedicine.com; 2008 Accessed 15.05.08. Chemical burns

Diagnosis and Prevention of Bullous Diseases

6

Supriya S. Venugopal and Dedee F. Murrell

6.1 Introduction

Bullous diseases may be broadly divided into the inherited, autoimmune, and infectious types. This chapter will deal with each in turn: how to diagnose and how to, where possible, prevent these from occurring or worsening.

6.2 Inherited Bullous Diseases

6.2.1 Epidermolysis Bullosa

Epidermolysis bullosa is a blistering disease occurring at birth or shortly after birth, characterized by the tendency to develop blisters spontaneously or after sustaining minimal trauma. There are many different types of epidermolysis bullosa. The three main inherited subtypes (Table 6.1), classified according to the level at which skin cleavage occurs, include:

- Epidermolysis bullosa simplex (EBS)
- Junctional epidermolysis bullosa (JEB)
- Dystrophic epidermolysis bullosa (DEB)

EBS is characterized by intradermal skin cleavage above the basement membrane at the level of the keratinocytes. In JEB, blister formation occurs at the level of the lamina lucida, and DEB is characterized by blister formation in the sublamina densa.[65] The classification

D.F. Murrell (✉)
Department of Dermatology,
St. George Hospital, University of NSW Medical School,
Sydney, NSW, Australia
e-mail: d.murrell@unsw.edu.au

of EB has been upgraded[67] and at the time of writing this chapter the terminology was being further revised and upgraded to include some additional syndromes.[68]

EBS is a blistering disorder affecting the basal layer of the epidermis. Most cases are caused by mutations in the genes encoding keratin 5 (K5) and keratin 14 (K14) and are characterized by cytolysis within the basal layer of the epidermis.[163] Patients with the Dowling-Meara type of EB simplex (EBS-DM) can have severe blistering at birth, but this tends to markedly improve as the patient grows older and by early adulthood, patients rarely develop blisters.[135] Additional features are hyperkeratosis of the palms and soles, and herpetiform grouping of blisters.[36] In EBS-DM, some of the keratin filaments are organized into dense, circumscribed clumps that sometimes connect with either hemidesmosomes or desmosomes.[12] Transmission electron microscopy (TEM) is highly specific for the diagnosis of the EBS-DM, though it has variable sensitivity.[104,213]

There are multiple important considerations with respect to the ultrastructural findings in autosomal recessive EBS (R-EBS) and autosomal recessive EBS associated with muscular dystrophy (EBS-MD). In R-EBS, there may be an ablation of K14 expression and also a lack of visible keratin filaments in basal but not suprabasal keratinocytes.[112,214] Autosomal recessive EBS is associated with the following findings: a lack of integration of keratin filaments with hemidesmosomes, neuro muscular disease, and mutation of the plectin gene.[64,147]

JEB is an autosomal recessive disorder characterized by blisters that develop within the lamina lucida. Clinical manifestations aid in subtype classification in particular, generalized (Herlitz, H-JEB) type, which is lethal, and a generalized but less severe (non-Herlitz, nH-JEB) type.[68] H-JEB is caused by mutations in one of the three genes encoding the anchoring filament

Table 6.1 The major EB types, subtypes, and the associated targeted proteins (Fine et al.[68])

Major EB type	Major EB subtypes	Targeted proteins
Epidermolysis bullosa simplex (EBS)	Suprabasal	Plakophilin-1
	Basal	Desmoplakin
		Keratins 5 and 14; plectin; a6b4 integrins
Junctional epidermolysis bullosa (JEB)	JEB-Herlitz	Lam332
	JEB-other	Lam 332; Col XVII; a6b4 integrins
Dystrophic epidermolysis bullosa (DEB)	Dominant	Collagen VII
	Recessive	Collagen VII
Kindler syndrome	–	Kindlin 1

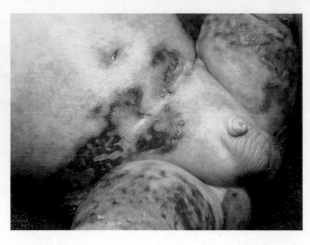

Fig. 6.1 H-JEB with groin involvement exacerbated by nappies

components of laminin 5, now referred to as *Lam332* (*LAMA3*, *LAMB3*, and *LAMC2*).[137] nH-JEB is caused by less deleterious mutations in the aforementioned genes or mutations in the gene that encodes type XVII collagen or *BP180*, known as *COL17A1*.[111,136,137] Classical sites of involvement include the buttocks, mouth, back of the scalp, and periungual areas.[52] Absent or dystrophic nails, enamel hypoplasia, laryngeal edema or stenosis, profound growth retardation, anemia, and the presence of exuberant granulation tissue, particularly on the trunk and on periorificial and periungual sites, are also features. Epidermolysis bullosa, usually but not necessarily in the lamina lucida, associated with pyloric atresia (EB-PA), manifests with neonatal blistering and gastric anomalies. EB-PA is known to be caused by mutations in the hemidesmosomal genes *ITGA6* and *ITGB4*, encoding the alpha6 and beta4 integrin polypeptides, respectively.[157]

Herlitz JEB skin demonstrates a split at the dermal–epidermal junction with minimal dermal inflammation (Fig. 6.1). Immunofluorescence mapping (IFM) and electron microscopy (EM) studies confirm the level of cleavage to be through the lamina lucida. Hemidesmosomes may be significantly reduced, small, and lacking normal subbasal plates.[189] More severely affected patients may display absence or marked reduction in density of the subbasal dense plate along the dermoepidermal junction. In addition, a reduction in hermidesmosome count is associated with a rudimentary or embryonic-appearing ultrastructure. Severely affected

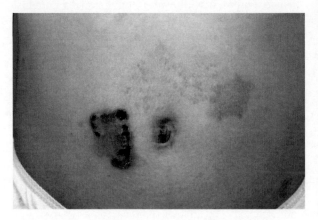

Fig. 6.2 Grouped blistering and postinflammatory change in EBS-DM

individuals are associated with either the absence of hemidesmosomes or have reduced numbers of hemidesmosomes lacking subbasal dense plates.[66]

Laminin 5 is a glycoprotein comprising three subunits: alpha 3, beta 3, and gamma 2. These subunit chains are encoded by the following genes: *LAMA3* (localized to chromosome 18q),[15] *LAMB3* (at 1q32), and *LAMC2* (at 1q25–31),[194] respectively. These have been proposed as candidate genes in Herlitz disease. Studies have demonstrated that mutations in any one of these three genes may be associated with the Herlitz phenotype.[1,116,165] Mutations in *LAMB3* have also been shown to underlie non-Herlitz JEB,[136,137] and recently mutations in the genes encoding (b) 4 integrin and the 180-kDa bullous pemphigoid (BP) antigens have also been demonstrated (Fig. 6.2).[136,137,195]

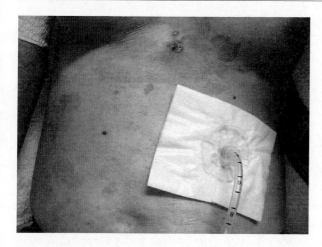

Fig. 6.3 Gastrostomy in RDEB-HS to prevent malnutrition, osteoporosis. Protective nonstick dressing to prevent blistering

DEB may be inherited in an autosomal dominant (DDEB) and an autosomal recessive manner (RDEB). Mutations in the type VII collagen gene (*COL7A1*) gene result in both RDEB and DDEB.[47] RDEB is further subclassified into:

- RDEB-GS: Generalized Severe type
- RDEB-nGS: Generalized non severe type
- Inversa RDEB
- Centripetal RDEB
- Pruriginosa RDEB
- Pretibial RDEB

The generalized severe type (RDEB-GS) is characterized by generalized lesions and scarring of the hands and feet, leading to fusion of the digits pseudosyndactyly and severe mucosal involvement. The milder RDEB-nGS type can be localized or generalized, in contrast with RDEB-GS is associated with very mild or no pseudo-syndactyly, and less frequent extra-cutaneous involvement (Fig. 6.3).[67]

The precise diagnosis of EB is crucial for molecular diagnosis and is the key for prevention using prenatal diagnosis. There are three main modalities for the diagnosis of EB. These include:

- Transmission electron microscopy (TEM)
- Immunofluorescence antigenic mapping
- Genetic studies

Ultrastructural examination demonstrates the level of skin cleavage, allowing discrimination of epidermolytic, junctional, and dermolytic types of EB. Immunofluorescence antigenic mapping (IFM) is a convenient and rapid method for classification and involves the localization of previously defined components within certain ultrastructural regions of the dermoepidermal junction.

TEM allows direct visualization and quantification of specific ultrastructural features. TEM was first used as a diagnostic tool in EB in the early 1960s by Pearson[154,155] which allowed for the first accurate method of distinguishing between the various types of EB. Further developments and refinement of TEM methods have allowed for the diagnosis of further subclassification in the major types of EB. TEM may help establish a definitive diagnosis not only of major variants of EB, but also of main subtypes.[11] TEM is performed on tissue that is stained with uranyl acetate, lead citrate, and osmium tetroxide. The tissue is visualized under EM with a specific focus on the level of skin cleavage present. TEM also allows measurement of the number of keratin tonofilaments, hemidesmosones, subbasal dense plates, and anchoring fibrils.[154,155]

Alternative methods to the diagnosis of EB include IFM, first described by Hintner et al.[98] IFM has been aided by the discovery of several individual basement membrane zone (BMZ) antibodies. IFM is a powerful diagnostic tool for EB when combined with immunohistochemical mapping of these BMZ monoclonal antibodies. IFM determines the precise level of skin cleavage of a specimen by determining the site of binding by a series of antibodies directed to these BMZ antigens, with known ultrastructural binding sites.[63]

There are many reasons for favoring the use of IFM compared with TEM in modern dermatological practice in the diagnosis of EB. Yiasemides et al.[213] concluded that TEM and IFM were appropriate first-line techniques of choice in the diagnosis of EB. The study concluded that despite the lack of statistical significance, IFM consistently had higher sensitivity, specificity, and predictive values in the diagnosis of all three subtypes of EB compared with TEM. There are also several other reasons to favor the use of IFM as opposed to TEM. TEM requires a long training period and sample preparation is more laborious, often taking days to weeks to complete. As a result of skills shortage, TEM is not readily available in all hospitals and laboratories. In addition, interpretation of the skin biopsy using TEM may lead to greater mistakes in diagnosis. This is due to the relatively small area of the specimen sample that is visualized, which may result in the blister being missed. This may also result in the overestimation or underestimation of the number of fibrils and other structural components in EB. At high magnifications, artifactual spaces may be misinterpreted for cleavage sites. Other diagnostic misinterpretations include reporting nonspecific dense bundles of keratin filaments as clumped tonofilaments (i.e., resulting in the diagnosis of EBS-DM).[213]

Due to the variance in the ultrastructural findings in the various subsets of EB, TEM faces difficulties in the accurate diagnosis of the various different subgroups in EB. This is perhaps one of the main reasons why TEM appears to be less accurate in subset diagnosis of EB compared with IFM. Morphometric analysis in JEB demonstrates marked desmosomal heterogeneity.[190] In more severe recessive generalized DEB cases, morphometric analysis has shown a total absence of anchoring fibrils.[35]

Immunohistochemical staining of collagen IV in formalin fixed and paraffin-embedded samples followed by examination under a light microscope is a more rapid alternative to TEM. EBS variants are diagnosed by the presence of collagen IV staining at the floor of the blister. The positive staining in the roof of the blister establishes the diagnosis of dystrophic variants of EB. The present technique identifies collagen IV within the lamina densa and subsequently does not allow differentiation between EB simplex and junctional EB.[23]

6.2.1.1 Prevention of EB

Prenatal genetic diagnosis (PND) has most frequently been performed for the following subtypes of EB, as they are the most severe[59-61,138,180]:

- Recessive dystrophic EB – generalized severe
- Herlitz junctional EB
- Junctional EB associated with congenital pyloric atresia

However, in some countries there are differing ethical paradigms which have allowed PND for "milder" forms of EB, since these may not be perceived to be "mild" by the patients themselves or their carers. These include non-Herlitz JEB[141] and dominant dystrophic EB[118] and disorders in the EB umbrella, skin fragility ectodermal dysplasia and Kindler syndrome.[59-61,68]

Prenatal diagnosis for EB was initially done by examination of a fetal skin biopsy with EM and/or immunohistochemistry.[55,56,91,92,171] In the 1990s, the genes responsible for respective EB subtypes and the family-specific mutations were identified, as mentioned above. This led to the feasibility of DNA-based PND using fetal DNA extracted from amniocentesis at 12–15 weeks initially and later from chorionic villous sampling at about 10 weeks. Direct assessment of previously identified pathogenic mutations or the use of indirect linkage markers have been the methods used for the majority of DNA-based PND in RDEB.[180] Mutational analysis of the type VII collagen gene, COLA1 or haplotype analysis using a number of well-described informative polymorphisms within or flanking COL7A1, if the mutation(s) has/have not been identified are some of the assessment methods used.[138]

Fetal skin biopsy has several disadvantages and has been superseded by molecular diagnosis. A fetal skin biopsy can only be obtained later in gestation, usually 16 weeks or more, and is associated with a relatively high rate of miscarriage.[66] Mutation detection using fetal amniocytes or chorionic villous sampling can be performed earlier and as they are less invasive and have lower risks of miscarriage. However, fetal skin biopsy remains an option in those rare cases in which mutations cannot be identified and linked markers are not available to be used for prenatal diagnosis. Very few obstetricians have experience with fetal skin biopsies, however. Prenatal diagnosis can be greater than 98% accurate and is highly beneficial in pregnancy screening for mutations or informative markers.[158] Analyzing the sequence traces with the aid of computer software, rather than by hand, is mandatory nowadays to reduce human errors. Analysis of fetal skin biopsies and DNA-based prenatal tests allow the diagnosis of an affected fetus to be made once pregnancy is established, and can result in considerable emotional and physical distress for the parents contemplating the prospect of termination.[59-61]

Preimplantation genetic diagnosis (PGD) is a technique involving a single cell biopsy from the six-to-ten cell blastomere stage of the fertilized embryo proceeded by DNA mutational analysis.[86] Less DNA is needed if genome wide markers are used.[59-61] Diseasefree embryos are then implanted into the uterus, thereby avoiding any pregnancy termination procedures usually associated with conventional PND methods.

Mothers who decide to give birth to a baby known to have EB or at high-risk of EB can prevent some of the blistering associated with birth trauma in these infants by undergoing a planned Caesarian section rather than a normal vaginal delivery.

6.3 Autoimmune Bullous Diseases

Autoimmune bullous diseases are associated with autoimmunity against structural components which maintain cell–cell and cell-matrix adhesion in the skin and mucous membranes.[139] They include those where the skin blisters at the BMZ (BP, herpes gestationis, mucous membrane pemphigoid [MMP], linear IgA dermatosis [LAD], epidermolysis bullosa acquisita [EBA], bullous lupus and dermatitis herpetiformis [DH]) and those where the skin blisters within the epidermis (pemphigus vulgaris [PV], pemphigus foliaceus [PF] and other subtypes of pemphigus[88]).

Due to the considerable overlap in the clinical presentation of these conditions, diagnosis of autoimmune bullous skin conditions can be challenging. Detection of tissue-bound and circulating serum autoantibodies and characterization of their molecular specificity is an important modality for diagnosis. In the past decade, there have been several advances in diagnostic modalities for autoimmune bullous skin conditions.

6.3.1 Pemphigus

Pemphigus is a word derived from the Greek work "pemphix" meaning bubble or blister and is a life-threatening autoimmune blistering disease, characterized by intraepithelial blister formation.[95,96,102,124] Circulating autoantibodies directed against intercellular adhesion structures result in the loss of adhesion between the keratinocytes.[5,17] The incidence of pemphigus is approximately 1 in 100,000 people.[186] The variants of pemphigus are determined according to the level of intraepidermal split formation. There are five main variants of pemphigus. These include PV, PF, pemphigus erythematosus, drug-induced pemphigus, and paraneoplastic pemphigus (PNP).

The hallmark of pemphigus is acantholysis, an intradermal split formation due to the loss of adhesion between epidermal keratinocytes. This may result in the development of the Tzanck phenomenon (the rounding of single epidermal cells due to the loss of cell–cell attachment). Inflammatory cell infiltrates of the involved skin are generally absent. PF and PV are usually characterized by suprabasilar loss of adhesion leaving a single layer of basal keratinocytes attached to the dermoepidermal basement membrane (tombstone pattern). PF is associated with a superficial split formation in the subcorneal layer.

Tissue-bound IgG or IgA in a characteristic netlike intercellular distribution pattern within the epidermis, commonly associated with precipitation of C3 is demonstrated on direct immunofluorescence microscopy. Indirect immunofluorescence microscopy, the gold standard in pemphigus, reveals the presence of serum autoantibodies against desmosomal antigens. Pemphigus sera show a characteristic netlike intercellular staining of IgG with human skin as a substrate. Other substrates such as monkey esophagus, guinea pig esophagus, or rat bladder epithelium may be used in the diagnosis of PNP.[110]

Immunoserological tests such as enzyme-linked immunosorbent assay (ELISA) confirm the diagnosis of pemphigus and results can be used to determine disease activity. The development and commercial use of ELISA has provided higher sensitivity and specificity in making the diagnosis of pemphigus subtypes.[105] ELISA alone is insufficient to diagnose the condition. Immunoserological tests can provide valuable information on the clinical course of pemphigus, and can also be used as a diagnostic and prognostic indicator in the management of pemphigus.

Desmoglein 3[5,7] and desmoglein 1[37,57] are the targets for autoantibodies in PV and PF, respectively. In active PV, immunoblot analysis with recombinant Dsg3 demonstrated that anti-Dsg3 of the IgG4, IgA, and IgE subtypes predominate; however, chronic remittent PV is characterized by IgG1 and IgG4 autoantibodies.[22,88,120,185]

PV is the most common variant of pemphigus with an incidence of 0.1–0.5 per 100,000 population, and higher among Jewish patients.[3] The diagnosis of PV is made using four major criteria. These consist of:

- Clinical findings
- Light microscopic findings
- Direct immunofluorescence findings
- Indirect immunofluorescence findings[95,143]

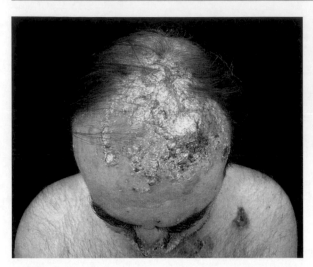

Fig. 6.4 Erosions and crusting of the scalp in a patient with pemphigus vulgaris (PV)

PV is the most common subtype of pemphigus (Fig. 6.4). It is a potentially life-threatening autoimmune vesiculobullous disorder characterized by non-scarring, fragile vesicles and bullae involving the mucosae with varying cutaneous involvement. PV usually presents in adults and can affect anywhere in the body but predominantly affects the buccal and labial mucosa. This condition is characterized by Nikolsky's sign: the application of slight pressure on the blisters resulting in their spread to neighboring areas. Histological studies of PV lesions usually demonstrate acantholysis in the suprabasilar part of the epidermis. Typical findings include IgG and/or C3 binding to the intracellular cement substance (ICS) in the mid-lower or entire epidermis of perilesional skin or mucosa on DIF.[2,125,176,177] PV is associated with autoantibodies to 130-kDa glycoprotein Dsg3 and secondary development of antibodies to 160-kDa glycoprotein Dsg1 antigens, when the skin is involved.[186] Acetylcholine receptors on keratinocytes have also been reported as a possible further target antigen in PV.[82,181,196]

PF generally has a benign clinical course and most frequently presents on the scalp, face, and upper trunk and is characterized by erythema, scaling, and crusting lesions and spares the mucus membranes.[186] An endemic version of PF, fogo selvagem (FS), is endemic to an Indian reservation in Brazil. The cause of this may be environmental and in particular may be due to saliva components of insects which may initiate the spread of the disease; the exact cause is not known but

as it has also been reported in unrelated people moving in to the reservation, not just those from the indigenous population there, it suggests an environmental agent.[49] Penicillamine is also a known causative agent in PF.[26] Other drugs and environmental agents/chemicals may be associated with triggering PV. Exposure to pesticides and occupational exposure to metal vapor were associated with an increased risk of pemphigus.[31] Brenner et al.[32] discussed the importance of various exogenic factors in triggering pemphigus including drugs, particularly those containing thiol and phenol groups, calcium channel blockers, ultraviolet radiation, burns, X-rays, neoplasms, nutritional factors, emotional stress, hormones and pregnancy, viruses and vaccinations. There are a number of cases in which exposure to viral disease, in particular herpes simplex, Epstein Barr virus, cytomegalovirus or human herpes viruses, have been associated with PV or PF.

Pemphigus erythematosus or Senear-Usher syndrome is a localized variant of PF. It is characterized by the presence of a malar erythema, similar to the rash of lupus erythematosus, also extending to sunexposed areas of the scalp, face, and upper trunk.[186] Histological and immunopathological studies confirm the diagnosis of PF. Histopathological examination of PF lesions show subcorneal acantholytic bullae. Binding of IgG and/or C3 to the ICS in the upper stratum malphigii is demonstrated on (DIF) studies of perilesional skin.[176]

PNP, a rare autoimmune bullous disease related to underlying neoplasia, is characterized by severe, painful mucosal erosions and polymorphous skin lesions.[10] PNP occurs in patients with underlying malignancies such as non-Hodgkin's lymphoma, chronic lymphocytic leukemia, and thymoma.[8] PNP is associated with autoantibodies to Dsg1, desmoglein3 (Dsg3) and plakins, a characteristic that differentiates this from the other variants of pemphigus.[41] Histopathologic hallmarks include acantholysis and interface dermatitis or keratinocyte necrosis.[100] PNP is characterized by the development of autoantibodies directed against multiple antigens, predominantly of the plakin family of intermediate filament-associated proteins and the desmogleins of the cadherin family in desmosomes.[6,24,89,164]

PV is strongly associated with the human leukocyte antigen (HLA) serotypes HLA-DR4 and HLA-DR6.[188] Ahmed et al.[4] reported low levels of autoantibody in 48% of healthy relatives of PV patients, and the inheritance of antibody positivity was linked to the DR4 and

DR6 haplotype. Greater than 95% of PV patients possess one or both of these haplotypes.[191] However, population studies report the differing prevalence of alleles in various ethnic groups and concluded that in the non-Jewish population, eight alleles were positively associated and one allele was negatively associated with PV.[123] The two candidate alleles, most likely to contribute to disease susceptibility in the non-Jewish population, included DRB1*0402 and DQB1*0503. DRB1*0402 was determined to be the sole allele likely to confer susceptibility to PV in Ashkenazi Jewish patients.

The global knowledge of PV is quickly advancing; however, there is a dearth of multicenter trials focused on effective strategies for the treatment of pemphigus and multiplicity of outcome measures used.[133] In 2005, the International Pemphigus Definitions Group proposed a consensus statement which provided clear definitions of pemphigus.

The consensus statement on disease endpoints and therapeutic response for pemphigus[142] divides pemphigus disease activity into the following categories:

1. Early endpoints
   (a) Baseline
   (b) Control of disease activity
   (c) End of consolidation phase
2. Late end points
   (a) Complete remission off therapy
   (b) Complete remission on therapy
      – Minimal therapy
      – Minimal adjuvant therapy
      – Partial remission off therapy
      – Partial remission on minimal therapy
3. Relapse/flare
4. Treatment failure

Early endpoints provide a useful clinical indicator for clinicians regarding the commencement of differing treatment regimes. The *baseline* is classified as the day that the treating practitioner initiates treatment. *Control of disease activity* is defined as the time at which there is cessation of new lesions in conjunction with the healing of preexisting lesions. In the majority of cases the expected time period in this stage is weeks. The *end of the consolidation phase* is the time period in which no new lesions have developed over a minimum period of 2 weeks. This phase is also characterized by the healing of most lesions, and most medical practitioners would consider the weaning of steroids.

Late endpoints of disease activity may be reached with or without therapy. *Complete remission off therapy* is characterized by the absence of new lesions over a 2-month period post cessation of therapy. *Minimal therapy* constitutes treatment with less than or equal to, 10 mg/day of prednisone or the equivalent and/or the use of minimal adjuvant therapy for a duration of at least 2 months. *Minimal adjuvant therapy* comprises half the dose required to be defined as treatment failure. *Partial remission off therapy* is classified as development of lesions post cessation of treatment that heal within 1 week without treatment. The patient must be off systemic therapy for 2 months to be classified in this category. Patients may suffer a partial remission on minimal therapy when they develop new lesions that heal within a week whilst receiving minimal therapy. Topical steroids also constitute minimal therapy.

A *relapse/flare* is defined by the development of three or more new lesions which persist without healing for greater than a week or by the extension of preexisting established lesions. Treatment failure results when there is no change in disease activity despite treatment on therapeutic doses of systemic steroids and other agents whose doses and durations were agreed by international consensus.[142]

6.3.2 Neonatal Pemphigus and Prevention

Neonatal PV is an autoimmune disease secondary to transplacental transference of IgG antibodies.[51] The first neonatal PV case was reported in 1975 after a woman with PV gave birth to a newborn who exhibited a positive direct immunofluorescence staining to epidermal acantholytic cells in a Tzanck preparation.[175] Pemphigus antibodies have been detected in fetal cardiac blood[83] and cord blood[199] in other stillborns.

Pregnancy may precipitate PV or aggravate PV which has been in remission. The timing of conception should probably be targeted to a period of clinical remission, with low IF titers and the choice and dosage of maternal medications should take into account possible fetal effects.[174]

Patients with PV tend to develop their skin lesions during the first or second trimester or immediately postpartum.[113] The improvement of PV during the third trimester may be due to rising endogenous corticosteroid production by the chorion and consequent immunosuppression.[200]

Transplacental transmission of maternally derived intercellular substance reactive IgG antibodies to the fetus, may result in clinical manifestation of PV in the neonate. This is supported by findings of circulating pemphigus antibodies in fetal plasma and its deposition in fetal skin, having the characteristic skin lesions of PV.[199]

The serum titer of pemphigus antibodies does not appear to influence neonatal outcome and there is no definite correlation between severity of the maternal disease and the neonatal outcome.[94] The treatment of choice is oral corticosteroids and plasmapheresis should be reserved for severe cases resistant to high dose corticosteroid therapy. Because of the significant risk of fetal loss, regular fetal monitoring, along with ultrasonography, is recommended.[94]

Vaginal delivery is the method of choice. Although local trauma sustained during a natural delivery can extend and impair recovery, Caesarean sections are generally discouraged because both the disease process and corticosteroid therapy can impair wound healing. Breast-feeding is not contraindicated but local lesions can occur and there is the theoretical possibility of passive transfer of PV IgG antibodies from mother to baby.[80]

There are several case reports of the cutaneous side effects of penicillamine, in particular PF, and is also implicated in patients with rheumatoid arthritis and systemic sclerosis.[202] Reports of pemphigoid are less common.

Mashiah and Brenner[134] have reported various environmental and pharmacological aetiological factors in pemphigus. The acronym PEMPHIGUS was proposed to summarize these factors: PEsticides, Malignancy, Pharmaceuticals, Hormones, Infectious agents, Gastronomy, Ultraviolet radiation, and Stress.[33] Drugs reported to induce pemphigus are divided into three main groups according to their chemical structure:

- Drugs containing a sulfhydryl radical, thiol drugs, including penicillamine, captopril, gold sodium thiomalate, penicillin, and piroxicam, and others.
- Phenol drugs, containing phenolic compounds, including rifampicin, levodopa, aspirin, heroin, and others.
- Nonthiol nonphenol drugs, including some of the calcium channel blockers, angiotensin converting

enzyme inhibitors, and nonsteroidal anti-inflammatory drugs (NSAIDs), in addition to dipyrone, and glibenclamide.[29,33,81]

Also recently reported has been the triggering of localized pemphigus by imiquimod used to treat nonmelanoma skin cancer.[40,129]

Garden materials and pesticides are an important cause of contact pemphigus.[27] Infectious diseases and immunizations have been implicated in inducing or exacerbating pemphigus, including viruses of the Herpetoviridae family.[32]

Certain foods have also been purported to induce or trigger pemphigus, in particular foods containing an allium, phenol, thiol, or urshiol group.[28,193] Several studies point to the possible contribution of emotional stress as a precipitating factor in pemphigus,[25,31] and pemphigus has long been considered a photosensitive disease.[109]

Acantholysis in pemphigus may be due to the induction of interleukin-1a and tumor necrosis factor-a release by keratinocytes resulting in the regulation and synthesis of complement and proteases like plasminogen activator.[34,87]

PV is uncommon in neonates and children and is a disease predominantly of the third to sixth decades of life.[152] PV in neonates is caused by maternal autoimmune disease with transplacental transmission of IgG antibodies.[44,166,197] It is controversial whether therapy with corticosteroids, azathioprine, or plasmapheresis in affected pregnant women is of benefit to the neonate.[174] In adults with P V, autoantibodies to Dsg 3 lead to mucosal blistering, whereas blistering of the skin is usually caused by autoantibodies to Dsg 1.[9] In contrast to the skin of adults, antibodies to Dsg 3 may induce blisters in the skin of neonates.[170]

There are several reported cases of neonatal PV. Neonatal PV is generally associated with a good prognosis and is due to transplacental transmission of IgG autoantibodies.[44,166] In addition, the autoantibodies to Dsg 3 predominantly belong to the IgG4 subclass.[152] The pathogenic process leading to blistering in adults with PV is autoantibodies to Dsg3, whereas in neonates it is associated with autoantibodies to Dsg1.[9] This is because the IgG4 anti-Dsg1 antibodies can cross the placenta and therefore the manifestation is in the skin rather than mucous membranes. In PV, maternal autoantibody titers appear to correlate well with disease activity in the newborn and mother. This is in contrast to the correlation in those with FS.[48] Alvarez et al.[169] reported that this entity shares similar clinical and immunopathological features with the nonendemic form of PF seen in the rest of the world. The majority of the mothers with FS showed moderately low titers of PF autoantibodies and the babies' cord sera showed low titers or no autoantibodies. Therefore, it was concluded that the placenta may function as an "in-vivo immunoadsorbent" of pathogenic antibodies. However, Avalos-Diaz et al.[14] demonstrated the reproduction of clinical, histological, and immunological features of PF in neonatal mice after intraperitoneal injection of anti-Dsg1 autoantibodies from the cord blood of a baby with PF. The exact mechanism of neonatal protection in PF is unknown.

There are several proposed theories for the absence of clinical disease in the newborn with mothers with PF. Wu et al.[211] demonstrated that protection against blisters induced by PF antibodies is provided by desmoglein 3 expression in the superficial epidermis in neonates. Hence in the rare cases of neonatal PF, the infants may lack the normal neonatal expression of desmoglein 3 in the upper epidermis, or the mothers may produce antidesmoglein 3 antibodies. Ishii et al.[106] reported a patient with PF in whom PV subsequently developed. This case suggests that mothers who deliver infants with bullous pathology may have undergone an antigenic shift and may be producing antidesmoglein 3 antibodies as well.

6.3.3 Bullous Pemphigoid

BP was first described by Lever in 1953 as a subepidermal blistering disease. Its immunohistological features include dermal–epidermal junction separation, an inflammatory cell infiltrate in the upper dermis, and BMZ-bound autoantibodies.[124] These autoantibodies show a linear staining at the dermal–epidermal junction, activate complement, and recognize two major hemidesmosomal antigens, BP230 (BPAG1) and BP180 (BPAG2 or type XVII collagen).[130]

BP typically affects the elderly, with most cases occurring in patients greater than 60 years of age. Its incidence is approximately 6.1–7/million in European countries.[41,187] BP is the most common autoimmune blistering disease and typically presents with lesions on the trunk, proximal extremities, and flexural surfaces, and involves the oral mucosa in 20% of cases.[41] There is ongoing research into the possibility that BP is associated with increased incidence of digestive tract, bladder and lung malignancies. However these associations may be age related rather than directly due to BP. Other autoimmune disorders such as rheumatoid arthritis, Hashimoto's thyroiditis, dermatomyositis, lupus erythematosus, and autoimmune thrombocytopenia have been described.[96] There are several clinical variants of BP and these include[187]:

- Erythematous and oedematous BP
- Vesicular BP
- Localized BP
- Seborrheic pemphigoid
- Vegetating BP
- Dyshidrosiform pemphigoid
- Nodular BP
- Cicatricial pemphigoid (mucus membrane pemphigoid)
- Localized scarring pemphigoid
- Disseminated scarring pemphigoid
- Herpes gestationis (pemphigoid gestationis)

The gold standard for diagnosis is direct immunoelectron microscopy and ELISA assays for BP 230 and BP 180, but these two tests are not routinely available in many countries. More recently, ELISA assays for BP 230 and BP 180 with bacterially derived recombinant proteins have been developed, which have been shown in recent studies to increase the sensitivity in diagnosing B P.

Light microscopy is useful in initial classification; however in the early stages of the disease or in atypical cases of BP, this technique is not diagnostic. The findings on light microscopy include subepidermal blister formation with a dermal inflammatory infiltrate predominantly composed of neutrophils and eosinophils. In the early phases of BP, subepidermal clefts and eosinophilic spongiosis are present.[124]

DIF demonstrates the deposition of IgG and C3 at the BMZ.[54] BP may be differentiated by the separation of skin layers at the dermoepidermoid junction using salt split skin, where autoantibodies bind to the upper portion of the split, as they are binding within the hemidesmosome and lamina lucida.[41]

Indirect immunoflourescence (IIF) is used to detect autoantibody titers and is a useful diagnostic technique for the diagnosis and evaluation of disease activity in BP. The major pathogenic epitope is the noncollagenous extracellular domain (NC 16A) of the

180-kDa transmembrane hemidesmosomal protein (BPAG2). The extracellular portion of BP antigen 180 contains 15 collagenous and 16 noncollagenous domains containing different antigenic sites recognized by autoantibodies from several blistering diseases including BP, MMP, and linear immunoglobulin a disease.[217] IIF studies are positive for circulating IgG antibodies in 60–80% of patients and the antibodies bind to the epidermal side of saline separated normal human skin.[96] Several studies have reported that the circulating antibody titers detected by IIF are not a reliable indicator of disease activity. Moreover, it is reported that IIF titers of BP patients' sera mainly reflect the amount of circulating anti-BPAG1 antibodies rather than of the pathogenic anti-BPAG2 antibodies.[153] Autoantibodies to BP antigen 180 and BP antigen 230 are detected in the sera using immunoblot and immunoprecipitation studies in 60–100% of cases.[96] IIF is sufficient for the serological diagnosis of BP in most cases however in cases that are negative on IIF, immunoblot studies may reveal circulating antibodies, particularly to BPAg2.[77]

Recently, the measurement of circulating pathogenic antibodies in BP patients has been commercially possible using an ELISA kit using the NC16A domain recombinant protein (BP180 ELISA kit).[192] concluded that the ELISA index measured by this commercially available kit correlated better with disease activity than the IIF titers, and may be a useful tool to evaluate the disease activity and to assess the effectiveness of the treatment of BP. The combination of BP230 ELISA and BP180 ELISA is a highly sensitive method for the diagnosis of BP.[215] A recent study by Sitaru et al.[184] investigated the ELISA system using NC16A tetramers instead of monomers, and found it to be a sensitive and specific tool for the diagnosis and monitoring of BP and PG. The sensitivity and specificity of the new antitetrameric NC16A ELISA were 89.9 and 97.8% respectively. The study also concluded that the levels of circulating autoantibodies against BP180 paralleled disease activity in the pemphigoid patients.

Alternatively, BP may be diagnosed by investigation of the blister fluid. Although the blister fluid is not a more sensitive substrate than serum, obtaining the fluid involves a less traumatic procedure than venepuncture, making it particularly applicable to children and elderly patients. This may be a useful adjunct method for detecting BMZ antibody titer, subclass, and complement fixing activity in BP.[216]

6.3.3.1 Prevention of Bullous Pemphigoid

In 1970, drug-induced BP was first reported secondary to salicylazosulfapyridine in an 11-year-old child.[16] The association between drugs and BP is being increasingly reported in the literature including frusemide, penicillins, sulfasalazine, and ibuprofen.[178]

Shachar et al.[178] postulated that nonimmunological mechanisms involve splitting at the dermoepidermal junction in drug-induced BP, independent of autoantibodies or other immune factors. Immunological mechanisms are generally of two types. Firstly, the drug produces an antigenic stimulus or, secondly, the drug has a direct regulatory effect on the immune system and results in immune dysregulation and autoantibody production.

Calcium channel blockers may result in drug induced BP. Brenner et al. concluded that drug induced BP may be as a result of induced alterations in calcium concentrations.[30] The study found that normal human skin explants cultured in the presence of nifedipine at different concentrations resulted in intraepithelial splitting (pemphigus type) which showed cell–cell dyshesion among the keratinocytes and subepithelial splitting (pemphigoid type) displaying dermoepidermal cleft formation. The study also concluded that the type of pathological change was donor-specific and not concentration-related.[30] This study has not been reproduced elsewhere, however.

Several case reports have been published linking penicillamine as a causative factor for BP.[127,131,202] There is strong evidence to suggest that drug-induced pemphigoid reverses with cessation of the offending medications and hence clinicians must be vigilant when drug-induced pemphigoid is suspected.

6.3.4 Pemphigoid Gestationis

Pemphigoid gestationis, previously referred to as herpes gestationis, is a pregnancy-associated nonviral autoimmune subepidermal blistering disease. It is not related to herpes virus infections; the old term herpes gestationis rather describes the occurrence of herpetiform lesions as part of the clinical picture of this condition.[58,179] Gestational pemphigoid is also known as "herpes gestationis" or "pemphigoid gestationis." It typically occurs during the second or third trimesters of pregnancy and resolves after delivery. It clinically presents with urticarial plaques, which develop into tense vesicles in the periumbilical area. The lesions may generalize and typically reappear in subsequent pregnancies. This condition is immunologically identical to BP.

Linear deposition of C3 and, less frequently, of immunoglobulin G along the cutaneous BMZ, detected on direct immunofluorescence microscopy are immunopathological hallmarks of pemphigoid gestationis.[179] Indirect complement fixation immunofluorescence identifies circulating immunoglobulin G autoantibodies, termed herpes gestationis factor and is identified in the sera of the majority of pemphigoid gestationis patients. Deposition of immunoreactants to the upper portion of the lamina lucida, directly beneath the plasma membrane of basal keratinocytes is evident on immunoelectronmicroscopy.[179] The 16th noncollagenous A domain of BP antigen 180 is the major target of autoantibodies in pemphigoid gestationis.[43,79,128,182] The antigenic sites are clustered within the membrane-proximal portion of this domain.[43,128,182,183] ELISA using recombinant BP antigen 180 is a sensitive tool for the detection and monitoring of levels of autoantibodies in pemphigoid gestationis.[183]

Gestational pemphigoid may be rarely associated with a choriocarcinoma, hydatiform mole, or premature birth. It is clinically important to differentiate PG from polymorphic urticarial plaques of pregnancy (PUPPP). Both conditions have similar presentations and have differing fetal and maternal prognostic implications. Powell et al.[162] found NC16a ELISA as highly sensitive and highly specific in differentiating PG from PUPPP, and a valuable tool in the serodiagnosis of PG.

6.3.5 Mucous Membrane Pemphigoid

MMP, formerly known as cicatricial pemphigoid, is a heterogeneous group of autoimmune subepidermal blistering diseases associated most commonly with autoantibodies to BP 180 and less frequently with those to laminin 5 or type VII collagen. In addition, a few cases have been described with autoantibodies to the b4 subunit of a6b4 integrin.[126]

MMP is an autoimmune bullous disease that primarily affects mucous membranes leading to a scarring phenotype. This is in contrast to BP where healing predominantly occurs without scarring. Patients can be classified as low or high risk. Low-risk patients have lesions which are limited to the oral mucosa and skin. High-risk patients have involvement of other mucosal surfaces resulting in significant morbidity. MMP patients produce autoantibodies to two recognized components of the dermoepidermal BMZ: BP180 and laminin 5 (Lam332).[18] IgG reactivity to Lam332 of the MMP and BP sera was not significantly associated with IgG reactivity against other autoantigens of the BMZ, such as BP180 or BP230. Thus, the established Lam332 ELISA may be a valuable novel diagnostic and prognostic parameter for MMP.[18]

6.3.6 Epidermolysis Bullosa Acquisita

EBA is an acquired bullous disease characterized by immunoglobulin G (IgG) autoantibodies that react with type VII collagen in the anchoring fibrils, resulting in bullae formation at the dermoepidermal junction.[210] The autoantibodies specifically bind to the 145-kDa amino-terminal domain (NC1).[122,208] EBA is a rare disease with an incidence of 0.17–0.26/million people in Western Europe and usually presents in the fourth to fifth decades of life, but has been reported in childhood.[20,84,218] Roenigk et al.[172] was the first to set the initial diagnostic criteria for EBA.

The etiology of EBA is unknown; however an autoimmune pathogenesis is postulated.[209,210] Bullous systemic lupus erythematosus (SLE) compared with EBA also display autoantibodies against type VII collagen.[73] The association of EBA and bullous SLE with HLA major histocompatibility (MHC) class II cell surface antigen, HLA-DR2 further supports the autoimmune hypothesis for EBA (Fig. 6.5).[74,96]

There are two main phenotypes. These include the classic noninflammatory mechanobullous type and the inflammatory type. Patients with the classic noninflammatory mechanobullous type have marked skin fragility with blisters and erosions at trauma sites. Healing results in scarring and milia. The inflammatory type[71] can be difficult to differentiate from BP, cicatricial pemphigoid, and chronic bullous dermatosis of childhood.[151] Previous studies have reported that at least 50% of patients with EBA show a BP-like clinical presentation and 10% of patients with the clinical presentation of BP may actually have EBA.[71]

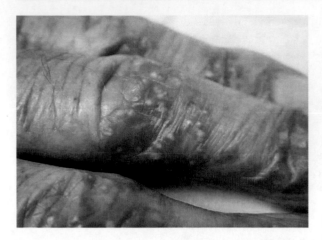

Fig. 6.5 Milia and atrophic scarring on the dorsal fingers in classical epidermolysis bullosa acquisita (EBA). Sites exposed to chronic trauma have most of the blistering

On direct and indirect immunofluorescence testing, linear IgG and C3 deposits on the basement membrane are found in both BP and EBA.[62] Dermal–epidermal separation with sodium chloride or suction can be a useful technique demonstrating IgG deposits at the DEJ, but immunoblotting confirms the diagnosis.[103,115] Direct immunoelectron microscopy is the gold standard of diagnosis and demonstrates IgG deposits either within or below the lamina densa of the BMZ.[41]

Blisters in EBA and bullous systemic lupus erythematosus (BSLE) are due to defective adhesion of the lamina densa subregion of the epithelial basement membrane to the underlying dermis. Previous studies of a small number of EBA patients show recognition by autoantibodies of proteolytic fragments containing the 145-kDa noncollagenous domain of type VII collagen. Interference with the adhesion function of type VII collagen may occur due to antibodies binding to fibronectin homology regions within the 145-kDa noncollagenous domain and contribute to lamina densadermal dysadhesion in epidermolysis bullous acquisita and bullous SLE.[75]

Lapiere et al. identified four major immunodominant epitopes localized within the amino-terminal, noncollagenous (NC-1) domain in patients with EBA. Sera from patients with bullous SLE (BSLE) revealed a similar pattern of epitopes to EBA, suggesting that the same epitopes could serve as autoantigens in both blistering conditions. Chen et al.[42] recently described that the pathogenic antibodies in EBA have been shown to bind to the cartilage matrix domain (CMP) of type

VII collagen. This study also showed that passive transfer of EBA autoantibodies directed against the CMP subdomain into mice are pathogenic and recommended that further fine mapping of the pathogenic epitope to a smaller region with the 227 AA CMP subdomain may also facilitate the development of effective peptide therapy for EBA.

6.3.7 Dermatitis Herpetiformis

DH is a relatively rare skin disorder with an estimated incidence of 1:10,000 in the United Kingdom and typically presents in patients in their third or fourth decades. In Anglo-Saxon and Scandinavian populations the prevalence is between 10 and 39 per 100,000. DH is much less common in blacks and Asians. Men are slightly more likely to be affected than females with a ratio of approximately 3:2.[46]

The typical lesions in DH include intensely pruritic eruptions of erythematous papules or vesicles distributed symmetrically along extensor surfaces. The areas most commonly affected are the extensor surfaces of the elbows and knees, and the buttocks and scalp. The diagnosis of DH is based on clinical presentation, biopsy for hematoxylin and eosin, and direct immunofluorescence.[198] Definitive diagnosis of DH depends on the direct immunofluorescence finding of granular or fibrillar IgA deposits along the BMZ.[161] In DH, dermal papillary edema and neutrophil infiltration are seen. A biopsy of an intact vesicle demonstrates a subepidermal blister with neutrophils. The hallmark finding on direct immunofluorescence testing in DH is granular deposition of IgA in the dermal papillae of perilesional skin.[70,146,220] DH typically has a chronic course with exacerbations and remissions. DH can be associated with a glutensensitive enteropathy which is identical to Celiac disease (CD). Most affected patients are asymptomatic however may develop steatorrhea, abnormal D -xylose absorption, or anemia caused by iron or folate deficiency.[114]

Two-thirds of patients have a small intestinal enteropathy with villous atrophy as seen in CD. However, the remaining third also show evidence of gluten sensitivity in the intestine. Gluten challenge in these patients results in villous atrophy. The initial treatment of the rash is gluten withdrawal in combination with one of the following three drugs: dapsone, sulphapyridine, or sulphamethoxypyridazine.[69] Despite DH being a skin manifestation of CD, many patients with DH may not complain of gastrointestinal symptoms.[146]

Patients with DH have a high incidence of autoimmune disorders including thyroid disease, pernicious anemia, and insulin-dependent diabetes, and should be screened for these conditions on a yearly basis. There is also an increased incidence of lymphoma.[69] DH patients can suffer from both B-Cell and T-cell lymphomas. Hervonen et al.[97] concluded that patients adhering to a strict gluten-free diet had a reduced incidence of lymphoma.

DH must be considered as a differential diagnosis for patients with a diagnosis of eczema, unresponsive to treatment. Eczema generally presents in early childhood, characterized by intraepidermal vesicles and bullae at sites of spongiosis.[19,159] Screening for DH can be performed by testing for tissue transglutaminase antibodies or antiendomysial antibodies (AEmA).[38,156] However, the gold standard is a skin biopsy for routine histologic examination and direct immunofluorescence.[76] In summary, key findings that can confirm a diagnosis of DH include: clinical findings, DIF detection of typical junctional IgA deposits, and positive serum tests for coeliac disease. Any two of these three findings are consistent with DH.[21] Adherence to a strict gluten-free diet requiring avoidance of foods containing wheat, rye, or barley can prevent outbreaks of DH.[69]

6.3.8   Linear IgA Dermatosis

LAD, an acquired subepidermal blistering skin disease, presents with vesicular or bullous skin lesions, often with herpetiform arrangement, and is associated with intense burning and pruritus. It can be differentiated from DH and BP by the linear deposits of IgA in the BMZ. The disease is not associated with a gluten-sensitive enteropathy. Histopathological findings include subepidermal blisters and intrapapillary microabscesses.

There are two clinical phenotypes reported: adult and childhood LAD (chronic bullous dermatosis of childhood). Childhood LAD usually remits in 64% of subjects by the age of 6–8 years.[50] The adult type of LAD predominantly presents in the fourth decade or later, has a slight female predisposition, and a remission rate of 48%.[204]

LAD is caused by the presence of IgA autoantibodies against different dermoepidermal antigens and is characterized by a homogeneous linear band of IgA deposition along the BMZ.[167] Frequently recognized antigens are a 180-kDa protein, presumably BP antigen II, a 120-kDa, and a 97-kDa molecule, related proteins associated with breakdown products of collagen type XVII.[219,221] The following antigenic proteins are also reported: BP230,[78] collagen VII[90,209] and antigens of molecular weights of 100, 110–120, 145, 160–180, 200, 220, 230, 255, and 285 kDa.[53,205,212]

LAD1 and LADB97, BP 230, LAD 285, and collagen VII are the target antigens.[99,132] EM studies have shown that serum from patients with LAD binds to the lamina lucida as well as the sublamina densa regions.[107] IgA autoantibodies also bind to the NC16 transmembrane epitope as well as the COL15 and Ecto 2 epitopes, located at the carboxyl terminus of the ectodomain in BP 180.[41,219] The gold standard for diagnosis of LAD is direct immunofluorescence showing linear deposits of IgA along the BMZ.[39]

6.3.8.1   Prevention

Collier et al.[45] stated that there were no contraindications to pregnancy in patients with LAD, and recommended that therapy be reduced or ceased whenever possible during pregnancy, with particular emphasis on counseling regarding the possibility of relapse post partum.

Medications reported to induce LAD include amiodarone, ampicillin, captopril, cefamandole, cyclosporine, diclofenac, glibenclamide, interferon-[gamma], interleukin 2, lithium, penicillin G, phenytoin, piroxicam, somatostatin, sulfamethoxazole/trimethoprim, and vigabatrin.[117,160] Up to two-thirds of LAD cases may be drug-induced, and vancomycin is the offending drug in approximately half of the drug-induced LAD cases.[160] Vancomycin-induced LAD (VILAD) has a heterogeneous clinical presentation. It may be difficult to differentiate VILAD from other common blistering disorders, such as BP or DH.[121] VILAD can present with targetoid erythema multiforme-like lesions, papules, vesicles, and bullae, predominantly located on the extremities (90%) and trunk (77%).[144]

Histological findings in VILAD include subepidermal bullae with a predominately neutrophilic infiltrate and basal cell vacuolization and these features distinguish it from other blistering conditions such as PF or PV.[144] Clinical differentials for VILAD include erythema multiforme, Stevens-Johnson syndrome (SJS), and toxic epidermal necrolysis. VILAD can be distinguished morphologically from these conditions by the absence of interface changes and keratinocyte necrosis.[140,148]

Perilesional skin biopsy DIF in VILAD reveals strong linear deposition of IgA along the BMZ, whereas BP is characterized by a linear IgG deposition along the BMZ. VILAD cannot be differentiated from idiopathic LAD, but the differing clinical course of these diseases suggests differing pathogenesis.[144] Spontaneous remission post vancomycin withdrawal has been observed in previously reported cases of VILAD. Based on available evidence, autoantibody mediated bullae formation is postulated as the pathogenesis of VILAD.[121,168,206]

6.3.9 Other Drug-Induced Bullous Diseases

6.3.9.1 Toxic Epidermal Necrolysis

Stevens-Johnson syndrome (SJS) and toxic epidermal necrolysis (TEN) are rare, life-threatening, bullous cutaneous diseases generally considered as immune-mediated reactions to drugs resulting in severe cutaneous adverse reactions (SCAR), characterized by epidermal necrosis, extensive detachment of the epidermis, erosions of mucous membranes, and severe constitutional symptoms.[85]

The majority of TEN cases are related to chemicals systemically administered as drug therapy. The drugs implicated in most series were antibacterial sulfonamides, anticonvulsants, allopurinol, pyrazolone derivatives, and, less frequently, other NSAIDs.[93] The SCAR study included 245 patients with TEN and SJS in Europe and confirmed the responsibility of the "classical culprit" drugs: antibacterial sulfonamides (cotrimoxazole); aromatic anticonvulsants (phenobarbital, phenytoin, carbamazepine); some antibiotics (aminopenicillins, quinolines, cephalosporins); some NSAIDs (tenoxicam, piroxicam), chlormezanone, and allopurinol.[173] Most of these drugs are therapeutic and may not be avoided, as the overall risk of SCAR is low. However, if there are early signs of SCAR, then these drugs are the likeliest causes and should be ceased. They should then be avoided completely in future, as these are potentially life-threatening drug reactions. Wearing a medicalert bracelet with the name of the culprit is worthwhile as a preventative to being given the SCAR-inducing drug again.

6.4 Infective Causes

Herpes simplex virus (HSV), also known as Human Herpes virus, has two strains: HSV1 and HSV2 and typically causes blisters in the skin, mucus membranes or the genitals. HSV becomes latent after the primary infection in the cell bodies of the nerves in the area of the primary infection. Transmission of the virus occurs with contact of carriers with active HSV. The vectors for HSV transmission include saliva, semen, vaginal fluid, and shed skin from active lesions. Herpes may also be transmitted to an infant during childbirth, which may result in aseptic meningitis. HSV1 may be prevented by simple measures such as not kissing when active lesions are present, and HSV2 can be prevented by barrier contraception and avoidance of sex when the blisters are active; however viral shedding may occur even without blisters.

Erythema multiforme (EM) is a disease of multiple etiologies and often recurs. It results in a polymorphic eruption caused by exposure to medication or various infections, in particular HSV.[13,119] The most common predisposing factor for EM is HSV. Other causes include mycoplasma and fungal disease. The medications predisposing to EM, outlined in the SCAR study, include: antibacterial sulfonamides, anticonvulsants (phenobarbital, phenytoin, carbamazepine, and valproic acid), oxicam NSAIDs, chlormezanone, allopurinol, and acetaminophen in countries other than France, imidazole antifungal agents, corticosteroids for systemic use, aminopenicillins, cephalosporins, quinolones, and tetracyclines.[173]

Differences in case selection in terms of subsets of EM studied may have partly resulted in wide variations in the detection of HSV DNA (36–75%) by polymerase chain reaction (PCR) in EM.[145] Kokuba et al.[119] state that HSV associated erythema multiforme pathology includes a delayed-type hypersensitivity component and is mechanistically distinct from drug-induced erythema multiforme. Diagnostic tests for HSV-induced erythema multiforme include serum hematology and biochemistry tests, blood and vesicle cultures, punch biopsy for histological examination, and PCR.

Oral acyclovir is used to suppress erythema multiforme associated with HSV. EM is not prevented if oral acyclovir is administered after a herpes simplex recurrence is evident, and it is of no value after erythema multiforme has occurred. There is some question whether prevention of erythema multiforme may be achieved with continuous topical treatment with acyclovir to sites affected by recurrent herpes.[101]

Herpes zoster (HZ), commonly known as shingles, is a disease caused by the varicella zoster virus (VZV) and is characterized by a painful, vesicular skin rash. The virus may remain dormant in the nerve cell bodies and trigger latent infections, typically in a dermatomal distribution. It particularly affects immunocomprised patients, resulting in significant morbidity.

Clinical findings are often sufficient to diagnose HZ. Atypical presentations may be confirmed on viral culture, direct immunoflourescence assay or PCR. Laboratory techniques can be particularly helpful when differentiating between VZV and zosteriform herpes simplex.[201]

Oxman et al.[130] found that use of the zoster vaccine, live attenuated Oka/Merck VZV vaccine, reduced the incidence of postherpetic neuralgia by 66% and HZ by 51%, and concluded that the vaccine markedly reduced the morbidity and postherpetic neuralgia associated with HZ in patients older than 60. Also, the treatment of HZ with oral acyclovir can reduce residual pain after 6 months in almost 50% of immunocompetent adults.[108] Wood et al.[207] found that acyclovir reduced zoster-related pain duration and prevalence by half. Combined acyclovir and prednisone therapy can improve quality of life in relatively healthy patients older than 50 years of age with localized HZ.[203]

Orf virus is an exanthemous disease caused by a parapox virus predominantly affecting sheep and goats. Orf is a zoonotic disease and may be transmitted to humans via direct contact from the infected animals. Infection in humans results in a self-limiting and benign course in immunocompetent individuals resulting in purulent papules with localized symptoms. Prevention of the Orf virus can be achieved by using gloves and good personal hygiene, particularly when working with infected animals.[149]

Acknowledgment   The authors would like to thank Ms. Kezia Gaitskell of Oxford University Medical School for proofreading of this manuscript.

References

1. Aberdam D, Galliano MG, Vailly J, et al Herlitz's junctional epidermolysis bullosa is linked to mutations in the gene (LAMC2) for the gamma 2 subunit of nicein/kalinin (laminin 5). Nat Genet. 1994;6:299–304
2. Ahmed AR, Graham J, Jordan RE, Provost TT. Pemphigus: current concepts. Ann Intern Med. 1980;92:396–405
3. Ahmed AR, Yunis EJ, Khatri K. Major histocompatibility complex haplotype studies in Ashkenazi Jewish patients with Pemphigus Vulgaris. Proc Natl Acad Sci USA. 1991; 87:7658–7662
4. Ahmed AR, Mohimen A, Yunis EJ, et al Linkage of pemphigus vulgaris antibody to the major histocompatibility complex in healthy relatives of patients. J Exp Med. 1993; 177:419
5. Amagai M, Klaus-Kovtun V, Stanley JR. Auto-Ab against a novel epithelial cadherin in pemphigus vulgaris, a disease of cell adhesion. *Cell.* 1991;67:869–877
6. Amagai M, Nishikawa T, Nousari HC, et al Antibodies against desmoglein 3 (pemphigus vulgaris antigen) are present in sera from patients with paraneoplastic pemphigus and cause acantholysis in vivo in neonatal mice. J Clin Invest. 1998;102:775–782
7. Amagai M, Hashimoto T, Komai A, et al Usefulness of enzyme-linked immunosorbent assay using recombinant desmogleins 1 and 3 for serodiagnosis of pemphigus. Br J Dermatol. 1999;140:351–357
8. Anhalt GJ. Paraneoplastic pemphigus. Adv Dermatol. 1997;12:77–96
9. Anhalt GJ. Making sense of antigens and antibodies in pemphigus. J Am Acad Dermatol. 1999;40:763–766
10. Anhalt GJ, Kim SC, Stanley JR, et al Paraneoplastic pemphigus. N Engl J Med. 1990;323:1729–1735
11. Anton-Lamprecht I. The skin. In: Papadimitriou JM, Henderson DW, Spagnolo V, eds. Diagnostic Ultrastructure of Non-Neoplastic Diseases. 5th ed. Edinburgh: Churchill and Livingstone; 1992
12. Anton-Lamprecht I, Schnyder UW. Epidermolysis bullosa herpetiformis Dowling-Meara: a report of a case and pathomorphogenesis. Dermatologica. 1982;164:221–235
13. Aurelian L, Kokuba H, et al Understanding the pathogenesis of HSV-associated erythema multiforme. Dermatology. 1998;197(3):219–222
14. Avalos-Diaz E, Olague-Marchan M, Lopez-Swiderski A, Herrera-Esparza R, Diaz LA. Transplacental passage of maternal pemphigus foliaceus autoantibodies induces neonatal pemphigus. J Am Acad Dermatol. 2000;43(6): 1130–1134
15. Baudoin C, Miquel C, Blanchet-Bardon C, et al Herlitz junctional epidermolysis bullosa keratinocytes display heterogeneous defects of nicein/kalinin gene expression. J Clin Invest. 1994;93:862–869

16. Bean SF, Good RA, Windhorst DB. Bullous pemphigoid in an 11-year-old boy. Arch Dermatol. 1970;102:205–208

17. Bedane C, Prost C, Thomine E, et al Binding of autoantibodies is not restricted to desmosomes in pemphigus vulgaris: comparison of 14 cases of pemphigus vulgaris and 10 cases of pemphigus foliaceus studied by western immunoblot and immunoelectron microscopy. Arch Dermatol Res. 1996;288: 343–352

18. Bekou V, Thoma-Uszynski S, Wendler O, et al Detection of laminin 5-specifi c auto-antibodies in mucous membrane and bullous pemphigoid sera by ELISA. J Invest Dermatol. 2005;124(4):732–740

19. Beltrani VS, Boguneiwicz M. Atopic dermatitis. Dermatol Online J. 2003;9:1

20. Bernard P, Vaillant L, Labeille B, et al Incidence of distribution of subepidermal autoimmune skin diseases in three French regions. Arch Dermatol. 1995;131:48–52

21. Beutner EH, Baughman RD, Austin BM, Plunkett RW, Binder WL. A case of dermatitis herpetiformis with IgA endomysial antibodies but negative direct immunofluorescent findings. J Am Acad Dermatol. 2000;43: 329–332

22. Bhol K, Ahmed AR, Aoki V, Mohimen A, Nagarwalla N, Natarajan K. Correlation of peptide specificity and IgG subclass with pathogenic and nonpathogenic autoantibodies in pemphigus vulgaris: a model for autoimmunity. Proc Natl Acad Sci USA. 1995;92:5239–5243

23. Bolte C, Gonzalez S. Rapid diagnosis of major variants of congenital epidermolysis bullosa using a monoclonal antibody against collagen type I V. Am J Dermatopathol. 1995; 17(6):580–583

24. Borradori L, Trueb RM, Jaunin F, et al Autoantibodies from a patient with paraneoplastic pemphigus bind periplakin, a novel member of the plakin family. J Invest Dermatol. 1998;111:338–340

25. Brenner S, Bar-Nathan EA. Pemphigus vulgaris triggered by emotional stress. J Am Acad Dermatol. 1984; 11:524–525

26. Brenner S, Wolf R, Ruocco V. Drug-induced pemphigus. I. A survey. Clin Dermatol. 1993;11(4):501–505

27. Brenner S, Wolf R, Ruocco V. Contact pemphigus: a subgroup of induced pemphigus. Int J Dermatol. 1994; 33:843–845

28. Brenner S, Ruocco V, Wolf R, De Angelis E, Lombardi ML. Pemphigus and dietary factors. In vitro acantholysis by allyl compounds of the genus Allium. Dermatology. 1995;190: 197–202

29. Brenner S, Bialy-Golan A, Ruocco V. Drug-induced pemphigus. Clin Dermatol. 1998;163:393–397

30. Brenner S, Ruocco V, Bialy-Golan A, et al Pemphigus and pemphigoid-like effects of nifedipine on in vitro cultured normal human skin explants. Int J Dermatol. 1999; 38(1):36–40

31. Brenner S, Tur E, Shapiro J, et al Pemphigus vulgaris: environmental factors. Occupational, behavioral, medical, and qualitative food frequency questionnaire. Int J Dermatol. 2001;40:562–569

32. Brenner S, Sasson A, Sharon O. Pemphigus and infections. Clin Dermatol. 2002;20:114–118

33. Brenner S, Mashiah J, Tamir E, Goldberg I, Wohl Y. Pemphigus: an acronym for a disease with multiple etiologies. Skinmed. 2003;2:163–167

34. Brenner S, Ruocco V, Ruocco E, Srebrnik A, Goldberg I. A possible mechanism for phenol-induced pemphigus. Skinmed. 2006;5(1):25–26; quiz 27–28

35. Bruckner-Tuderman L. Collagen VII and bullous disorders of the skin. Dermatology. 1994;189:16–20

36. Brust MD, Lin AN. Epidermolysis bullosa: practical management and clinical update. Dermatol Nurs. 1996; 8(2):81–89

37. Calvanico NJ, Martins CR, Diaz LA. Characterization of pemphigus foliaceus antigen from human epidermis. J Invest Dermatol. 1991;96(6):815–821

38. Caproni M, Cardinali C, Renzi D, Calabro A, Fabbri P. Tissue transglutaminase antibody assessment in dermatitis herpetiformis. Br J Dermatol. 2001;144:196–197

39. Cauza K, Hinterhuber G, Sterniczky B, et al Unusual clinical manifestation of linear IgA dermatosis: a report of two cases. J Am Acad Dermatol. 2004;51:112–117

40. Champagne G, Roca M, Martinez A. Successful treatment of a high-grade intraepithelial neoplasia with imiquimod, with vulvar pemphigus as a side effect. Eur J Obstet Gynecol Reprod Biol. 2003;109:224–227

41. Chaudhari P, Marinkovich MP. What's new in blistering disorders? Curr Allergy Asthma Rep. 2007;7(4):255–263

42. Chen M, Doostan A, Bandyopadhyay P, et al The cartilage matrix protein subdomain of type VII collagen is pathogenic for epidermolysis bullosa acquista. Am J Pathol. 2007; 170(6):2009–2018

43. Chimanovitch I, Schmidt E, Messer G, et al IgG1 and 0IgG3 are the major immunoglobulin subclasses targeting epitopes within the NC16A domain of BP180 in pemphigoid gestationis. J Invest Dermatol. 1999;113:140–142

44. Chowdhury MMU, Natarajan S. Neonatal pemphigus vulgaris associated with mild oral pemphigus vulgaris in the mother during pregnancy. Br J Dermatol. 1998;139: 500–503

45. Collier PM, Kelly SE, Wojnarowska F. Linear IgA disease and pregnancy. Acad Dermatol. 1994;30(3):407–411

46. Cotell S, Robinson ND, Chan LS. Autoimmune blistering skin diseases. Am J Emerg Med. 2000;18(3):288–299

47. Dang N, Klingberg S, Marr P, Murrell DF. Review of collagen VII sequence variants found in Australasian patients with dystrophic epidermolysis bullosa reveals nine novel COL7A1 variants. J Dermatol Sci. 2007;46(3): 169–178

48. Diaz LA, Sampaio SA, Rivitti EA, et al Endemic pemphigus foliaceus (fogo selvagem). I: Clinical features and immunopathology. J Am Acad Dermatol. 1989;20:657–659

49. Diaz LA, Arteaga LA, Hilario-Vargas J, et al Antidesmoglein-1 antibodies in onchocerciasis, leishmaniasis and Chagas disease suggest a possible aetiological link to Fogo Selvagem. J Invest Dermatol. 2004;123:1045–1051

50. Dippel E, Orfanos CE, Zouboulis C. Linear IgA dermatosis presenting with erythema annulare centrifugum lesions: report of three cases in adults. J Eur Acad Dermatol Venereol. 2001;15(2):167–170

51. Dugan EM, Anhalt GJ, Diaz LA. Pemphigus. In: Jordan RE, ed. Immunologic Diseases of the Skin. Norwalk, CN: Appleton and Lange; 1991:279–291

52. Eady RA, Tidman MJ. Junctional epidermolysis bullosa. In: Wojnarowska F, Briggaman RA, eds. Management of Blistering Diseases. London: Chapman and Hall Medical; 1992:213–224

53. Egan CA, Zone JJ. Linear IgA bullous dermatosis. Int J Dermatol. 1999;38:818–827
54. Egan CA, Lazarova Z, Darling TN, Yee C, Yancey KB. Anti-epiligrin cicatricial pemphigoid: clinical findings, immunopathogenesis, and significant associations. Medicine. 2003;82(3):177–186
55. Elias S. Use of fetoscopy for the prenatal diagnosis of hereditary skin disorders. Curr Probl Dermatol. 1987;16:1–3
56. Elias S, Emerson DS, Simpsos JL, Shulman LP, Holbrook KA. Ultrasound guided fetal skin sampling for prenatal diagnosis of genodermatoses. Obstet Gynecol. 1994;83: 337–341
57. Emery DJ, Diaz LA, Fairley JA, Lopez A, Taylor AF, Giudice GJ. Pemphigus foliaceus and pemphigus vulgaris autoantibodies react with the extracellular domain of desmoglein-1. J Invest Dermatol. 1995;104(3): 323–328
58. Engineer L, Bhol K, Ahmed AR. Pemphigoid gestationis: a review. Am J Obstet Gynecol. 2000;183:483–491
59. Fassihi H, Eady RA, Mellerio JE, et al Prenatal diagnosis for severe inherited skin disorders: 25 years' experience. Br J Dermatol. 2006;154(1):106–113
60. Fassihi H, Renwlckb PJ, Blackb C, McGrath JA. Single cell PCR amplification of microsatellites flanking the COL7A1 gene and suitability for preimplantation genetic diagnosis of Hallopeau-Siemens recessive dystrophic epidermolysis bullosa. J Dermatol Sci. 2006;42: 241–248
61. Fassihi H, Grace J, Lashwood A, et al Preimplantation genetic diagnosis of skin fragility-ectodermal dysplasia syndrome. Br J Dermatol. 2006;154(3):546–550
62. Fassihi H, Grace J, Lashwood A, et al Preimplantation genetic diagnosis of skin fragility-ectodermal dysplasia syndrome. Br J Dermatol. 2006;154(3):546–550
63. Fine JD. Laboratory tests for epidermolysis bullosa. Dermatopathol Clin. 1994;12:123–132
64. Fine JD, Stenn J, Johnson L, et al Autosomal recessive epidermolysis bullosa simplex: generalized phenotypic features suggestive of junctional or dystrophic epidermolysis bullosa, and association with neuromuscular diseases. Arch Dermatol. 1989;125:931–938
65. Fine JD, Bauer EA, Briggaman RA, et al Revised clinical and laboratory criteria for subtypes of inherited epidermolysis bullosa. A consensus report by the Subcommittee on Diagnosis and Classification of the National Epidermolysis Bullosa Registry. J Am Acad Dermatol. 1991;24:119–135
66. Fine JD, Bauer EA, Mcguire J, Moshell A. Non molecular diagnostic testing of epidermolysis bullosa: current techniques, major findings, and relative sensitivity and specificity. In: Fine JD, Bauer EA, McGuire J, Moshell A, eds. Epidermolysis Bullosa, Clinical, Epidemiologic, and Laboratory Advances and the Findings of the National Epidermolysis Bullosa Registry. Baltimore, MD: The John Hopkins University; 1999
67. Fine JD, Eady RA, Bauer EA, et al Revised classification for inherited epidermolysis bullosa: report of the second International Consensus Meeting on diagnosis and classification of epidermolysis bullosa. J Am Acad Dermatol. 2000;42:1051–1066
68. Fine J D, Eady RA, Bauer EA, Bauer J, Bruckner-Tuderman L, Heagerty A, Hintner H, Hovnanian A, Jonkman MF, Leigh I, McGrath JA, Mellerio JE, Murrell DF, Shimizu H, Uitto J, Vahlquist A, Woodley D, Zambruno G. Revised Consensus for Definitions of Epidermolysis Bullosa. *J Am Acad Dermatol* 58(June): 931–950, 2008 (in press Dec 2007; advance on line March 2008)
69. Fry L. Dermatitisherpetiformis. Baillieres Clin Gastroenterol. 1995;9(2):371–393
70. Fry F. Dermatitis herpetiformis: problems, progress, and prospects. Eur J Dermatol. 2002;12:523–531
71. Gammon WR, Briggaman RA, Wheeler CE. Epidermolysis bullosa acquisita presenting as an inflammatory bullous disease. F Am Acad Dermatol. 1982;7:382–387
72. Gammon WR, Briggaman RA, Woodley DT, et al Epidermolysis bullosa acquisita-a pemphigoid-like disease. J Am Acad Dermatol. 1984;11:820–832
73. Gammon WR, Woodley DT, Dole KC, Briggaman RA. Evidence that basement membrane zone antibodies in bullous eruption of systemic lupus erythematosus recognized epidermolysis bullosa acquista auto antigens. J Invest Dermatol. 1985;84:472–476
74. Gammon WR, Heise ER, Burke WA, Fine JD, Woodley DT, Briggaman RA. Increased frequency of HLA-DR2 in patients with autoantibodies to epidermolysis bullosa acquista antigen; evidence that the expression of autoimmunity to type VII collagen is HLA class II allele associated. J Invest Dermatol. 1988;91:228–232
75. Gammon WR, Murrell DF, Jenison M, et al Autoantibodies to type VII collagen recognize epitopes in a fibronectin-like region of the noncollagenous (NC1) domain. J Invest Dermatol. 1993;100:618–622
76. George DE, Browning JC, George DF, Browning JC, Hsu S. Medical pearl: dermatitis herpetiformis – potential for confusion with eczema. J Am Acad Dermatol. 2006; 54(2):327–328
77. Ghohestani R, Kanitakis J, Nicolas JF, Cozzani E, Claudy A. Comparative sensitivity of indirect immunofluorescence to immunoblot assay for the detection of circulating antibodies to bullous pemphigoid antigens 1 and 2. Br J Dermatol. 1996;135(1):74–79
78. Ghohestani RF, Nicolas JF, Kanitakis J, Claudy A. Linear IgA bullous dermatosis with IgA antibodies exclusively directed against the 180- or 230-kDa epidermal antigens. J Invest Dermatol. 1997;108:854–858
79. Giudice GJ, Emery DJ, Zelickson BD, Anhalt GJ, Liu Z, Diaz LA. Bullous pemphigoid and herpes gestationis autoantibodies recognize a common non-collagenous site on the BP180 ectodomain. J Immunol. 1993;151:5742–5750
80. Goldberg NS, DeFeo C, Krishenbaum N. Pemphigus vulgaris and pregnancy: risk factors and recommendations. J Am Acad Dermatol. 1993;28:877–879
81. Goldberg I, Kashman Y, Brenner S. The induction of pemphigus by phenol drugs. Int J Dermatol. 1999;38: 888–892
82. Grando SA. Autoimmunity to keratinocyte acetylcholine receptors in pemphigus. Dermatology. 2000;201(4): 290–295
83. Green D, Maize JC. Maternal pemphigus vulgaris with in vivo bound antibodies in the stillborn fetus. J Am Acad Dermatol. 1982;7:388–392
84. Hakimian J, Koransky J, Murrell DF. Childhood Epidermolysis Bullosa Acquista. *Proceedings of the 54th Annual American Academy of Dermatology*. Washington; 1996
85. Halevy S, Ghislain PD, Mockenhaupt M, Fagot JP, Bouwes Bavinck JN, Sidoroff A, Naldi L, Dunant A, Viboud C,

Roujeau JC, EuroSCAR Study Group. Allopurinol is the most common cause of Stevens-Johnson syndrome and toxic epidermal necrolysis in Europe and Israel. J Am Acad Dermatol. 2008;58(1):25–32

86. Handyside AH, Kontogianni EH, Hardy K, Winston RML. Pregnancies from biopsied human preimplantation embryos used by Y specific DNA amplification. Nature. 1990; 344:768–770

87. Hashimoto K, Wun TC, Baird J, Lazarus GS, Jensen PJ. Characterization of keratinocyte plasminogen activator inhibitors and demonstration of the prevention of pemphigus IgG-induced acantholysis by a purified plasminogen activator inhibitor. J Invest Dermatol. 1989;92(3): 310–314

88. Hashimoto T, Konohana A, Nishikawa T. Immunoblot assay as an aid to the diagnoses of unclassified cases of pemphigus. Arch Dermatol. 1991;127:843–847

89. Hashimoto T, Amagai M, Watanabe K, et al Characterization of paraneoplastic pemphigus autoantigens by immunoblot analysis. J Invest Dermatol. 1995;104:829–834

90. Hashimoto T, Ishiko A, Shimizu H, et al A case of linear IgA bullous dermatosis with IgA anti-type VII collagen autoantibodies. Br J Dermatol. 1996;134:336–339

91. Heagerty AH, Kennedy AR, Gunner DB, Eady RA. Rapid prenatal diagnosis and exclusion of epidermolysis bullosa using novel antibody probes. J Invest Dermatol. 1986;86(5): 603–605

92. Heagerty AH, Eady RA, Kennedy AR, et al Rapid prenatal diagnosis of epidermolysis bullosa letalis using GB3 monoclonal antibody. Br J Dermatol. 1987;117(3):271–275

93. Heimbach DM, Engrav LH, Marvin JA, et al Toxic epidermal necrolysis: a step forward in treatment. JAMA. 1987; 257:2171–2175

94. Hern S, Vaughan Jones SA, Setterfield J, et al Pemphigus vulgaris in pregnancy with favourable fetal prognosis. Clin Exp Dermatol. 1998;23(6):260–263

95. Hertl M. Humoral and cellular autoimmunity in autoimmune bullous skin disorders. Int Arch Allergy Immunol. 2000; 122:91–100

96. Hertl M. Autoimmune bullous skin disorders. In: Autoimmune Disease of The Skin. Pathogenesis, Diagnosis, Management. New York, Springer Wien; 2005

97. Hervonen K, Vornanen M, Kautiainen H, Collin P, Reunala T. Lymphoma in patients with dermatitis herpetiformis and their first-degree relatives. Br J Dermatol. 2005; 152(1):82–86

98. Hintner H, Stingl G, Schuler G, et al Immunofluorescence mapping of antigenic determinants within the dermal-epidermal junction in mechanobullous diseases. J Invest Dermatol. 1981;76:113–118

99. Hirako Y, Niishizawa Y, Sitaru C, et al The 97k-Da (LABD97) and 120-kDa (LAD-1) fragments of bullous pemphigoid antigen 180/type XVII collagen have different N-termini. J Invest Dermatol. 2003;121:1554–1556

100. Horn TD, Anhalt GJ. Histologic features of paraneolastic pemphigus. Arch Dermatol. 1992;128:1091–1095

101. Huff JC. Acyclovir for recurrent erythema multiforme caused by herpes simplex. J Am Acad Dermatol. 1988;18: 197–199

102. Huilgol SC, Black MM. Management of the immunobullous disorders. II. Pemphigus. Clin Exp Dermatol. 1995;20: 283–293

103. Inauen P, Hunziker TH, Gerber H, et al Childhood epidermolysis bullosa acquisita. Br J Dermatol. 1994;131: 898–900

104. Ishida-Yamamoto A, McGrath JA, Chapman SJ, et al Epidermolysis Bullosa simplex (Dowling-Meara type) is a genetic disease characterized by an abnormal keratin-filament network involving keratins K5 and K14. J Invest Dermatol. 1991;97:959–968

105. Ishii K, et al Characterization of autoantibodies in pemphigus using antigen-specifi c enzyme linked immunosorbent assays with baculovirus expressed recombinant desmogleins. J Immunol. 1997;159:2010–2017

106. Ishii K, Amagai M, Ohata Y, et al Development of pemphigus vulgaris in a patient with pemphigus foliaceus antidesmoglein antibody profile shift confirmed by enzyme-linked immunosorbent assay. J Am Acad Dermatol. 2000;42: 859–861

107. Ishiko A, Shimizu H, Masunaga T, et al 97-kDa linear IgA bullous dermatosis (LAD) antigen localizes to the lamina lucida of the epidermal basement membrane. J Invest Dermatol. 1996;106:734–738

108. Jackson JL, Gibbons R, Meyer G, Inouye L. The effect of treating herpes zoster with oral acyclovir in preventing postherpetic neuralgia. A meta-analysis. Arch Intern Med. 1997;157(8):909–912

109. Jacobs SE. Pemphigus erythematosus and ultraviolet light. A case report. Arch Dermatol. 1965;91:139–141

110. Jiao D, Bystryn JC. Sensitivity of indirect immunofluorescence, substrate specifi city and immunoblotting in the diagnosis of pemphigus. J Am Acad Dermatol. 1997;37: 211–216

111. Jonkman MF, De Jong MCJM, Heeres K, et al 180-kD bullous pemphigoid antigen (BP180) is deficient in generalized atrophic benign epidermolysis bullosa. J Clin Invest. 1995;95:1345–1352

112. Jonkman MF, Heeres K, Pas HH, et al Effects of keratin 14 ablation on the clinical and cellular phenotype in a kindred with recessive epidermolysis bullosa simplex. J Invest Dermatol. 1996;107:764–769

113. Kaplan RP, Callen JP. Pemphigus-associated diseases and induced pemphigus. Clin Dermatol. 1983;1:42–71

114. Katz SI. Dermatitis herpetiformis. In: Freedberg IM, Eisen AZ, Wolff K, et al, eds. Fitzpatrick's Dermatology in General Medicine. New York, NY: McGraw-Hill; 1999

115. Kirtschig G, Wojnarowska F, Marsden RA, et al Acquired bullous diseases of childhood: re-evaluation of diagnosis by indirect immunofluorescence examination on 1 M NaCl split skin and immunoblotting. Br J Dermatol. 1994;130: 610–616

116. Kivirikko S, McGrath JA, Abderam D, et al A homozygous nonsense mutation in the alpha 3 chain gene of laminin 5 (LAMA3) in lethel (Herlitz) junctional epidermolysis bullosa. Hum Mol Genet. 1995;4:959–962

117. Klein PA, Callen JP. Drug-induced linear IgA bullous dermatosis after vancomycin discontinuance in a patient with renal insufficiency. J Am Acad Dermatol. 2000;42: 316–323

118. Klingberg S, Mortimore R, Parkes J, et al Prenatal diagnosis of dominant dystrophic epidermolysis bullosa, by COL7A1 molecular analysis. Prenat Diagn. 2000;20(8): 618–62

119. Kokuba H, Aurelian L, et al Herpes simplex virus associated erythema multiforme (HAEM) is mechanistically distinct from drug-induced erythema multiforme: interferon-gamma is expressed in HAEM lesions and tumor necrosis factor-alpha in drug-induced erythema multiforme lesions. J Invest Dermatol. 1999;113(5):808–815

120. Kricheli D, David M, Frusic-Zlotkin M. The distribution of pemphigus vulgaris IgG subclasses and reactivity with desmoglein 3 and 1 in pemphigus patients and first degree relatives. N J Dermatol. 2000;143:337–342

121. Kuechle MK, Stegemeir E, Maynard B, et al Drug-induced linear IgA bullous dermatosis: report of six cases and review of the literature. J Am Acad Dermatol. 1994;30: 187–192

122. Lapiere JC, Woodley DT, Parente MG, et al Epitope mapping of type VII collagen. Identification of discrete peptide sequences recognized by sera from patients with acquired epidermolysis bullosa. J Clin Invest. 1993;92:1831–1839

123. Lee E, Lendas KA, Chow S, et al Disease relevant HLA class II alleles isolated by genotypic, haplotypic, and sequence analysis in North American Caucasians with pemphigus vulgaris. Hum Immunol. 2006;67(1–2):125–139

124. Lever WF. Pemphigus. Medicine. 1953;32:1–123

125. Lever WF. Pemphigus and pemphigoid. J Am Acad Dermatol. 1979;1:2–31

126. Leverkus M, Bhol K, Hirako Y, et al Cicatricial pemphigoid with circulating autoantibodies to beta4 integrin, bullous pemphigoid 180 and bullous pemphigoid 230. Br J Dermatol. 2001;145(6):998–1004

127. Levy RS, Fisher M, Alter NA. Penicillamine: review and cutaneous manifestations. J Am Acad Dermatol. 1983;8: 548–558

128. Lin MS, Gharia M, Fu CL, et al Molecular mapping of the major epitopes of BP180 recognized by herpes gestationis autoantibodies. Clin Immunol. 1999;92:285–292

129. Lin R, Ladd DJ, Powell DJ, Way BV. Localized pemphigus foliaceus induced by topical imiquimod. Arch Dermatol. 2004;140:889–890

130. Liu Z. Bullous pemphigoid: using animal models to study the immunopathology. J Invest Dermatol Symp Proc. 2004; 9(1):41–46

131. Mackenzie-Wood A, Kirkham B, Hart K, Murrell DF. Second Case of Bullous Pemphigoid like Eruption Induced by D-Penicillamine. Mini Consults in Dermatology Volume VI, American Academy of Dermatology. Mosby-Year Book; 1999

132. Marinkovich MP, Taylor TB, Keene DR, et al LAD-1, the linear IgA bullous dermatosis autoantigen, is a novel 120-kDa anchoring filament protein synthesized by epidermal cells. J Invest Dermatol. 1996;106:734–738

133. Martin LK, Murrell DF. Treatment of pemphigus: the need for more evidence. Arch Dermatol. 2008;144(1):100–101

134. Mashiah J, Brenner S. Medical pearl: first step in managing pemphigus – addressing the etiology. J Am Acad Dermatol. 2005;53(4):706–707

135. McGrath JA, Ishida-Yamamoto A, Tidman MJ, Heagerty AHM, Schofield OMV, Eady RAJ. Epidermolysis bullosa simplex (Dowling-Meara). A clinicopathological review. Br J Dermatol. 1992;126:421–430

136. McGrath JA, Gatalica B, Crhistiano AM, et al Mutations in the 180kD bullous pemphigoid antigen (BPAG2), a hemidesmosomal transmembrane collagen (COL17A1), in generalised atrophic benign epidermolysis bullosa. Nat Genet. 1995;11:83–86

137. McGrath JA, Pulkkinen L, Christiano AM, et al Altered laminin 5 expression due to mutations in the gene encoding the beta 3 chain (LAMB3) in generalised atrophic benign epidermolysis bullosa. J Invest Dermatol. 1995;104: 467–474

138. McGrath JA, Dunnill MG, Christiano AM, et al First trimester DNA-based exclusion of recessive dystrophic epidermolysis bullosa from chorionic villous sampling. Br J Dermatol. 1996;134(4):734–739

139. Mihai S, Sitaru C. Immunopathology and molecular diagnosis of autoimmune bullous diseases. J Cell Mol Med. 2007;11(3):462–481

140. Mofid MZ, Costarangos C, Bernstein B, et al Drug-induced linear immunoglobulin A bullous disease that clinically mimics toxic epidermal necrolysis. J Burn Care Rehabil. 2000;21:246–247

141. Murrell DF, Pasmooij AM, Pas HH, et al Retrospective diagnosis of fatal BP180-deficient non-Herlitz junctional epidermolysis bullosa suggested by immunofluorescence (IF) antigen-mapping of parental carriers bearing enamel defects. J Invest Dermatol. 2007;127(7):1772–1775

142. Murrell DF, Amagai M, Barnadas MA, et al Consensus statement on definitions of disease endpoints and therapeutic response for pemphigus. JAAD. 2008;58(6):1043–1046

143. Mutasim DF. Autoimmune bullous diseases: diagnosis and management. Dermatol Nurs. 1999;11:15–21

144. Neughebauer BI, Negron G, Pelton S, Plunkett RW, Beutner EH, Magnussen R. Bullous skin disease: an unusual allergic reaction to vancomycin. Am J Med Sci. 2002;323(5): 273–278

145. Ng PP, Sun YJ. Detection of herpes simplex virus genomic DNA in various subsets of erythema multiforme by polymerase chain reaction. Dermatology. 2003;207(4):349–353

146. Nicolas ME, Krause PK, Gibson LE, Murray JA. Dermatitis herpetiformis. Int J Dermatol. 2003;42:588–600

147. Niemi K-M, Sommer H, Kero M, et al Epidermolysis bullosa simplex associated with muscular dystrophy with recessive inheritance. Arch Dermatol. 1988;124:551–554

148. Nousari HC, Kimyai-Asadi A, Caeiro JP, et al Clinical, demographic, and immunohistologic features of vancomycin-induced linear IgA bullous disease of the skin. Medicine. 1999;78:1–8

149. Nuemberger S, Driscoll A, Gabel P, et al Orf virus infection in humans-New York, Illinois, California and Tennessee 2004–2005. JAMA. 2006;55:65–68

150. Oxman MN, Levin MJ, Johnson GR, et al A vaccine to prevent herpes zoster and postherpetic neuralgia in older adults. N Engl J Med. 2005;253(22):2271–2284

151. Park SB, Cho KH, Youn JL, Hwang DH, Kim SC, Chung JH. Epidermolysis bullosa acquisita in childhood-a case mimicking chronic bullous dermatosis of childhood. Clin Exp Dermatol. 1997;22(5):220–222

152. Parlowsky T, Welzel J, Amagai M, Zillikens D, Wygold T. Neonatal pemphigus vulgaris: IgG4 autoantibodies to desmoglein 3 induce skin blisters in newborns. J Am Acad Dermatol. 2003;48(4):623–625

153. Pas HH, De Jong MC, Jonkman MF, Heeres K, Slijper-Pal IJ, Van der Meer JB. Bullous pemphigoid: serum antibody titre and antigen specifi city. Exp Dermatol. 1995;4: 372–376

154. Pearson RW. Studies on the pathogenesis of epidermolysis bullosa. J Invest Dermatol. 1962;39:551–575

155. Pearson RW, Spargo B. Electron microscopic studies of dermal-epidermal separation in human skin. J Invest Dermatol. 1961;36:213–224

156. Peters MS, McEvoy MT. IgA antiendomysial antibodies in dermatitis herpetiformis. J Am Acad Dermatol. 1989;21: 1225–1231

157. Pfendner E, Uitto J. Plectin gene mutations can cause epidermolysis bullosa with pyloric atresia. J Invest Dermatol. 2005;124(1):111–115

158. Pfendner EG, Nakano A, Pulkkinen L, Christiano AM, Uitto J. Prenatal diagnosis for epidermolysis bullosa: a study of 144 consecutive pregnancies at risk. Prenat Diagn. 2003;23(6):447–456

159. Phelps RG, Miller MK, Singh F. The varieties of eczema: clinicopathologic correlation. Clin Dermatol. 2003;25: 95–100

160. Plunkett RW, Chiarello SE, Beutner EH. Linear IgA bullous dermatosis in one of two piroxicam-induced eruptions: a distinct direct immunofluorescence trend revealed by the literature. J Am Acad Dermatol. 2001;45:691–696

161. Powell GR, Bruckner AL, Weston WL. Dermatitis herpetiformis presenting as chronic urticaria. Pediatr Dermatol. 2004;21(5):564–567

162. Powell AM, Sakuma-Oyama Y, Oyama N, et al Usefulness of BP180 NC16a enzyme-linked immunosorbent assay in the serodiagnosis of pemphigoid gestationis and in differentiating between pemphigoid gestationis and pruritic urticarial papules and plaques of pregnancy. Arch Dermatol. 2005;141(6):705–710

163. Premaratne C, Klingberg S, Glass I, Wright K, Murrell D. Epidermolysis bullosa simplex Dowling-Meara due to an arginine to cysteine substitution in exon 1 of keratin 14. Australas J Dermatol. 2002;43(1):28–34

164. Proby C, Fujii Y, Owaribe K, et al Human autoantibodies against HD1/plectin in paraneoplatic pemphigus. J Invest Dermatol. 1999;112:153–156

165. Pulkkinen L, Christiano AM, Gerecke D, et al A homozygous nonsense mutation in the beta 3 chain gene of laminin 5 (LAMB3) in Herlitz junctional epidermolysis bullosa. Genomics. 1994;24:357–360

166. Rabinowitz LG, Esterly NB. Inflammatory bullous diseases in children. Dermatol Clin. 1993;11:565–581

167. Rao CL, Hall RP. III, Linear IgA dermatosis and chronic bullous disease of childhood. In: Freedberg IM, Eisen AZ, Wolff K, Austen KF, Goldsmith LA, Katz SI, eds. Dermatology in General Medicine. New York: McGraw-Hill; 2003

168. Richards SS, Hall S, Yokel B, et al A bullous eruption in an elderly woman. Vancomycin-associated linear IgA dermatosis (LAD). Arch Dermatol. 1995;131:1447–1451

169. Rocha-Alvarez R, Friedman H, Campbell IT, Souza-Aguiar L, Martins-Castro R, Diaz LA. Pregnant women with endemic pemphigus foliaceus (fogo selvagem) give birth to disease-free babies. J Invest Dermatol. 1992;99:78–82

170. Rock B, Martins CR, Theofilopoulos AN, et al The pathogenic effect of IgG4 autoantibodies in endemic pemphigus foliaceus (fogo selvagem). N Eng J Med. 1989;320: 1463–1469

171. Rodeck CH, Eady RA, Gosden CM. Prenatal diagnosis of epidermolysis bullosa letalis. Lancet. 1980;1(8175): 949–952

172. Roenigk HH, Ryan JG, Bergfeld WF. Epidermolysis bullosa acquista: Report of three cases and review of all published cases. Arch Dermatol. 1971;103:1–10

173. Roujeau JC, Kelly JP, Naldi L, et al Medication use and the risk of Stevens-Johnson syndrome or toxic epidermal necrolysis. N Engl J Mcd. 1995;333:1600–1607

174. Ruach M, Ohel G, Rahav D, Samueloff A. Pemphigus vulgaris and pregnancy. Obstet Gynecol Surv. 1995;50(10): 755–760

175. Ruocco V, Rossi A, Astarita C, et al A congenital acantholytic bullous eruption in the newborn infant of a pemphigus mother. Ital Gen Rev Dermatol. 1975;12:169–174

176. Scott JE, Ahmed AR. The blistering diseases. Med Clin North Am. 1998;82:1239–1283

177. Scully C. A review of mucocutaneous disorders affecting the mouth and lips. Ann Acad Med Singap. 1999;28: 704–707

178. Shachar E, Bialy-Golan A, Srebrnik A, Brenner S. "Two-step" drug-induced bullous pemphigoid. Int J Dermatol. 1998;37(12):938–939

179. Shimanovich I, Bröcker EB, Zillikens D. Pemphigoid gestationis: new insights into the pathogenesis lead to novel diagnostic tools. Br J Obstet Gynaecol. 2002;109: 970–976

180. Shimizu H, Suzumori L. Prenatal diagnosis as a test for genodermatoses: its past, present and future. J Dermatol Sci. 1999;19:1–8

181. Sison-Fonacier L, Bystryn JC. Heterogeneity of pemphigus vulgaris antigens. Arch Dermatol. 1987;123:1507–1510

182. Sitaru C, Powell J, Shimanovich I, et al Pemphigoid gestationis: maternal sera recognise epitopes restricted to the N-terminal portion of the extracellular domain of BP180 not present on its shed ectodomain. Br J Dermatol. 2003; 149:420–422

183. Sitaru C, Powell J, Messer G, Brocker EB, Wojnarowska F, Zillikens D. Immunoblotting and enzyme-linked immunosorbent assay for the diagnosis of pemphigoid gestationis. Obstet Gynecol. 2004;103(4):757–763

184. Sitaru C, Dahnrich C, Probst C, et al Enzyme-linked immunosorbent assay using multimers of the 16th non-collagenous domain of the BP180 antigen for sensitive and specific detection of pemphigoid autoantibodies. Exp Dermatol. 2007;16(9):770–777

185. Späth S, Riechers R, Borradori L, Zillikens D, Bdinger L, Hertl M. Detection of autoantibodies of various subclasses (IgG1, IgG4, IgA, IgE) against desmoglein 3 in patients with acute onset and chronic pemphigus vulgaris. Br J Dermatol. 2001;144:1183–1188

186. Stanley JR. Pemphigus. In: Freedberg IM, ed. Fitzpatrick's Dermatology in General Medicine. 6th ed. New York: McGraw Hill; 1999:654–666

187. Stanley JR. Bullous pemphigoid. In: Freedberg IM, ed. Fitzpatrick's Dermatology in General Medicine. 6th ed. New York: McGraw Hill; 1999:574–580

188. Szafer F, Brautbar C, Tzfoni E, et al Detection of disease-specifi c restriction fragment length polymorphisms in pemphigus vulgaris linked to the DQw1 and DQw3 alleles of the HLA-D region. Proc Natl Acad Sci USA. 1987; 84: 6542

189. Tidman M, Eady RA. Hemidesmosomes heterogeneity in junctional epidermolysis bullosa revealed by morphometric analysis. J Invest Dermatol. 1986;86:51–56
190. Tidman M, Eady RA. Diagnosis and diagnostic techniques. In: Wojnarowska F, Briggaman RA, eds. Management of Blistering Diseases. London: Chapman and Hall; 1990
191. Todd JA, Acha-Orbea H, Bell JI, et al A molecular basis for MHC class II–associated autoimmunity. Science. 1988; 240:1003
192. Tsuji-Abe Y, Akiyama M, Yamanaka Y, Kikuchi T, Sato-Matsumura KC, Shimizu H. Correlation of clinical severity and ELISA indices for the NC16A domain of BP180 measured using BP180 ELISA kit in bullous pemphigoid. J Dermatol Sci. 2005;37(3):145–149
193. Tur E, Brenner S. Diet and pemphigus. In pursuit of exogenous factors in pemphigus and fogo selvagem. Arch Dermatol. 1998;134:1406–1410
194. Vailley J, Szepetowski P, Pedeutour F, et al The genes for nicein/kalinin 125kDa and 100kDa subunits, candidates for junctional epidermolysis bullosa, map to chromosome 1q32 and 1q25–q31. Genomics. 1994;21:286–288
195. Vidal F, Aberdam D, Miquel C, et al Integrin beta 4 mutations associated with junctional epidermolysis bullosa with pyloric atresia. Nat Genet. 1995;10:229–234
196. Vu TN, Lee TX, Ndoye A, et al The pathophysiological significance of nondesmoglein targets of pemphigus autoimmunity. Development of antibodies against keratinocyte cholinergic receptors in patients with pemphigus vulgaris and pemphigus foliaceus. Arch Dermatol. 1998;134(8): 971–980
197. Waananakul S, Pongprasit P. Childhood pemphigus. Int J Dermatol. 1999;38:29–35
198. Warren SJ, Cockerell CJ. Characterization of a subgroup of patients with dermatitis herpetiformis with nonclassical histologic features. Am J Dermatopathol. 2002;24(4): 305–308
199. Wasserstrum N, Laros RK Jr. Transplacental transmission of pemphigus. JAMA. 1983;249(11):1480–1482
200. Weinberg ED. Pregnancy-associated depression of cell-mediated immunity. Rev Infect Dis. 1984;6:814–831
201. Weinberg JM. Herpes zoster: epidemiology, natural history, and common complications. J Am Acad Dermatol. 2007;57 (6):130–135
202. Weller R, White MI. Bullous pemphigoid and penicillamine. Clin Exp Dermatol. 1996;21(2):121–122
203. Whitley RJ, Weiss H, Gnann JW Jr, et al Acyclovir with and without prednisone for the treatment of herpes zoster. A randomized, placebo-controlled trial. The National Institute of Allergy and Infectious Diseases Collaborative Antiviral Study Group. Ann Intern Med. 1996;125(5): 376–383
204. Wojnarowska F, Marsden RA, Bhogal B, Black MM. Chronic bullous disease of childhood, childhood cicatricial pemphigoid, and linear IgA disease of adults. A comparative study demonstrating clinical and immunopathologic overlap. J Am Acad Dermatol. 1988;19:792–805
205. Wojnarowska F, Whitehead P, Leigh IM, Bhogal BS, Black MM. Identification of the target antigen in chronic bullous disease of childhood and linear IgA disease of adults. Br J Dermatol. 1991;124:157–162
206. Wojnarowska F, Allen J, Collier P. Linear IgA disease: a heterogenous disease. Dermatology. 1994;189:52–56
207. Wood MJ, Kay R, Dworkin RH, Soong SJ, Whitley RJ. Oral acyclovir therapy accelerates pain resolution in patients with herpes zoster: a meta-analysis of placebo controlled trials. Clin Infect Dis. 1996;22:341–347
208. Woodley DT. Epidermolysis bullosa acquista. Prog Dermatol. 1988;22:1
209. Woodley DT, Briggaman RA, O'Keefe EJ, Inman AO, Queen LL, Gammon WR. Identification of the skin basement-membrane autoantigen in epidermolysis bullosa acquisita. N Engl J Med. 1984;310:1007–1013
210. Woodley DT, Burgeson RE, Lunstrum G, et al Epidermolysis bullosa acquisita antigen is globular carboxyl terminus of type VII procollagen. J Clin Invest. 1988;81:683–687
211. Wu H, Wang ZH, Yan A, et al Protection against pemphigus foliaceus by desmoglein 3 in neonates. N Engl J Med. 2000;343:31–35
212. Yamane Y, Sato H, Higashi K, Yaoita H. Linear immunoglobulin A (IgA) bullous dermatosis of childhood: identification of the target antigens and study of the cellular sources. Br J Dermatol. 1996;135:785–790
213. Yiasemedes E, Walton J, Marr P, Villaneuva EV, Murrell DF. A comparative study between transmission electron microscopy and immunofluorescence mapping in the diagnosis of epidermolysis bullosa. Am J Dermatopathol. 2006;28(5):387–394
214. Yiasemides E, Trisnowati N, Su J, Dang NN, Klingberg S, Marr P, Chow CW, Orchard D, Varigos G, Murrell DF: Clinical heterogeneity in recessive epidermolysis bullosa due to mutations in the keratin 14 gene, KRT14. Clin Exp Dermatol. Nov 2008; 33(6):689–97
215. Yoshida M, Hamada T, Amagai M, et al Enzyme-linked immunosorbent assay using bacterial recombinant proteins of human BP230 as a diagnostic tool for bullous pemphigoid. J Dermatol Sci. 2006;41(1):21–30
216. Zhou S, Wakelin SH, Allen J, Wojnarowska F. Blister fluid for the diagnosis of subepidermal immunobullous diseases: a comparative study of basement membrane zone autoantibodies detected in blister fluid and serum. Br J Dermatol. 1998;139(1):27–32
217. Zillikens D. Acquired skin disease of hemidesmosomes. J Dermatol Sci. 1999;20:134–154
218. Zillikens D, Wever S, Roth A, Hashimoto T, Brocker EB. Incidence of autoimmune subepidermal blistering dermatosis in a region of central Germany. Arch Dermatol. 1995; 131:957–958
219. Zillikens D, Herzele K, Georgi M, et al Autoantibodies in a subgroup of patients with linear IgA disease react with the NC16A domain of BP180. J Invest Dermatol. 1999; 113: 947–953
220. Zone JJ. Skin manifestations of celiac disease. Gastroenterology. 2005;128:S87–S91
221. Zone JJ, Taylor TB, Meyer LJ, Petersen MJ. The 97 kDa linear IgA bullous disease antigen is identical to a portion of the extracellular domain of the 180 kDa bullous pemphigoid antigen, BPAG 2. J Invest Dermatol. 1998;110: 207–210

Diagnosis and Prevention of Atopic Eczema

Stefan Wöhrl

7.1 Introduction

Atopic eczema (AE) is a chronic, highly prevalent, inflammatory skin disease with a characteristic phenotype and distribution pattern. A variety of terms have been created to describe this characteristic phenotype. The historic terms "neurodermitis" and "neurodermatitis"[1] were replaced later by the term "atopic dermatitis" and finally "AE."[2] The term AE will be used in this chapter because it is the proposed term in the World Allergy Organization (WAO) guideline of 2004.[2] AE often occurs together with allergic rhinoconjunctivitis and bronchial asthma. These three entities are referred to as "atopic diseases" or "allergic diseases." The atopic diseases have the highest levels of incidence in the first decades of life.[3] Typically, AE is the earliest symptom in the life of infants, then continues to allergic rhinoconjunctivitis and, finally, ends with allergic bronchial asthma. The term "atopic march" was coined for this natural course of the disease complex.[4]

Over the past decades, the prevalence of AE has steadily increased to affect now about 1 out of 10 young children and 2 out of 100 adults in the Western societies.[5] A large worldwide study with more than 50 participating countries showed that the increase of atopic diseases has become less steep in recent years but is still on the rise.[5] How can this be explained? Although it has been observed for a long time that the predisposition for atopic diseases is highly inherited,[6] human genes cannot have changed within the past century and other factors have to be involved. "Western lifestyle" has often been accused as one of the causes of the "allergy epidemic."[7] The "hygiene hypothesis" postulates that the neonatal immune system needs microbial and parasitic infection for full maturation and that the much-too-clean environment of childhood nowadays shifts the immune system from tolerance toward allergy to environmental allergens.[8] Although attractive, this theory has been challenged lately.[9] Others speculated that modern housing conditions lead to increased allergen exposition and that this contributes to higher rates of sensitization to indoor allergens such as storage and house dust mites in 33% or to cat dander in 13% of the patients suffering from AE when compared with nonatopic controls (25% and 4%, respectively).[10]

So, environmental conditions have changed. Both abnormal immunologic response to harmless allergens and inadequate epidermal barrier function lead to the development of AE; "Western lifestyle," for example, directly changed environmental factors affecting the skin. The frequency of daily personal washing has increased dramatically in the past decades. The average use of water for this purpose increased from 11 L in 1961 to 51 L in 1997.[11] Using soap and other detergents during washing aggravates the situation and has also increased. The use of soap and personal wash detergents in the UK increased from £76 million in 1981 to £453 million (inflation adjusted) in 2001 while the population remained nearly stable.[12]

S. Wöhrl
Division of Immunology, Department of Dermatology, Allergy and Infectious Diseases (DIAID), Medical University of Vienna, Vienna, Austria
e-mail: stefan.woehrl@meduniwien.ac.at

R.A. Norman (ed.), *Preventive Dermatology in Infectious Diseases*, DOI 10.1007/978-0-85729-847-8_7, © Springer-Verlag London Limited 2012

7.2 Pathophysiology

7.2.1 Skin Physiology

The skin is the largest organ and serves as a barrier between the interior and the exterior world. It protects the body from desiccation and from xenobiotics. The epidermal barrier function has been visualized as a "brick wall" with the corneocytes – the flattened keratinocytes of the upper epidermis – serving as the bricks and the lipid lamellae as cement[13] (Fig. 7.1).[12,14] The lipid lamellae are secreted by the corneocytes and are composed mainly of ceramides, cholesterol, fatty acids, and cholesterol esters.[15] These substances form the so-called "cornified envelope" and surround the corneocytes. The main function of the lipid lamellae is the prevention of water loss. The integrity of these lamellae can be reduced by washing the skin with mild detergents, e.g., soaps. Other important structures are the corneodesmosomes, modified desmosomes of the *Stratum corneum*. They lock the corneocytes together. Corneodesmosomes provide the *Str. corneum* with the strength to resist against shearing forces.[12] These structures can be visualized as iron rods (Fig. 7.1). Upon normal epidermal turnover, the corneodesmosomes are cleaved in the upper corneal layer by endogenous serine proteases such as the *Str. corneum chymotryptic enzyme* to facilitate epidermal shedding. A fine balance has to be kept for maintaining epidermal homeostasis. Exaggerated corneodesmolysis by endogenous or *Staphylococci* and house dust mite enzymes leads to epidermal thinning and decreased barrier function, decelerated endogenous cleavage to squamation.

Cork et al.[12] speculate that skin thickness is an important key to explain the mystique behind the predilection sites of AE. The eyelids are reported to have the lowest skin thickness, followed by genitals, flexural forearm and the posterior auricular region.[12] The thickness of the elbow flexures is unknown but the ones of the palms and soles are the thickest. Skin thickness is also associated with percutaneous penetration of topically applied drugs like corticosteroids. Neonatal skin is not fully mature in respect of barrier function and percutaneous penetration is elevated in compare with adult skin.[16]

7.2.2 Genetics

There is a strong genetic background for all kinds of atopic diseases. Until recently, the focus has been on the immunologic side. In 1999, Taïeb[14] hypothesized that genes involved in the epidermal barrier function might also play an important role in the etiology of AE. In a very important study, Palmer et al.[17] showed that two loss-of-function deletions in the gene encoding for filaggrin are associated with a high risk for suffering from AE. Around 49% of the European population are heterozygous carriers for this allele.[18] Interestingly, carriers of the mutated allele are not only at higher risk for AE but also for bronchial asthma. A recent meta-analysis of nine studies on filaggrin

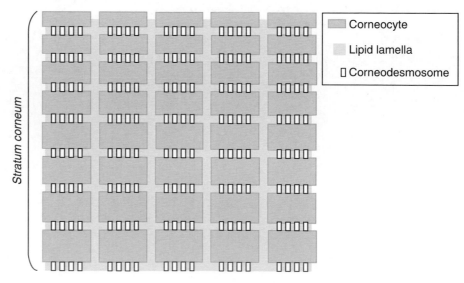

Fig. 7.1 The "brick wall" model of the upper epidermis (Modified after Taïeb[14] and Cork et al [12]: in this model, the corneocytes – the flattened keratinocytes of the upper epidermis – are visualized as bricks and the lipid lamella, almost a synonym for the "cornified envelope," as cement. The main function of the lipid lamella is to waterproof the epidermis. The corneodesmosomes are visualized as iron rods that provide resistance to shearing forces)

mutations in AE pinned the odds ratio for carriers down to four when compared with noncarriers.[18]

Also other factors contribute to the reduced barrier function of atopic skin; for example, the normal un-inflamed skin of AE patients contains less ceramide and sphingosine than that of nonatopic controls.[15]

7.2.3 Immunology and Allergy

7.2.3.1 Immunology

Although the breakdown of the skin barrier is an important aspect in the initiation phase of AE, there has been the long-term clinical observation that using potent immunosuppression (e.g., cyclosporine) stops skin inflammation and leads to long-term remission.

The immunologic response to antigens in atopic patients differs from nonatopic controls. Atopics have a pronounced immunological response of Th2 cells to external antigens with a characteristic cytokine profile, namely interleukin-4 (IL-4), IL-5, IL-9, and IL-13. IL-4 differentiates naïve T-helper 0 cells (Th0) into Th2[1] and together with IL-13 promotes isotype-switching of B-cells to IgE production.[19] IL-4 upregulates Fc e [epsilon] receptor I expression on dendritic cells facilitating allergen uptake in dendritic cells and allergen presentation to other immunologic cell types. Finally, it suppresses the production of Th1-type cytokines like IFN-g (gamma) and IL-12.[20] IL-5 attracts and stimulates the growth of eosinophils. These are the reasons for the elevated serum IgE levels and the eosinophilia in differential blood counts from patients suffering from atopic diseases.

Interestingly, AE lesions are biphasic in nature. Th2 cytokines predominate in acute AE lesions, whereas the Th1 cytokines IFN- g (gamma) and IL-12 outweigh in chronic eczema.[21]

Regulatory T-cells are key players in self-tolerance and tolerance to environmental antigens such as allergens. Their upregulation is a key feature of regaining tolerance to allergens with specific immunotherapy.[22] Verhagen et al.[23] showed that regulatory T-cells are missing in AE skin lesions.

7.2.3.2 Allergy

Sensitization with specific IgE to food and aeroallergens is an important contributor to symptom severity in atopic patients. Food is the major allergen in infants of up to 2 years and may cause skin rashes in around 35% of pediatric AE patients.[24] Milk protein, hen's egg, soy, wheat, peanut, tree nut, fish, and shellfish are the most important food allergens. Among them, milk is the predominant allergen in infants. The prognosis for food allergy in young children is good. Eighty percent will outgrow their symptoms by their fifth birthday with the exception of peanut allergy, which persists in 80% of the patients.[24] Three-and-a-half to 4% of adult Americans have specific IgE to food allergens.[24] Contrasting AE as the main manifestation of food allergy in young children, food-allergic adults tend to suffer from other type-1 allergic manifestations like urticaria, angioedema, gastrointestinal symptoms, or anaphylaxis.

Sensitization to aeroallergens like birch, grass, and ragweed pollen as well as house dust mite and cat dander comes into fore from the age of 2 years and above. The degree of sensitization to house dust, mite, and fungal allergens was shown to correlate with symptom severity in AE patients.[25] Patients with a primary sensitization to pollen aeroallergens may cross-react to the same allergenic components in food laying the base for typical syndromes (e.g., the "oral allergy syndrome " to apples and tree nuts in birch-pollen–allergic patients or the "mugwort-celery-spice" syndrome in patients sensitized to profilins).[26]

A subset of severely affected AE patients has specific IgE against the superoxide manganese dismutase, an inducible human stress enzyme. It is one of several described self-antigens that were termed "atopy related autoantigens."[20] Patients with high levels of self-IgE-autoantibodies suffer from a more severe disease than those without and belong to the subgroup with an onset in early childhood.[27] The human superoxide manganese dismutase cross-reacts with that from the skin-colonizing yeast *Malassezia sympodialis*. A high colonization with *Malassezia sympodialis* was described as an important trigger for AE.[28]

7.2.4 Disease-Aggravating Factors

7.2.4.1 Stress and Itch

Patients with AE suffer from chronic itch that typically intensifies periodically. Scratch marks are a frequent clinical sign of severely affected patients. Pruritus has several pathophysiological dimensions:

- The central "neurogenic" itch is generated in the central nervous system in response to circulating pruritogens as in cholestasis or in response to intraspinal morphines.[29]
- "Psychogenic" itch is also produced in the central nervous system and aggravated by emotional stress.[20] The immune system of patients with AE reacts to psychological stress with a higher elevation of IL-4, IL-5, and CLA+, a T cell activation marker, than healthy controls.[30] This means that psychological stress influences an atopic immune system in a more pronounced way than a healthy one.
- The peripheral "pruritoreceptive itch" is generated in inflamed skin.[29]

Itch is mediated by sensory peripheral nerves. Sensory peripheral nerves can be activated by histamine type 1, 2, and 3 receptors as well as by Substance P. Mast cells are an important booster of pruritus by releasing histamine but also other mediators such as tryptase and mast cell chymase.[31] Their number is increased in lesional as well as nonlesional skin of atopic patients.[32] Dermal contacts between mast cells and peripheral nerve fibers as well as the number of nerval fibers themselves are increased in atopic skin.[33] The latter can be (partly) explained by elevated levels of the nerve-growth promoting neurotrophins in the serum of patients with AE.[34]

IL-31 is a recently described cytokine. Its overexpression in transgenic mice leads to severe pruritus and AE-like dermatitis.[35] IL-31 expression is increased in the epidermis of atopic patients when compared with healthy controls.[36] Interestingly, the IL-31 serum levels do not differ between both patients groups.

7.2.4.2 Superinfection with Staphylococci and Herpes Virus

Exacerbations of AE are often accompanied by infection with *Staphylococcus aureus*.[37] The bacterium *S. aureus* is not part of the normal skin *flora* and only 36% of healthy nonatopic children are colonized in their nostrils, the natural reservoir.[38] In contrast, more than 90% of inflammatory and 76% of noninflammatory AE skin lesions are colonized with *S. aureus*.[39] *S. aureus* produces several enterotoxins that can serve

as superantigens.[40] A subset of AE patients also produces measurable specific IgE against these superantigens.[41] *S. aureus* produces ceramidase, further aggravating the lack of ceramides in atopic skin (see Sect. 7.2.1). Also, *staphylococcal* enterotoxin leads to rapid upregulation of the pruritogenic IL-31 in atopic patients aggravating their itch sensation[42] (see Sect. 7.2.4.1).

Also, innate immunity is reduced in AE patients. Human skin expresses antibacterial peptides that inhibit bacterial growth of *Staphylococci,* so-called cathelicidins and b (beta)-defensins. It was shown that the production of both peptides is reduced in lesional as well as nonlesional skin of AE patients.[43] Cathelicidins also provide resistance to viral infection. AE patients with a very low epidermal cathelicidin activity are prone to recurrent, severe infections with herpes viruses, the so-called "eczema herpeticum."[44]

7.3 Diagnosis of Atopic Eczema

7.3.1 Clinical Presentation

The case presentation of AE is age-dependent. While infants typically suffer from facial eczema and a cradle cap – an eczema of the scalp – toddlers and adolescents tend to suffer from flexural eczema as cardinal symptoms. Eyelid eczema is another characteristic presentation in 21% of young adults.[45] Other typical variants are neck and hand eczema as well as the so-called "atopic winter feet." More clinical features of AE in adults are listed Table 7.1.[46]

The clinical spectrum of AE is very broad, ranging from very mild variants presenting as fingertip eczema ("pulpitis sicca") to a generalized erythromatous rash.[47] In difficult cases, scratch marks can be observed as a sign of the severe pruritus.

7.3.2 Diagnostic Criteria

According to the 2004 WAO definition, "atopic dermatitis" should be referred to as "AE."[2] The term AE should stay restricted to patients with elevated total IgE of >150 kU/L and sensitization to aero- and/or food-allergens proved either by skin tests or by

Table 7.1 Diagnostic features of AE according to Hanifin and Rajka[46]

Major criteria: 3 of 4 present	Pruritus
	Typical morphology and distribution of skin lesions
	Chronic or chronically relapsing dermatitis
	Personal or family history of atopy
Minor criteria: 3 of 23 present	Xerosis
	Ichthyosis/palmar hyperlinearity/keratosis pilaris
	Immediate (type I) skin test reactivity
	Elevated serum IgE
	Early age of onset
	Tendency toward cutaneous infections/impaired cell-mediated immunity
	Tendency toward nonspecific hand or foot dermatitis
	Nipple eczema
	Cheilitis
	Recurrent conjunctivitis
	Dennie–Morgan infraorbital fold
	Keratoconus
	Anterior subcapsular cataracts
	Orbital darkening
	Facial pallor/erythema
	Pityriasis alba
	Anterior neck folds
	Itch when sweating
	Intolerance to wool and lipid solvents
	Perifollicular accentuation
	Food intolerance
	Course influenced by environmental/emotional factors
	White dermographism/delayed blanch

Table 7.2 Diagnostic criteria for diagnosing AE according to the UK working party[48]

Major criterion: one of one present	Itchy skin condition in the preceding 12 months
Minor criteria: three of five present	Onset <2 years
	History of flexural involvement
	History of a generally dry skin
	Personal history of other atopic disease or atopic disease in first degree relatives when age of patient <4 years
	Visible dermatitis as per photographic protocol

measuring specific serum IgE. According to current data, 80% of adult AE patients are monosensitized to at least one allergen and should be classified as AE.[20] Formerly, this type of AE was called "extrinsic atopic dermatitis."[1] The other 20% of patients can be classified as suffering from "nonatopic eczema,"[2] formerly known as "intrinsic atopic dermatitis."[1] It remains to be seen whether this classification will find acceptance in the dermatologic community.

Currently, there are no definitive criteria for the diagnosis of AE. In 1980, Hanifin and Rajka[46] were the first to set up rules for the definition of AE. They based their definition on extensive dermatological criteria. Three out of four main and 3 out of 28 minor criteria must be fulfilled for the diagnosis of AE (Table 7.1).[46] The UK working party developed much simpler criteria depending on the presence of just one main and three out of five minor criteria (Table 7.2).[48] Although

the approach of the UK criteria is much simpler, both ways of defining AE show good agreement on comparison.[49] Hence, for daily practice, use of the UK criteria seems to be sufficient and is recommended by the British National Institute for Health and Clinical Excellence (NICE) guidelines on the management of AE in children of up to 12 years.[50]

7.3.3 Allergologic Workup

The allergologic workup should begin with a careful dermatological examination. Several clinical scoring systems have been published for objectivation (e.g., SCORAD – score atopic dermatitis [1993]). A careful history-taking should give special regard to a family history for atopic diseases, to a worsening of the eczema after exposure to certain foods, to exposure to environmental allergens such as pets or job related allergens, and to hints of other atopic diseases such as bronchial asthma.

The performance of skin prick tests and/or the measurement of specific IgE should be performed to assess the sensitization to type-1 environmental and food allergens as well as the measurement of total serum IgE. Under special circumstances, skin prick tests with fresh food may be performed as "prick to prick tests." A lung function must be performed whenever bronchial asthma is suspected.

In daily practice, the clinical relevance of sensitization to foods often remains unresolved. Food challenge is the gold standard for the confirmation of the clinical relevance of the sensitization in the patient. It can be performed open label or, in severe cases, as double blind, placebo-controlled, food challenge.

The atopy patch test (APT) is derived from the patch test performed for assessing contact dermatitis with type-4 allergens. It was developed with the aim to make oral food challenges superfluous. In an APT, a type-1 allergen is tested either in the form of a commercial extract or as fresh food (e.g., milk) in Finn chambers (Epitest Ltd Oy, Tuusula, Finland) on either the back or the lateral upper arm. The current European guideline recommends using preferably fresh food whenever possible.[51] The sensitivity of APTs with fresh food is higher.[52] While the specificity of the APT is good, the sensitivity is low, so that its value in daily practice is still a matter of debate.[53]

Alternative medicine is quite popular among AE patients.[54] Some methods of questionable validity are offered by health professionals and nonprofessionals alike. Some of them can cause considerable harm to patients, especially if they are leading to wrong recommendations (e.g., unnecessary elimination diets). The measurement of serum IgG levels to food allergens is one such method. Its clinical value has not yet been demonstrated and should therefore not be performed in AE patients.[55]

7.3.4 Differential Diagnoses

The most important differential diagnoses to AE are other variants of eczema. In adults, irritant eczema often occurs in combination with AE, such as nummular and dyshidrotic (pompholyx) eczema. Palmoplantar psoriasis must be differentiated from AE in patients with exclusive eczema of the palms and soles. Chronic eczema can lead to type-4 sensitization and contact allergy that should be considered as a differential diagnosis.[56]

Scabies infection must be considered, especially if other family members are also affected. In newborns with a cradle cap, seborrheic dermatitis is an important differential diagnosis.

Cutaneous T cell lymphomas should be considered in elderly patients with very chronic eczematous lesions, in particular when they are reappearing at the same sites after several courses of topical corticosteroid treatment.

Genetic disorders must be considered in young patients as they can mimic AE. Ichthyosis vulgaris is the most common keratinization disorder. One in 250 UK school children is affected. Patients present with dry skin, flexural ichthyosis, and palmar hyperlamellosis. Interestingly, they carry the same mutations in the filaggrin gene that put patients at risk for AE.[57]

Netherton syndrome is a rare congenital syndrome characterized by ichthyosiform erythroderma, hair shaft abnormalities, and atopic diathesis. It could be linked to a defect in the SPINK5 gene, a serine protease.[58] The recently described IPEX syndrome is caused by a very rare mutation of the FoxP3 gene that is essential for a normal function of regulatory T cells. As a consequence, these patients lack the tolerance-inducing regulatory T-cells. The phenotype is characterized by an eczematous rash, the early onset of multiple autoendocrinopathies such as type-1 diabetes and highly elevated IgE levels.[59]

In patients with eosinophilia and elevated serum IgE levels, parasite infections should be considered as a differential.

7.4 Prevention

7.4.1 Primary Prevention ("Fighting the Cause")

Primary prevention strategies are meant for those who are not yet affected. This can be achieved either by avoiding known risks or by promoting "health-sustaining" conditions. In the context of preventing AE, the main strategy has been to avoid exposure to potent allergens (e.g., cat as a major indoor allergen and milk as a prominent food allergen)[3] as well as other known risk factors such as cigarette smoke.[60]

The most direct approach of dietary allergen avoidance is breast-feeding. European[61] and American[62] guidelines recommend 4–6 months of exclusive breast-feeding in children at risk (with a first degree relative suffering from an allergic disease). If breast-feeding is not possible, the same guidelines recommend using hydrolyzed cow's milk formulas. There is only little evidence that delaying the introduction of complementary foods beyond the age of 6 months prevents the occurring of atopic disease.[62] Elimination diets impose significant harm to small infants by withholding essential dietary nutrients. A thorough allergologic work-up is a "must" before recommending elimination diets to parents and food-challenges are needed in cases of doubt. Beyond the age of 3, food allergy is generally outgrown and elimination diets are usually not needed in adolescent or adult AE.[63,64]

Dietary restrictions in pregnancy to protect the fetus and for the lactating mother had never been recommended in the European guidelines[61] and, due to the lack of evidence, have also been abandoned in the 2008 American guidelines.[62]

The situation is more complex for nonfood allergens. While the avoidance of cats seem to reduce the arising of allergic asthma,[65,66] primary prevention from house dust mite exposure does not prevent the arising of allergy because children living at high altitudes – where there are practically no house dust mites – develop allergies in the same way as those in the lowlands.[67]

The second aspect of primary prevention, promoting "health-sustaining conditions," does not seem to be met by what is called the Western lifestyle.[68] Children growing up under more natural anthroposophical lifestyle (e.g., avoidance of vaccination and conventional medication, consumption of more traditional food) within Western societies have a lower prevalence of AE and allergic asthma than controls.[69] Another protective factor is early attendance at daycare facilities which has been attributed as a surrogate marker for more episodes of viral infections.[3] Growing up among livestock farming is an even stronger preventive environment.[72] The change of living conditions when migrating from a country with a low prevalence of allergies to a highly developed country with a high prevalence of allergies increases the risk of atopic diseases.[70] De-worming of Gabonese school children led to a higher skin prick test-reactivity to house dust mites.[71]

These observations have been placed in the context of the "hygiene hypothesis"; resulting in another active intervention approach. Children with a high colonization of commensal and hardly pathogenic germs such as *Lactobacilli, Bifidobacteria* and *Mycobacteria* have a low rate of atopic diseases. Alimentation with the addition of these bacteria in the form of "probiotics" led to a reduction of allergic asthma, rhinoconjunctivitis[73,74] and AE.[75] However, most of these data come from one group and could not be reproduced sufficiently elsewhere. It is possible that components of "probiotics" such as CpG motifs will be safer, better defined, and have stronger effects in the near future.

For a prevention of allergic sensitization, preventive allergen vaccinations in nonsensitized infants were proposed before a sensitization occurs, in analogy to preventive vaccination for viral diseases.[76] Valenta's group demonstrated that they could induce allergy-protecting "blocking IgG" antibodies with a genetically modified birch protein that was unable to induce the potentially "anaphylactogenic IgE" antibodies.[77] They argue that a preventive allergy vaccination to the most common type-1 allergens could be useful to prevent allergies in all newborns. However, type-1 allergy causes significant morbidity but hardly any mortality. Hence, the necessity to prevent type-1 allergy has a much lower clinical priority than the prevention of potentially life-threatening viral infectious like measles. Currently, the medical community is judging the benefit–risk ratio of a broad allergy vaccination in not-yet allergic infants as an unfavorable one. Maybe this will change sometime in the future.

In contrast to the very clear recommendations concerning breast-feeding and using hydrolyzed cow's milk formulas, all other data on primary prevention strategies are much less clear and the evidence was not validated high enough to include any of these possible intervention methods into the joint American/European PRACTALL guidelines.[63,64]

7.4.2 Secondary Prevention ("Preventing Disease Progression")

Only a few possibilities have been tested to stop disease progression in already sensitized individuals. It was shown convincingly that specific immunotherapy (allergy shots) can stop disease progression, reduce the morbidity of allergic asthma and rhinoconjunctivitis, and reduce the acquisition of new allergies.[78,79] Sublingual immunotherapy seems to work in the same way although it has a weaker effect. In contrast, patients with AE did not benefit from specific immunotherapy and, until recently, specific immunotherapy was not recommended in patients with AE. Two recent studies came up showing a reduction of AE-severity after treating eczema patients sensitized to house dust mite with specific immunotherapy.[80,81]

For patients suffering from AE and concomitant allergic rhinoconjunctivitis and/or asthma, the situation is clear. They should undergo specific immunotherapy for their rhinoconjunctivitis and/or asthma but must be informed that the effect of the specific immunotherapy on AE is yet not clear. For patients with AE and a sensitization to house dust mite and no other atopic diseases more data are needed before specific immunotherapy can be recommended unequivocally.

7.4.3 Tertiary Prevention ("Preventing Complications and Permanent Disabilities")

The treatment of patients with chronic AE is challenging. A stepwise approach depending on the symptom severity was developed by a joint American/European initiative endorsing members of the American Academy of Immunology (AAAI) and the European Academy of Allergy and Immunology (EAACI) called PRACTALL for "practical allergy" (Fig. 7.2).[63,64]

7.4.3.1 Topical Therapy

Skin Care

Dry skin is a prominent feature of AE. Hence, the regular use of emollients two times a day is the basic treatment for AE patients.[50,56] Emollients should be applied continuously even if the patient is currently in remission for the prevention of relapses.[63,64] Addition of low concentrations of urea (up to 4%) can increase the rehydrating effect. "Topical emollients are preferentially applied directly after a bath or shower, when the skin is still slightly humid, after gentle drying."[56] Skin hydration can be ameliorated by using bath oils. Hot water, especially showering, and swimming in water with high chlorine concentrations worsens the xerosis in the same way as alcohol used for disinfection.

The lack of ceramides is an important factor in the increased transepidermal water loss of atopic skin. New emollients with physiological ceramide concentration (e.g., Atopiclair®, Sinclair) have shown some promising effect by increasing the rehydrating effect in patients with mild-to-moderate AE.[82]

Detergents such as the ones used in soaps should be replaced by synthetic wash syndets (synthetic detergents) with a neutral or mild acidic pH 6.0–5.5.[63,64] Dry skin is prone to micro-fissures, easing the entry of bacteria. Wet dressings can help in treating severely affected lesions.[47]

Rough clothing or wool is known to cause irritation and should be avoided.[63,64] Activities leading to increased perspiration like some sports can exacerbate AE. Cigarette smoke is another known irritant. Further hints for counseling AE patients on the avoidance of nonspecific irritants can be found in Table 7.3.[56]

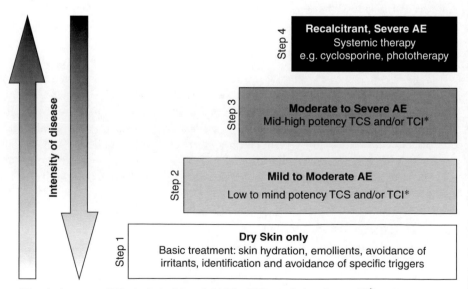

Fig. 7.2 Stepwise management of patients with atopic eczema (AE) according to the joint American/European PRACTALL guidelines[63,64]

AE = atopic eczema, TCI = topical calcineurin inhibitor, TCS = topical corticosteroid,* = > 2 years

Table 7.3 List for counseling AE patients[56]

Clothing: avoid skin contact with irritating fibers (wool, large-fiber textiles); do not use tight and too warm clothing to avoid excessive sweating
Tobacco: avoid exposure
Cool temperature in the bedroom; avoid too many bed covers
Increase emollient use with cold weather
Vaccines: normal schedule in noninvolved skin, including egg-allergic patients
Sun exposure: no specific restriction. Usually helpful because of improvement of epidermal barrier. Encourage summer holidays at high altitude or at beach resorts
Physical exercise, sports: no restriction. If sweating induces flares of AE, progressive adaptation to exercise. Shower and emollients after swimming pool

Allergy:
  Food allergens
    Maintain breast-feeding until 4–6 months if possible or use hydrolyzed formula and delay introduction of solid foods until the seventh month. Avoid foods possibly containing peanut (marked "vegetal fat"). Otherwise normal diet, unless an allergy workup has proven the need to exclude a specific food
 	
  Indoor aeroallergens
  House dust mites
    Use adequate ventilation of housing. Keep the rooms well-aerated even in winter
    Avoid wall-to-wall carpeting
    Remove dust with a wet sponge
    Avoid soft toys in bed (cot), except washable ones
    Wash bedsheets at a temperature higher than 55°C every 10 days
    Use bed and pillow encasings
 	
  Furred pets
    Advise to avoid preventively; if allergy is demonstrated, be firm on avoidance measures

Topical Corticosteroids

Although nearly all published guidelines consider topical corticosteroids (TCS) as the first-line treatment for AE, there is a lack of literature demonstrating the efficacy of this recommendation.[83] TCS are grouped according to their potency, which should be known to their prescribers[56]: group I: mild; group II: moderate; group III and IV: potent to very potent. Because side effects of TCS such as striae, telangiectasias, or atrophy are directly related to their strength, very potent TCS should only be used for a very short time and not on the face or intertriginous areas.[47] Systemic resorption of TCS has to be kept in mind in children of <2 years and in patients with severe flares.

Using TCS twice a day does not improve efficacy over a once-a-day regimen.[84] Interestingly, the type of corticosteroid used does not seem to be of much importance in terms of efficacy.[83] TCS are the treatment of choice for acute flares.[83] Once control over the current fl are has been reached, some authors proposed that a twice-weekly application on skin sites prone to relapse can help to maintain long-term control.[85] Recently, the term "proactive therapy" has been introduced for this preventive treatment concept and studies were performed with some corticosteroids and the topical calcineurin inhibitor tacrolimus.[86]

Topical Calcineurin Inhibitors

In the United States and Europe, pimecrolimus (Elidel®, Novartis) cream (1%) and tacrolimus (Protopic®, Astellas) ointment (0.03%) are approved for the treatment of AE in children of more than 2 years and of adults. Tacrolimus ointment (0.1%) is only approved for use in adults.[63,64] Both drugs have shown their efficacy in numerous studies.[83] The clinical potency of tacrolimus is comparable with a TCS of intermediate activity[87] while pimecrolimus is less active.[88] The most observed side effect of both is a transient, mild, burning sensation on the application site.[56]

Since the United States Food and Drug Administration (FDA) issued a "black box warning" on March tenth 2005 concerning the safety of the topical calcineurin inhibitors because of a lack of long-term safety data,[89] these valuable alternatives to TCS have been labeled as second-line therapy and their use is not recommended in infants younger than the age of 2. Many clinicians found the FDA warning overcautious and statements on the safety have been issued in response to the warning by multiple scientific societies. For example, the American Academy of Dermatology (AAD) states that "topical calcineurin inhibitors remain available for patients with atopic dermatitis."[90] Recent literature published after the FDA warning indicates that the overall safety profile of both drugs is still excellent even after long-term use.[91,92]

7.4.3.2 UV Light Therapy

The treatment of AE with UV light is a well-established standard second-line therapy.[63,64] A combination with TCS for the treatment of acute flares is possible. All treatment regimens have been used: broadband UVB (280–320 nm), narrow-band UVB (311–313 nm), UVA (320–400 nm), UVA_1 (340–400 nm), PUVA, and Balneo-PUVA.[56] Erythema and inflammation are limiting to this method. Due to the unknown long-term safety profile, phototherapy should be restricted to patients of 12 years and above.[63,64]

7.4.3.3 Antimicrobial Therapy

As already mentioned above (see Sect. 7.2.4.2), the atopic skin tends to be over-colonized by microbes like *Staphylococci* and some fungi.

Topical

The use of "intelligent clothing" consisting of silver-coated fabrics and specially coated silk textiles with antimicrobial have shown some promising effect in preliminary studies.[93] The PRACTALL guidelines recommend the use of chlorhexidine or triclosan to reduce the microbial load.[63,64] The use of topical antibiotics like erythromycin and fusidic acid has increased the abundance of resistant *Staphylococci*. Therefore, topical antibiotic therapy should not be extended over more than 2 weeks.[63,64]

Systemic

Severe exacerbations with widespread bacterial infection need a systemic antibiotic therapy. Usually, oral therapy with penicillinase-resistant penicillins or first or second generation cephalosporins for 7–10 days is sufficient. Clindamycin and fusidic acid are alternatives.

Acute eczema herpeticum is a dermatological emergency and hospitalization should be considered. Neck stiffness is a clue to meningeal involvement and lumbar puncture should be performed to exclude herpes meningitis. Acute eczema herpeticum should be treated with intravenous acyclovir.[94] For AE patients with recurrent eczema herpeticum a continuous suppression therapy with acyclovir or valacyclovir can reduce the frequency of episodes and should be recommended to these patients.[94]

Fungal infection is often found in patients with severe AE. However, it is yet not clear whether systemic antimycotic treatment reduces symptom severity and is not recommended.[63,64]

7.4.3.4 Dietary Restrictions

As mentioned above (allergy), dietary restrictions in children should only be recommended when food allergy has been proven by meaningful methods (see Sect. 7.3.3). Hints on counseling patients with proven allergies are found in Table 7.3.[56]

7.4.3.5 Antipruritic Treatment

Topical polidocanol at 1%, although known as a weak contact sensitizer, can be added to emollients and has a mild antipruritic effect. The pruritus of AE patients typically exacerbates at night. Hence, sleeplessness is a common problem. The treatment of choice is adjuvant sedation with first-generation antihistamines that are capable of crossing the blood–brain barrier and sedating central arousal functions mediated by histamine.[50] Typical drugs are diphenhydramine and hydroxycine.[95] Both drugs are available for children and in liquid form.

Doxepin is a tricyclic antidepressant with a pronounced antagonistic effect on histamine receptors. It is a strong sedating drug and another option for treating sleep disturbances. It is used at a dose of 10 mg for pediatric and 25 mg for adult AE patients.[95] Melatonin has also been suggested for mild cases.[95]

7.4.3.6 Systemic Immunosuppression

Cyclosporine

Cyclosporine A is a calcineurin inhibitor functioning in the same way as the topical immunomodulators. Treatment with cyclosporine leads to a reduction of the T-cell activating IL-2 and IFN-g (gamma) cytokines. In fact, it is a very potent drug for the treatment of AE and its clinical effectiveness has been demonstrated in numerous studies for children and adults with an excellent level of evidence.[96] It is a registered therapy for the treatment of AE and is recommended as first option for patients with AE refractory to conventional treatment.[97] The treatment can either be based on short-term high dose (3–5 mg/kg body weight) or on long-term low dose (2.5 mg/kg body weight) regimens.[63,64] The narrow therapeutic index and the known side effects such as renal toxicity or elevation of the blood pressure limit this therapy to severe cases.

Malignancies have been reported after high-dose, long-term treatment in transplant patients. A recent review on the long-term safety data of dermatologic patients revealed a higher risk for the development of basal cell carcinoma but not of other tumors.[98] The authors conclude that due to the overall beneficial benefit–risk ratio, cyclosporine can still be used at the lower dermatologic doses of 3–5 mg/kg body weight.[98]

Azathioprine

Azathioprine at 1–3 mg/kg body weight has some tradition as off-label therapy for recalcitrant AE.[56] The onset of action is rather slow. Myelosuppression, hepatotoxicity, and induction of skin malignancies, among others, are relevant side effects. Azathioprine is metabolized by the thiopurine methyltransferase. Around 11.5% of the population have a reduced or no activity in this enzyme caused mostly by three mutations.[99] Since this enzyme deficiency causes most toxicities, enzymatic or genetic testing must be performed before starting this therapy.[99]

Other Immunosuppression

Different other immunosuppressive modalities have been tried for the treatment AE: mycophenolate mofetil at 2 g/day has a better security profile than azathioprine but larger randomized trials are still missing.[56] Systemic corticosteroids are usually avoided because of the pronounced rebound effect in AE patients. Although a short-term course during an acute fl are might be useful in some cases, a long-term treatment should be avoided especially in children due to the problematic side-effect profile (osteoporosis, growth retardation, diabetes, cataracts). The so-called biologicals that have been so valuable for the treatment of psoriasis have been disappointing when tried anecdotally in AE and currently have no place in the treatment of atopic skin.[100]

7.4.3.7 Nonpharmacological Intervention Strategies

The goal of patient education is for patients to accept their diagnosis of AE, to increase their knowledge of the disease, and to reduce doctor shopping. Hints for counseling AE patients are found in Table 7.3.[56] Other guidelines from the UK regarding counseling of AE patients are available online.[101]

One excellently designed German study showed that an educational intervention (6 weekly standardized group sessions led by a multidisciplinary team consisting of dermatologists or pediatricians, psychologists, and dieticians who had undergone 40 h of special training) resulted in a reduction of objective eczema as well as subjective severity indexes when compared with a nonintervention control group.[102]

One American guideline covers recommendations on psychological approaches,[83] while such are lacking in other guidelines.[50,56,63,64] Behavior modification techniques and relaxation techniques showed some benefit in reducing scratching, although the data are contradictive.[103]

A recent Cochrane review[104] concludes that the level of evidence for the effectiveness for educational and psychological interventions in AE is low due to the small number and the inferior design of existing studies except for the one German study mentioned above.[102]

References

1. Novak N, Bieber T, et al Immune mechanisms leading to atopic dermatitis. *J Allergy Clin Immunol.* 2003;112(6 suppl): S128–S139
2. Johansson SG, Bieber T, et al Revised nomenclature for allergy for global use: Report of the Nomenclature Review Committee of the World Allergy Organization, October 2003. *J Allergy Clin Immunol.* 2004;113(5):832–836
3. Hamelmann E, Beyer K, et al Primary prevention of allergy: avoiding risk or providing protection? *Clin Exp Allergy.* 2008;38(2):233–245
4. Illi S, von Mutius E, et al The natural course of atopic dermatitis from birth to age 7 years and the association with asthma. *J Allergy Clin Immunol.* 2004;113(5):925–931
5. Asher MI, Montefort S, et al Worldwide time trends in the prevalence of symptoms of asthma, allergic rhinoconjunctivitis, and eczema in childhood: ISAAC phases one and three repeat multicountry cross-sectional surveys. *Lancet.* 2006; 368(9537):733–743
6. Van Eerdewegh P, Little RD, et al Association of the ADAM33 gene with asthma and bronchial hyperresponsiveness. *Nature.* 2002;418(6896):426–430
7. Prescott SL. Allergy: the price we pay for cleaner living? *Ann Allergy Asthma Immunol.* 2003;90(6 suppl 3):64–70
8. Liu AH. Hygiene theory and allergy and asthma prevention. *Paediatr Perinat Epidemiol.* 2007;21(suppl 3):2–7
9. Ring J, Krämer U, et al A critical approach to the hygiene hypothesis. *Clin Exp Allergy Rev.* 2004;4(suppl 2):40–44
10. Jovanovic S, Felder-Kennel A, et al Exposition und Sensibilisierung gegenüber Milben- und Katzenallergenen bei Kindern in Baden-Württemberg. *Gesundheitswesen.* 2003;65(7):457–463
11. Cork M, Murphy R, et al The rising prevalence of atopic eczema and environmental trauma to the skin. *Dermatol Pract.* 2002;10(3):22–26
12. Cork MJ, Robinson DA, et al New perspectives on epidermal barrier dysfunction in atopic dermatitis: gene-environment interactions. *J Allergy Clin Immunol.* 2006;118(1):3–21
13. Elias PM. Epidermal lipids, barrier function, and desquamation. *J Invest Dermatol.* 1983;80 suppl:44s–49s
14. Taïeb A. Hypothesis: from epidermal barrier dysfunction to atopic disorders. *Contact Derm.* 1999;41(4):177–180
15. Holleran WM, Takagi Y, et al Epidermal sphingolipids: metabolism, function, and roles in skin disorders. *FEBS Lett.* 2006;580(23):5456–5466
16. Chiou YB, Blume-Peytavi U. Stratum corneum maturation. *Skin Pharmacol Physiol.* 2004;17(2):57–66
17. Palmer CN, Irvine AD, et al Common loss-of-function variants of the epidermal barrier protein filaggrin are a major predisposing factor for atopic dermatitis. *Nat Genet.* 2006;38(4):441–446
18. Baurecht H, Irvine AD, et al Toward a major risk factor for atopic eczema: meta-analysis of filaggrin polymorphism data. *J Allergy Clin Immunol.* 2007;120:1406–1412
19. Lebman DA, Coffman RL. Interleukin 4 causes isotype switching to IgE in T cell-stimulated clonal B cell cultures. *J Exp Med.* 1988;168(3):853–862
20. Maintz L, Novak N. Getting more and more complex: the pathophysiology of atopic eczema. *Eur J Dermatol.* 2007; 17(4):267–283
21. Hamid Q, Boguniewicz M, et al Differential in situ cytokine gene expression in acute versus chronic atopic dermatitis. *J Clin Invest.* 1994;94(2):870–876
22. Larché M, Akdis CA, et al Immunological mechanisms of allergen-specific immunotherapy. *Nat Rev Immunol.* 2006; 6(10):761–771
23. Verhagen J, Akdis M, et al Absence of T-regulatory cell expression and function in atopic dermatitis skin. *J Allergy Clin Immunol.* 2006;117(1):176–183
24. Sampson HA. Update on food allergy. *J Allergy Clin Immunol.* 2004;113(5):805–819; quiz 820
25. Scalabrin DM, Bavbek S, et al Use of specific IgE in assessing the relevance of fungal and dust mite allergens to atopic dermatitis: a comparison with asthmatic and nonasthmatic control subjects. *J Allergy Clin Immunol.* 1999; 104(6):1273–1279
26. Werfel T, Ballmer-Weber B, et al Eczematous reactions to food in atopic eczema: position paper of the EAACI and GA²LEN. *Allergy.* 2007;62(7):723–728
27. Mothes N, Niggemann B, et al The cradle of IgE autoreactivity in atopic eczema lies in early infancy. *J Allergy Clin Immunol.* 2005;116(3):706–709
28. Scheynius A, Johansson C, et al Atopic eczema/dermatitis syndrome and Malassezia. *Int Arch Allergy Immunol.* 2002; 127(3):161–169
29. Greaves MW. Recent advances in pathophysiology and current management of itch. *Ann Acad Med Singap.* 2007;36(9): 788–792
30. Schmid-Ott G, Jaeger B, et al Different expression of cytokine and membrane molecules by circulating lymphocytes on acute mental stress in patients with atopic dermatitis in comparison with healthy controls. *J Allergy Clin Immunol.* 2001;108(3):455–462
31. Rukwied R, Lischetzki G, et al Mast cell mediators other than histamine induce pruritus in atopic dermatitis patients: a dermal microdialysis study. *Br J Dermatol.* 2000;142(6): 1114–1120
32. Badertscher K, Bronnimann M, et al Mast cell chymase is increased in chronic atopic dermatitis but not in psoriasis. *Arch Dermatol Res.* 2005;296(10):503–506
33. Järvikallio A, Harvima IT, et al Mast cells, nerves and neuropeptides in atopic dermatitis and nummular eczema. *Arch Dermatol Res.* 2003;295(1):2–7
34. Raap U, Werfel T, et al Circulating levels of brain-derived neurotrophic factor correlate with disease severity in the intrinsic type of atopic dermatitis. *Allergy.* 2006;61(12): 1416–1418
35. Dillon SR, Sprecher C, et al Interleukin 31, a cytokine produced by activated T cells, induces dermatitis in mice. *Nat Immunol.* 2004;5(7):752–760

36. Bilsborough J, Leung DY, et al IL-31 is associated with cutaneous lymphocyte antigen-positive skin homing T cells in patients with atopic dermatitis. *J Allergy Clin Immunol.* 2006;117(2):418–425

37. Abeck D, Mempel M. Kutane *Staphylococcus aureus* Besiedelung des atopischen Ekzems. *Hautarzt.* 1998;49(12): 902–906

38. Bogaert D, van Belkum A, et al Colonisation by *Streptococcus pneumoniae* and *Staphylococcus aureus* in healthy children. *Lancet.* 2004;363(9424):1871–1872

39. Leyden JJ, Marples RR, et al *Staphylococcus aureus* in the lesions of atopic dermatitis. *Br J Dermatol.* 1974;90(5): 525–530

40. Novak N, Bieber T. Pathogenese des atopischen Ekzems. *JDDG J Ger Soc Dermatol.* 2005;3(12):994–1005

41. Bunikowski R, Mielke M, et al Prevalence and role of serum IgE antibodies to the *Staphylococcus aureus*-derived superantigens SEA and SEB in children with atopic dermatitis. *J Allergy Clin Immunol.* 1999;103(1 Pt 1):119–124

42. Sonkoly E, Muller A, et al IL-31: a new link between T cells and pruritus in atopic skin inflammation. *J Allergy Clin Immunol.* 2006;117(2):411–417

43. Ong P Y, Ohtake T, et al Endogenous antimicrobial peptides and skin infections in atopic dermatitis. *N Engl J Med.* 2002;347(15):1151–1160

44. Howell MD, Wollenberg A, et al Cathelicidin deficiency predisposes to eczema herpeticum. *J Allergy Clin Immunol.* 2006;117(4):836–841

45. Schudel P, Wüthrich B. Klinische Verlaufsbeobachtungen bei Neurodermitis atopica nach dem Kleinkindesalter. Eine katamnestische Untersuchung anhand von 121 Fällen. *H ± G Zeitschrift für Hautkrankheiten.* 1985,60(6).479–486

46. Hanifin J, Rajka G. Diagnostic features of atopic dermatitis. *Acta Derm Venereol (Stockh).* 1980;92 suppl:44 s–47s.

47. Leung DY, Bieber T. Atopic dermatitis. *Lancet.* 2003; 361(9352):151–160

48. Williams HC, Burney PG, et al The U.K. Working Party's Diagnostic Criteria for Atopic Dermatitis. I. Derivation of a minimum set of discriminators for atopic dermatitis. *Br J Dermatol.* 1994;131(3):383–396

49. Jøhnke H, Vach W, et al A comparison between criteria for diagnosing atopic eczema in infants. *Br J Dermatol.* 2005; 153(2):352–358

50. Lewis-Jones S, Mugglestone MA. Management of atopic eczema in children aged up to 12 years: summary of NICE guidance. *Bmj.* 2007;335(7632):1263–1264

51. Turjanmaa K, Darsow U, et al EAACI/GA²LEN position paper: present status of the atopy patch test. *Allergy.* 2006;61(12):1377–1384

52. Berni Canani R, Ruotolo S, et al Diagnostic accuracy of the atopy patch test in children with food allergy-related gastrointestinal symptoms. *Allergy.* 2007;62(7):738–743

53. Mehl A, Rolinck-Werninghaus C, et al The atopy patch test in the diagnostic workup of suspected food-related symptoms in children. *J Allergy Clin Immunol.* 2006; 118(4): 923–929

54. Niggemann B, Gruber C. Unproven diagnostic procedures in IgE-mediated allergic diseases. *Allergy.* 2004;59(8): 806–808

55. Stapel SO, Asero R, et al Testing for IgG4 against foods is not recommended as a diagnostic tool: EAACI task force report. *Allergy.* 2008;63(7):793–796

56. Darsow U, Lübbe J, et al Position paper on diagnosis and treatment of atopic dermatitis. *J Eur Acad Dermatol Venereol.* 2005;19(3):286–295

57. Smith FJ, Irvine AD, et al Loss-of-function mutations in the gene encoding filaggrin cause ichthyosis vulgaris. *Nat Genet.* 2006;38(3):337–342

58. Lin SP, Huang S Y, et al Netherton syndrome: mutation analysis of two Taiwanese families. *Arch Dermatol Res.* 2007;299(3):145–150

59. Torgerson TR, Ochs HD. Immune dysregulation, polyendocrinopathy, enteropathy, X-linked: forkhead box protein 3 mutations and lack of regulatory T cells. *J Allergy Clin Immunol.* 2007;120(4):744–750

60. Lannerö E, Wickman M, et al Maternal smoking during pregnancy increases the risk of recurrent wheezing during the first years of life (BAMSE). *Respir Res.* 2006;7:3

61. Muraro A, Dreborg S, et al Dietary prevention of allergic diseases in infants and small children. Part III: critical review of published peer-reviewed observational and interventional studies and final recommendations. Pediatr Allergy Immunol. 2004;15(4):291–307

62. Greer FR, Sicherer SH, et al Effects of early nutritional interventions on the development of atopic disease in infants and children: the role of maternal dietary restriction, breastfeeding, timing of introduction of complementary foods, and hydrolyzed formulas. Pediatrics. 2008;121(1):183–191

63. Akdis CA, Akdis M, et al Diagnosis and treatment of atopic dermatitis in children and adults: European Academy of Allergology and Clinical Immunology/American Academy of Allergy, Asthma and Immunology/PRACTALL Consensus Report. J Allergy Clin Immunol. 2006;118(1):152–169

64. Akdis CA, Akdis M, et al Diagnosis and treatment of atopic dermatitis in children and adults: European Academy of Allergology and Clinical Immunology/American Academy of Allergy, Asthma and Immunology/PRACTALL Consensus Report. Allergy. 2006;61(8):969–987

65. Lowe LA, Woodcock A, et al Lung function at age 3 years: effect of pet ownership and exposure to indoor allergens. Arch Pediatr Adolesc Med. 2004;158(10):996–1001

66. Svanes C, Zock JP, et al Do asthma and allergy influence subsequent pet keeping? An analysis of childhood and adulthood. J Allergy Clin Immunol. 2006;118(3):691–698

67. Sporik R, Ingram JM, et al Association of asthma with serum IgE and skin test reactivity to allergens among children living at high altitude. Tickling the dragon's breath. Am J Respir Crit Care Med. 1995;151(5):1388–1392

68. von Mutius E, Weiland SK, et al Increasing prevalence of hay fever and atopy among children in Leipzig, East Germany. Lancet. 1998;351(9106):862–866

69. Flöistrup H, Swartz J, et al Allergic disease and sensitization in Steiner school children. J Allergy Clin Immunol. 2006;117(1):59–66

70. Ventura MT, Munno G, et al Allergy, asthma and markers of infections among Albanian migrants to Southern Italy. Allergy. 2004;59(6):632–636

71. van den Biggelaar AH, Rodrigues LC, et al Long-term treatment of intestinal helminths increases mite skin-test reactivity in Gabonese schoolchildren. J Infect Dis. 2004;189(5): 892–900

72. Flood JM, Weinstock HS, et al Neurosyphilis during the AIDS epidemic, San Francisco, 1985–1992. J Infect Dis. 1998;177(4):931–940

73. Kalliomaki M, Salminen S, et al Probiotics in primary prevention of atopic disease: a randomised placebo-controlled trial. Lancet. 2001;357(9262):1076–1079

74. Kalliomaki M, Salminen S, et al Probiotics and prevention of atopic disease: 4-year follow-up of a randomised placebo-controlled trial. Lancet. 2003;361(9372):1869–1871

75. Kalliomaki M, Salminen S, et al Probiotics during the first 7 years of life: a cumulative risk reduction of eczema in a randomized, placebo-controlled trial. J Allergy Clin Immunol. 2007;119(4):1019–1021

76. Niederberger V, Valenta R. Molecular approaches for new vaccines against allergy. Expert Rev Vaccines. 2006; 5(1):103–110

77. Niederberger V, Horak F, et al Vaccination with genetically engineered allergens prevents progression of allergic disease. Proc Natl Acad Sci USA. 2004;101(suppl 2): 14677–14682

78. Niggemann B, Jacobsen L, et al Five-year follow-up on the PAT study: specific immunotherapy and long-term prevention of asthma in children. Allergy. 2006;61(7):855–859

79. Jacobsen L, Niggemann B, et al Specific immunotherapy has long-term preventive effect of seasonal and perennial asthma: 10-year follow-up on the PAT study. Allergy. 2007;62(8): 943–948

80. Bussmann C, Maintz L, et al Clinical improvement and immunological changes in atopic dermatitis patients undergoing subcutaneous immunotherapy with a house dust mite allergoid: a pilot study. Clin Exp Allergy. 2007;37(9): 1277–1285

81. Werfel T, Breuer K, et al Usefulness of specific immunotherapy in patients with atopic dermatitis and allergic sensitization to house dust mites: a multi-centre, randomized, dose-response study. Allergy. 2006;61(2):202–205

82. Abramovits W, Boguniewicz M. A multicenter, randomized, vehicle-controlled clinical study to examine the efficacy and safety of MAS063DP (Atopiclair) in the management of mild to moderate atopic dermatitis in adults. J Drugs Dermatol. 2006;5(3):236–244

83. Hanifin JM, Cooper KD, et al Guidelines of care for atopic dermatitis, developed in accordance with the American Academy of Dermatology (AAD)/American Academy of Dermatology Association "Administrative Regulations for Evidence-Based Clinical Practice Guidelines". J Am Acad Dermatol. 2004;50(3):391–404

84. Hoare C, Li Wan Po A, et al Systematic review of treatments for atopic eczema. Health Technol Assess. 2000;4(37): 1–191

85. Van Der Meer JB, Glazenburg EJ, et al The management of moderate to severe atopic dermatitis in adults with topical fluticasone propionate. The Netherlands Adult Atopic Dermatitis Study Group. Br J Dermatol. 1999;140(6): 1114–1121

86. Wollenberg A, Bieber T. Proactive therapy of atopic dermatitis – an emerging concept. Allergy. 2009;64(2):276–278

87. Ashcroft DM, Dimmock P, et al Efficacy and tolerability of topical pimecrolimus and tacrolimus in the treatment of atopic dermatitis: meta-analysis of randomised controlled trials. BMJ. 2005;330(7490):516

88. Luger T, Van Leent EJ, et al SDZ ASM 981: an emerging safe and effective treatment for atopic dermatitis. Br J Dermatol. 2001;144(4):788–794

89. Thaçi D, Salgo R. The topical calcineurin inhibitor pimecrolimus in atopic dermatitis: a safety update. Acta Dermatovenerol Alp Panonica Adriat. 2007;16(2):58, 60–62

90. Berger TG, Duvic M, et al The use of topical calcineurin inhibitors in dermatology: safety concerns. Report of the American Academy of Dermatology Association Task Force. J Am Acad Dermatol. 2006;54(5):818–823

91. Remitz A, Harper J, et al Long-term safety and efficacy of tacrolimus ointment for the treatment of atopic dermatitis in children. Acta Derm Venereol. 2007;87(1):54–61

92. Ring J, Abraham A, et al Control of atopic eczema with pimecrolimus cream 1% under daily practice conditions: results of a >2000 patient study. J Eur Acad Dermatol Venereol. 2008;22(2):195–203

93. Ricci G, Patrizi A, et al Use of textiles in atopic dermatitis: care of atopic dermatitis. Curr Probl Dermatol. 2006;33:127–143

94. Rerinck HC, Kamann S, et al Eczema herpeticum: Pathogenese und Therapie. Hautarzt. 2006;57(7):586–591

95. Kelsay K. Management of sleep disturbance associated with atopic dermatitis. J Allergy Clin Immunol.2006;118(1): 198–201

96. Schmitt J, Schmitt N, et al Cyclosporin in the treatment of patients with atopic eczema – a systematic review and meta-analysis. J Eur Acad Dermatol Venereol. 2007;21(5): 606–619

97. Schmitt J, Schakel K, et al Systemic treatment of severe atopic eczema: a systematic review. Acta Derm Venereol. 2007;87(2):100–111

98. Behnam SM, Behnam SE, et al Review of cyclosporine immunosuppressive safety data in dermatology patients after two decades of use. J Drugs Dermatol. 2005;4(2): 189–194

99. Wise M, Callen JP. Azathioprine: a guide for the management of dermatology patients. Dermatol Ther. 2007;20(4): 206–215

100. Heymann WR. Antipsoriatic biologic agents for the treatment of atopic dermatitis. J Am Acad Dermatol. 2007;56(5): 854–855

101. National Institute for Health and Clinical Excellence. NICE guidance. At: <http://www.nice.org.uk/search/searchresults. jsp?keywords=eczema&searchType=all>; 2009 Accessed 04.04.09

102. Staab D, Diepgen TL, et al Age related, structured educational programmes for the management of atopic dermatitis in children and adolescents: multicentre, randomised controlled trial. BMJ. 2006;332(7547):933–938

103. Chida Y, Steptoe A, et al The effects of psychological intervention on atopic dermatitis. A systematic review and meta-analysis. Int Arch Allergy Immunol. 2007;144(1):1–9

104. Ersser SJ, Latter S, et al Psychological and educational interventions for atopic eczema in children. Cochrane Database Syst Rev. 2007;(3):CD004054

Prevention of Psoriasis

8

Gwynn Coatney and Robert A. Norman

8.1 Introduction

Psoriasis is one of the most common skin diseases and it affects millions of people all over the world. It is usually chronic in nature with onset and flare-ups being unpredictable. The disease course ranges from mild forms consisting of annoying symptomatology of itchy dry skin and unsightly scaling plaques to extreme cases that can induce disfigurement, prolonged suffering, and systemic manifestations such as arthritis and even an increased mortality. Psoriasis is very costly to treat and treatment itself can be a very time-consuming commitment. Some of the newest treatments can cost up to $25,000 a year and most treatments involve months of intensive treatment regimens.[13] In general, psoriasis is a major cause of social and physical discomfort that can also become a serious burden financially for patients affected by this inflammatory disease. Due to the widespread affliction and the severe nature of psoriasis special attention should be focused on preventing the disease.

8.1.1 Pathogenesis

Psoriasis is an immune-mediated inflammatory disorder, in which epithelial cells have an increased production and turnover rate. Normal skin takes almost a month to cycle from newly formed keratinocytes (from stem cells of the innermost or basal layer) upwards to the most superficial layer of the epidermis, the stratum corneum. In psoriasis this process is much faster, taking only 3–5 days to complete the cycle. The hyperproliferation of these cells is caused by an inflammatory response in the immune system. It is still unclear what causes this response in psoriasis, but it is known that the immune system erroneously activates T cells. T cells then activate inflammatory mediators, or cytokines like tumor necrosis factor-alpha (TNF-α), to trigger the increased proliferation of the epithelial cells.[11,24]

8.1.2 Prevalence/Incidence

Current estimates show that 2–3% of the world population is affected by psoriasis. Up to seven million people in the United States have this common cutaneous disease. It is also estimated that 150,000–200,000 new cases are diagnosed each year in the US. Psoriasis equally affects the male and female genders. There is a lower incidence of psoriasis seen in people with darker skin – Africans, Asians, and Inuits, and the disease is very rarely seen in North and South American Indians.[11,17,24]

8.1.3 Onset

The peak age of onset of psoriasis usually occurs in people in their third decade of life, but it can present anywhere from the neonatal period to people in their 70s. When the disease presents early in life it is more likely to develop into a more severe form and become chronic in nature.[24]

G. Coatney (✉)
Department of Family Medicine,
University of Medicine and Dentistry of New Jersey,
Stratford, NJ, USA
e-mail: gcoatney@hotmail.com

8.1.4 Severity/Types/Distribution

There are two major classifications of psoriasis, psoriasis vulgaris and pustular psoriasis (Table 8.1). Psoriasis vulgaris includes the acute guttate, chronic plaque, inverse and palmoplantar subtypes. Characteristically, these different types range from eruptive and inflammatory lesions to chronic and lichenified. Guttate psoriasis is seen in about 2% of all psoriasis cases and consists of small erythematous lesions that appear acutely. This subtype of psoriasis vulgaris can spontaneously resolve without treatment. Guttate psoriasis has a generalized distribution with the majority of lesions appearing on the trunk. A common presentation of guttate psoriasis occurs after an infection like streptococcal pharyngitis. The lesions appear diffusely on the skin, much like an exanthem-type rash. Plaque psoriasis is usually chronic in nature and is the most common type of psoriasis. Clinically, this subtype exhibits the classic lesions that most people associate with psoriasis. They are sharply demarcated, salmon pink to erythematous in color and have a loose silvery white scale. Lesions are classically concentrated on the elbows, knees, over the sacrum, on the scalp, and on the palms and soles of the hands and feet. The face and neck are rarely involved. These plaques are generally bilateral and symmetric. Inverse type of psoriasis chronically affects the skin-fold areas of the body including the groin region, under the breasts, and the axillae. These areas are moist, giving the psoriatic plaques a different appearance than seen in the classic presentation. The thick, scaly plaques are replaced with bright red and fissured lesions. The plaques of the palmoplantar type of psoriasis are distributed only on the palms and soles and usually demonstrate more hyperkeratotic and scaling type lesions.[8]

Pustular psoriasis has two subtypes, palmoplantar and generalized acute pustular psoriasis. Cases of pustular psoriasis are much less frequently seen than the psoriasis vulgaris types. Palmoplantar psoriasis usually appears later in life and has a higher incidence females, a ratio of almost 4:1. Palmoplantar pustulosis is a chronic condition where pustules in different stages of evolution and healing appear in groups only on the palms and soles of the hands and feet. Relapse and recurrence of the disorder is common. Generalized acute pustular psoriasis can be a dermatologic emergency. In this subtype the skin becomes diffusely erythematous and pustules appear in clusters within hours of initial onset. This condition is usually accompanied by fever, malaise and generalized weakness.

About 10% of those diagnosed with psoriasis are also diagnosed with psoriatic arthritis. The age of onset for psoriatic arthritis is 10–15 years later in life, averaging in the mid-30s. Psoriatic arthritis is most often found in the hands and feet, resulting in "sausage" digits, but can also affect larger joints. Finger and toenails are involved in 25% of psoriatic cases in general, and have a high correlation with psoriatic arthritis. Clinically the nail may include pitting, hyperpigmented spots under the nail plate and hyperkeratotic changes of the nail itself.[11,24]

Table 8.1 Types psoriasis

	Psoriasis vulgaris subtypes				Pustular subtypes	
Subtypes	Acute guttate	Chronic plaque	Inverse	Palmo-plantar	Generalized acute pustular	Palmo-plantar
Onset/duration	Acute	Chronic	Sub-acute to chronic	Chronic	Acute	Chronic
Distribution pattern	Diffuse, but mainly on the trunk	Bilateral, symmetric, elbows, knees, scalp, sacrum	In skin folds, under breast groin axillae	Palms of hands, soles of feet	Generalized and diffuse	Palms and soles
Characteristics	Erythematous, small, round-oval in shape	Salmon pink with a silvery scale, thick sharply demarcated	Bright red, fissured	Scaly-crusted thick	Base is erythematous with overlying clusters of pustules	Pustules are arranged in groups in clusters of different stages of healing

8.1.5 Genetics

Immunological factors contribute to the pathophysiology of psoriasis, but it is unknown whether psoriasis is caused by an immune system dysfunction or by genetic defects found in keratinocytes of the epidermis.[1] Many studies suggest that there is a genetic predisposition for psoriasis. The Lomholt study conducted on the Faroe Islands of Denmark found that 91% of those questioned with psoriasis had at least one first- or second-degree relative who were also inflicted with the disease.[18,23] Over 5,000 study subjects with psoriasis had family members also affected by the disease in a study done by Farber and Nall.[4,23] A study by Kavli showed that the prevalence of psoriasis increases with the number of relatives with the same disease.[14,23] Twin studies have been performed revealing that the heritability of psoriasis was estimated to be as high as 60–90%.[2,23] When one parent has psoriasis 8% of the offspring will develop the disease. When both parents have psoriasis 41% of their children will also have the disease. Psoriasis is inherited as a polygenic trait in which disease types, severity, and degree of skin involvement depends on several different alleles found on different genes. The human leukocyte antigen (HLA) types most frequently associated with psoriasis are HLA-B13, -B17, Bw57, and Cw6. Nearly half the patients with psoriatic arthritis will have HLA-B27, which is most commonly associated with ankylosing spondylitis.[24]

8.2 Risk Factors/Triggers

Most triggers for psoriasis are immunologic in nature. Physical trauma like harsh rubbing of the epidermis or scratching can elicit the lesions, known as Koebner's phenomenon. Infections have been known to precipitate outbreaks of psoriasis. For example, the first lesion of psoriasis can show up after a streptococcal infection. This is most often seen in the guttate type of psoriasis, and in children. Stress is an important risk factor causing flares in up to 40% of adults and children. In the Farber and Nall study one-third of the 5,600 psoriasis patients studied reported that stress or worry induced new areas of affected skin.[4,23]

Certain types of drugs have been associated with the onset and exacerbation of psoriasis. The most studied include beta blockers, calcium channel blockers, lithium, NSAIDs, and antimalarial medications.

Smoking cigarettes and drinking alcohol have a strong correlation with psoriasis. Combining the results of two studies performed in Germany, current smokers have a higher prevalence rate of psoriasis, when compared to those who have quit smoking or who have never smoked. The results indicating positive histories of both smoking and psoriasis were 3.8% vs. 2.7% and 2.8% respectively. One of these studies also showed that participants that drank more than 20 g of alcohol a day had a prevalence of psoriasis of 4.7%.[23] More specifically, 4.8% of the participants who drank a daily beer also had psoriasis, and of those who admitted to drinking at least three glasses of wine a week 6.4% also had the disease. The dermatology clinics of the University of Utah enrolled patients in the Utah Psoriasis Initiative (UPI), which studied the impact of smoking and obesity on psoriasis. Of the patients studied 37% admitted being current smokers. The prevalence of smoking in the UPI was higher than the general Utah population, which is 13%. It was also higher than in the nonpsoriatic population of Utah of which 25% are smokers.[9]

In the two separate research pursuits of Naldi and Kavli evidence was found that lack of a balanced diet or being deficient in certain vitamins and minerals are risk factors for psoriasis. Proper nutrition in general is important for a person's overall health and maintenance of immune system function. People who have a low consumption of fruit and vegetables, especially carrots, tomatoes or Beta carotene are more likely to have psoriasis.[20,14]

8.2.1 Disease Associations

There are many diseases associated with psoriasis. Some of the more common disorders include hypertension, cardiovascular diseases, obesity, inflammatory bowel disorders, depression, and cancer.[15,16]

Those who are overweight and obese or who have an increased body mass index (BMI) have been shown to have a higher incidence of psoriasis.[20] Looking again at the UPI, the percentage of patients that were obese and had psoriasis was double the number compared to the general Utah population that was obese and without psoriasis. This study found that the majority of their participants were of normal weight at the time of onset or diagnosis of psoriasis and transitioned into being obese. This suggests that obesity is not a risk factor for psoriasis, but a result of the disease.[9]

There is a strong relationship between Crohn's disease and psoriasis. This may be due to a common factor between inflammatory bowel disease and psoriasis; they both have increased levels of the inflammatory cytokine, tumor necrosis factor-a.[19]

Multiple television ads portray people with psoriasis and their embarrassment about their skin's appearance. Over the years many writers and poets have written about the disease and how it has a negative effect on their lives. It has long been known that psoriasis has a link to psychosocial disorders and decreased self-esteem.[22] An Italian study done in 2006 sent questionnaires to patients who were diagnosed with psoriasis. The goal of this study was to assess the degree of depressive symptomatology in psoriasis patients. A total of 2,391 people participated and it was found that 62% of those polled admitted to symptoms of depression.[3]

A retrospective survey has shown the correlation of psoriasis and cancer. The percentage of subjects of this study with no cancer history was 3.3% compared with 9.4% of the participants who had a positive cancer history. These results were obtained after controlling age, gender, and alcohol or tobacco use. Many studies have concluded that patients with psoriasis are at an increased risk for developing a specific type of cancer, lymphoma.[5,23]

Patients with psoriasis have an increased morbidity and mortality rate. A cohort study done by Dr. Gelfand and his colleagues used the United Kingdom's general practice research database (GPRD) to follow patients with psoriasis over a 15-year period. They compared three groups of patients. The first included over 130,000 patients with mild psoriasis, the second group was comprised of almost 4,000 patients with severe psoriasis, and the third group was considered the control group, patients not diagnosed with psoriasis. This last group included 5 times as many patients as the first two groups combined. To differentiate between mild and severe psoriasis the researchers classified the mild group as patients that had the diagnosis of psoriasis, but had no history of systemic therapy. Conversely the severe group was classified as patients with the diagnosis of psoriasis and also with history of being treated with systemic therapy. One objective of this study was to determine whether psoriasis is an independent risk factor for myocardial infarction (MI). Adjustments were made to the study regarding major cardiovascular risk factors such as hypertension, diabetes mellitus, hyperlipidemia, age, sex, smoking history, family history of MI, BMI, or previous personal history of MI. The incidence of MI for the control group and the mild psoriasis group was about 2%. The incidence of MI in the severe psoriasis group was 2.9%. Relative risk was also measured according to age. For a 30-year-old patient the relative risk for MI is 1.29 for mild psoriasis and 3.10 for severe psoriasis. The relative risk for MI in a 60-year-old is 1.08 for mild and 1.36 for severe psoriasis. This same study found that the group of patients with severe psoriasis had a death rate almost double of the control group. This ratio even persisted after controlling other comorbidities linked to mortality from the equation, including smoking status, BMI, heart disease, AIDs, cancer, renal disease, and others. An interesting observation showed that there was no significant difference when comparing the death rate of the group with mild psoriasis to the group without psoriasis. On average, patients with severe psoriasis died 3–4 years earlier than patients not diagnosed with and treated for the severe form of the disease.[6,7]

8.3 Treatments

Psoriasis is a chronic and recurrent disease that requires appropriate care and often includes systematic treatment.[12] A recent survey from the National Psoriasis Foundation polled 1,657 participants diagnosed with severe or moderate psoriasis to assess their level of treatment. This study found that almost 40% of those surveyed are currently receiving no treatment at all for their condition. In opposition, one quarter of those questioned with severe psoriasis were receiving either systemic therapy or phototherapy and 35% are being treated with only topical therapy (Table 8.2).[10,21]

8.3.1 Topicals

One of the longest treatments in use is Anthralin, a synthetic form of chrysarobin, which is a chemical compound found in the bark of the Araroba tree of South America. It can be a good treatment choice for the plaque type of psoriasis.

Table 8.2 Overview of treatments

Treatment	Examples	Treatment for	Use in conjunction with	Common side effects
Topicals	Anthralin, Dovonex, Taclonex, Tazorac	Mild-to-moderate plaque psoriasis, scalp	Topical steroids, phototherapy or oral medications used to treat psoriasis	Anthralin can stain the skin, Dovonex, Taclonex, and Tazorac can cause skin irritation
Phototherapy	UVB treatment, PUVA treatment with Psoralen	Mild-to-moderate plaque psoriasis, vitiligo	May be used together or alternate with topicals, orals, or biologics, but avoid with Taclonex and Tazorac	Redness/sunburn, irritated skin, blistering. Psoralen can cause nausea
Oral systemics	Cyclosporine, Soriatane, Methotrexate	Moderate-to-severe plaque psoriasis, Cyclosporine is good to treat nail involvement, Methotrexate can also treat psoriatic arthritis	Topical medications like Dovonex	Possibility of organ damage, most commonly the kidneys or liver
Biologics	Amevive, Enbrel, Humira, Remicade	Moderate to severe plaque those who did not clear with other treatments. Enbrel, Humira and Remicade can also be used to treat psoriatic arthritis	Can be used alternatively with phototherapy and oral medications like Methotrexate	Nausea, itching, chills, sore throat, dizziness, injection site irritation, headache, cough

Dovonex is a synthetic form of vitamin D3 which treats psoriasis by decreasing the rate of keratinocyte proliferation. It does not treat the inflammation aspect of the disease but it decreases the surface area of the lesions and helps in removing the scale. A scalp solution of Dovonex is also available. Recommendations say to apply the solution at night and wear a shower cap to bed. The solution can then be washed out in the morning. This cream or ointment has been shown to be safe and effective when used in combination with topical steroids and systemic treatments to combat more severe cases of psoriasis. Dovonex has also been shown to increase the effectiveness of phototherapy treatments when applied after the UV ray treatment.

Another topical treatment option is Taclonex, which is a combination of the same active ingredient found in Dovonex and a steroid. There is also a formulation that can be used on the scalp.

Tazorac is a topical therapy used for plaque psoriasis. It is a topical retinoid, or vitamin A derivative. Tazorac comes in two forms, gel and cream and each has two strengths, 0.05% and 0.1%. The gel is clear and fast-drying and the cream has a moisturizer that makes it a good choice for patients with drier, more sensitive skin. Both formulations work to slow the rapid proliferation of the epithelial cells. Tazorac can be combined with steroids to promote faster clearing time and can also reduce skin irritation and redness. Combining Tazorac with phototherapy has also been shown to get better results than using either treatment alone.

Topical steroids can be a great aid in the treatment of psoriasis. They can be used in combination with most other topical treatments but are not effective when used alone. They can help achieve the goal of clearing the psoriasis lesions at a faster rate. Their anti-inflammatory capabilities help reduce side effects of the medications, including irritation, itching, and redness. For resistant psoriasis plaques intralesional injections of steroids may be a good option.[21]

8.3.2 Systemic Therapy

Systemic therapy for psoriasis is usually reserved for moderate-to-severe psoriasis or for patients who have failed to become clear with topical or phototherapy treatment.

Cyclosporine, or Neoral, is an immune-suppressant. Its mechanism of action works to inhibit T cells. It is taken every day in either pill or liquid form. Good outcomes have been achieved when combining Cyclosporine and Dovonex topical therapy. By using both medications the dosage of Cyclosporine can be lowered and thus decreases potential side effects caused by high doses or chronic use of Cyclosporine.

The only oral retinoid approved for the treatment of psoriasis is called Soriatane. It is a synthetic form of vitamin A. Soriatane is a good treatment for the plaque, guttate, pustular and palmoplantar types of psoriasis. Oral retinoids like Soriatane result in clearer skin by modifying how keratinocytes multiply and the rate at which they divide and shed. Soriatane is taken once daily in pill form. It can be used in combination with Dovonex and has had great results when used in conjunction with phototherapy.

Methotrexate is another common oral systemic medication used to treat psoriasis. It is a medication that has been used to treat cancer since the 1950s and 20 years later was approved to treat psoriasis. Methotrexate is effective in treating psoriasis because the medication decreases epithelial cell growth. Unlike Cyclosporine and Soriatane, Methotrexate can also be used to treat psoriatic arthritis. Methotrexate is administered once a week either in pill or liquid form, or by injection. After the clearance of psoriasis lesions is obtained the dosage is tapered. Some patients may require a maintenance dose to prevent relapse.[21]

8.3.3 Biologics

Biologics are the newest treatments for psoriasis and psoriatic arthritis. The name for this group of medications is fitting, because these formulations are derived from human or animal proteins, not chemicals or synthetic compounds. Biologics are different from other psoriasis treatments because they are designed to work in the immune system; their goal is to block the disease in the early developmental stages. Biologics do this by targeting the overactive immune cells in the body. Some concentrate on T cells by preventing their activation or by stopping their migration in the immune response. Other biologic treatments bind to TNF-a and prevent it from initiating the proliferation of keratinocytes.

Amevive and Raptiva are two of the biologic preparations that work by blocking the activation of T cells, thereby decreasing inflammation and halting the immune response before TNF-a cells can cause rapid growth and turnover of epithelial cells. Amevive and Raptiva are FDA-approved for the treatment of moderate-to-severe plaque psoriasis in adults, but not psoriatic arthritis. Patients receiving Amevive receive an intramuscular shot at their doctor's office weekly for at least 12 weeks. If the goal of 75% clearance is not achieved a second 12 week course can be instituted. Raptiva can be self-injected by patients on a weekly basis.

The mechanism of action for Enbrel, Humira and Remicade consists of blocking TNF-a and interrupting the inflammatory cycle of psoriasis and psoriatic arthritis. Patients using Enbrel give themselves a subcutaneous injection once or twice weekly, those using Humira also inject subcutaneously, but only every other week. Remicade is given in a doctor's office and the treatment includes three separate 2-h infusions during the first 6 weeks of treatment. Every 8 weeks following another infusion is given. Enbrel, Humira, and Remicade are currently approved to treat moderate-to-severe plaque psoriasis and psoriatic arthritis in adults. They are also being used to treat rheumatoid arthritis, juvenile rheumatoid arthritis, and ankylosing spondylitis. Remicade is also approved for the treatment of Crohn's disease and ulcerative colitis. In the future Enbrel may be approved to treat psoriasis in children as well as adults.[21]

8.3.4 Phototherapy

Natural sunlight contains ultraviolet light bands A–C. Most ultraviolet light is absorbed by the earth's atmosphere, with mostly U VA reaching the earth's surface. UVB light can be beneficial to our skin in small doses by initiating vitamin D synthesis. Too much UVB exposure can be harmful by causing sunburn in human skin. UV treatments are being used in a controlled setting at dermatology offices to treat dermatologic conditions such as psoriasis and vitiligo. Many offices have stand-up units that emit the artificial rays and some have smaller handheld devices to treat localized areas. Exposure time starts at a few seconds and can be increased to 25 or 30 min increments. Phototherapy treatments are usually scheduled 3 times a week. Treatment times depend on the patient's skin type and the skin's ability to respond to the treatment and are gradually increased as the treatment progresses until clearing of the psoriasis lesions is achieved.

UVB phototherapy can be useful in treating psoriasis when supplied at a set length on a regular schedule. Broadband UVB treatment uses a wider range of UV wavelengths and the narrowband type of treatment uses a more specific range to treat psoriasis. Narrowband UVB has been shown to clear psoriasis faster and can achieve the treatment goal with less exposure time and with fewer treatments than broadband UVB. Unlike PUVA treatment, UVB can be used on adults as well as children.

PUVA is a type of phototherapy treatment that combines Psoralen and ultraviolet light A. Psoralen is a light-sensitizing medication and represents the "P" in the acronym. It comes in a pill form and a topical form. UVA is ineffective to treat psoriasis by itself, but when combined with Psoralen in PUVA therapy it can clear up to 85% of patients. PUVA works by slowing down the increased cell production. This treatment has most patients cleared by 25 treatments and has a good chance of inducing remissions. PUVA is a good treatment for moderate to severe cases.[21]

8.4 Prevention

8.4.1 Avoid Risk Factors/Triggers

Patients diagnosed with psoriasis or with a family history of the disease should avoid certain risk factors. Cold or dry climates can worsen symptoms and increase the severity of psoriasis. Avoid scratching and picking at the skin. Epidermal injuries or mechanical trauma such as cuts or scratches of the skin can invoke Koebner's phenomenon. In this event, psoriasis lesions appear on the skin at sites of induced trauma. Although it may sound almost impossible, psoriasis patients should be encouraged to avoid stress and anxiety. They may wish to consider learning meditation techniques, yoga, or participate in regular exercise in order to reduce stress and anxiety. Infections can induce types of psoriasis or flares. Regular office visits and antibiotic treatment when indicated can reduce occurrences.

Certain medications can also trigger psoriasis; therefore these medications should be avoided if possible. Potential patients should consult a physician before beginning any new medications that may induce psoriasis. Alcohol should be limited to two drinks a day for a man or one drink for a woman. People with a family history of psoriasis or a current diagnosis should quit smoking. According to studies, people who use tobacco are much more likely to develop psoriasis. Smoking has also been linked to making psoriasis outbreaks more severe and symptoms last longer.[9]

8.4.2 Diet

Multiple studies have shown that psoriasis can actually cause nutritional deficiencies in protein, iron, and folate. It has also been noted that gaining weight can cause flares or can worsen symptoms or psoriasis. Therefore, a low-fat diet with high protein content and green leafy vegetables can help prevent psoriasis flares. Eliminating or limiting caffeinated beverages and foods with high gluten content may reduce outbreaks.[20,21]

8.4.3 Side Effects of Treatments

Anthralin cream can stain surrounding unaffected skin and hair a brownish color. To prevent this adverse effect rub this medication only on areas of psoriasis and wipe excess cream away. Occlusive dressings should be used to prevent stains on clothing or bed linens. Patients with light hair should use caution if using Anthralin to treat scalp psoriasis because of the staining quality of the medication.

Dovonex has no major side effects when used correctly. The most common adverse reaction is skin irritation. To prevent this Dovonex can be mixed with petroleum jelly in increasing potencies until the skin becomes adjusted to the medication.

As with any topical steroid Taclonex should only be applied to any area of the skin for up to 4 weeks. It should also be omitted from use in the axillae, groin area, or face as there is increased sensitivity in those areas. The overuse of this medication can cause atrophy of the epidermis. Increased sun exposure should be limited when using this medication; therefore, no phototherapy treatment should be instituted to avoid unwanted side effects.

The most common side effect from using Tazorac is skin irritation. The best way to prevent this effect is to spot test the medication on a small area of skin before using on all the affected areas. Tazorac can make your skin more susceptible to sunburn. To avoid the adverse effects of using the medication in the sun the patients should be instructed to wear sunscreen or protective clothing when sun exposure is expected. Another option would be to wear the cream at night and wash it off in the morning before spending a day out in the sun.

Topical steroids can be great assets when treating psoriasis but those using topical steroids should be advised of the many possible adverse effects. The steroid strength should be chosen carefully by the treating physician, using low strengths on the face and groin, and the most potent on thick skin like elbows and knees. Overuse of steroids can cause skin to thin or change pigmentation. Topical steroids have also been known to induce acne. Psoriasis lesions may even become worse if steroid treatment suddenly ceases. It is recommended to slowly taper steroids when planning to discontinue use. Topical steroids, especially the more potent types should be avoided around the eyes. Cataracts and glaucoma can present after prolonged steroid exposure to the eyelids and skin around the orbit. Intralesional injections have few side effects if used sparingly and only on a few resistant lesions. Be careful not to inject the same area repeatedly which could lead to skin atrophy at the injection site and can even result in divots in the skin. To prevent these effects the treatment regimen involving steroids should be explained to patients. Patients should have regular visits to their dermatologist in order to closely monitor the frequency and duration of steroid use.[21]

8.4.4 Systemic Therapy: Oral Medications

Patients that are immunocompromised (HIV, history of malignancy, current radiation treatment, etc.), or those with hypertension or renal disease should not take Cyclosporine. To prevent side effects seen with Cyclosporine patients should be encouraged to have their blood pressure and kidney functions closely monitored while taking this medication. Before starting patients on this medication physicians should obtain a detailed list of medications and supplements the patient is taking as there are many cross-reactions with Cyclosporine. Patients should also avoid eating grapefruit or drinking grapefruit juice, because it decreases the excretion of the drug leading to increased levels of Cyclosporine in the blood. Conversely St. John's wort can decrease Cyclosporine levels in the blood so it should also be avoided.

A good medical history and exam should be obtained before starting a patient on Methotrexate. To prevent side effects the patient should have no history or current illness including blood disorders, anemia, peptic ulcers, any significant liver or kidney abnormalities, or excessive alcohol use. A close calculation of the total dosage amount should be recorded each time the patient has a doctor's visit. Once the cumulative dose exceeds 1.5 g there is an increased risk for irreversible liver damage. NSAIDs and medications containing sulfa should be avoided in patients taking Methotrexate to prevent harmful side effects.

Common side effects in Cyclosporine and Soriatane include bleeding or sensitive gums, changes in lipid levels in the blood, hair loss or excessive hair growth, and joint and muscle pains to name a few. These adverse reactions disappear when the medication dosages are lowered or stopped all together.

Soriatane and Methotrexate are known teratogenic drugs. They should be avoided at all costs in pregnant women or those who may become pregnant to prevent birth defects in the developing fetus. Women of child-bearing age can prevent the chance of harmful side effects to the fetus by getting regular pregnancy tests and remaining on two types of contraceptives during treatment. Cyclosporine is usually contraindicated in pregnant or breast-feeding women, but in cases of pustular psoriasis where the patient's life is threatened Cyclosporine may be the treatment of choice compared to the other options of Soriatane and Methotrexate.[21]

8.4.5 Prevention of Biologics Side Effects

All of the biologics are administered by injection. Irritation, pain, and inflammation at the site of injection are common side effects but these reactions have been proven to decrease after the initial dose. Other common side effects include sore throat, cough, nausea, headache, dizziness, and abdominal pain. To prevent patients from discontinuing treatment on their own due to adverse effects educate them on these potential side effects and how they will most likely decrease and cease if continuing to use the medication as directed. Biologics are still relatively new treatments for psoriasis. Long-term side effects are still being evaluated.

Because Amevive decreases the body's immune response, people with a history of malignancy, recurrent infections, or in an immunocompromised state (HIV) should not use this medication. Amevive decreases the amount of T cells in the body, even though patients with psoriasis have an increased amount of T cells some patients can exhibit lymphopenia. Weekly CBCs should be drawn to monitor white blood cell counts to prevent levels from dropping to dangerously low levels.

Patients with any active infection or history of recurrent infections should not use Enbrel, Humira, or Remicade. Those who have a history of multiple sclerosis or congestive heart failure should also not use these medications. A PPD skin test should be performed on patients before initiating treatment to rule out latent tuberculosis.[21]

8.4.6 Prevention of Phototherapy Adverse Effects

Prevention of UVB treatment side effects is simple. Before UV exposure, apply sunscreen to the areas that are free of psoriasis lesions. Patients should also avoid UV exposure in sensitive areas such as the groin and face and neck. As there are many prescription and over-the-counter medications that increase UV sensitivity patients should provide a detailed list of all medications and supplements they take on a regular basis to their dermatologist. Many UVB and PUVA therapy patients experience remission of their disease, but some patients may need to continue with a maintenance regimen to prevent relapse of psoriasis. The maintenance regimen could be once a week to once a month depending on how severe the case of psoriasis.

Oral Psoralen can cause nausea, pruritus, and erythema. To prevent these side effects patients should consider drinking ginger ale or eating at the same time the pill is taken for the nausea, and take a mild antihistamine to alleviate itching. If the adverse effects are unbearable the switch to topical Psoralen should be considered. Patients that have participated in more than 150 phototherapy treatments are at an increased risk for sun-induced keratoses and nonmelanoma skin cancers. These patients should have an annual full-body exam, even after phototherapy has stopped, performed by a dermatologist to catch and treat any precancerous lesions. To prevent cataracts and any other eye problems, UVA-blocking sunglasses should be worn for at least 12 h after taking Psoralen when going out in the sun. To help avoid risks associated with increased U VA exposure the number of treatments should be kept to a minimum. This can be achieved by combining phototherapy with other treatments. Anthralin or topical steroids can be added to treat persistent lesions. Dovonex can also be used in combination with U VA therapy, but needs to be applied after phototherapy because UVA can inactivate this medication.[21]

8.5 Conclusion

There is no cure for psoriasis but there are many ways to prevent the initial onset or exacerbations of the disease. Health education is an important aspect of psoriatic prevention and treatment. Patients should be informed about risk factors associated with psoriasis and about potential side effects associated with specific treatments. As stated earlier, psoriasis has a genetic link, and therefore may be unpreventable for some people. Those who have a family history of the disorder should pay special attention to their health in general, and to the health of their skin in particular in order to prevent initial psoriasis outbreaks or flares of previous incidents of the disease. For patients already suffering from the disease the treatment goal is to prevent exacerbations and flares to achieve the longest possible remission. Since the severity of psoriasis varies so much from case to case it is imperative to monitor it as closely as possible by maintaining regular appointments with primary care physicians or dermatologists. If prevention of the initial onset of psoriasis or preventing exacerbations of the disease is achieved a greater quality of life can be maintained.

References

1. Atochina O, Harn D. Prevention of psoriasis-like lesions development in fsn/fsn mice by helminth glycans. *Exp Dermatol*. 2006;15:461–468
2. Elder J, Nair R, Guo S, et al The genetics of psoriasis. *Arch Dermatol*. 1994;130:216–224
3. Esposito M, Saraceno R, Giunta A, et al An Italian study on psoriasis and depression. *Dermatology*. 2006;212:123–127
4. Farber E, Nall M. The natural history of psoriasis in 5,600 patients. *Dermatologica*. 1974;148:1–18
5. Gelfand JM, Berlin J, Van Voorhees A, et al Lymphoma rates are low but increased in patients with psoriasis. *Arch Dermatol*. 2003;139:1425–1429
6. Gelfand JM, Neimann AL, Shin DB, et al Risk of myocardial infarction in patients with psoriasis. *JAMA*. 2006;296: 1735–1741
7. Gelfand JM, Troxel AB, Lewis JD, et al The risk of mortality in patients with psoriasis: results from a population-based study. *Arch Dermatol*. 2007;143(12):1493–1499
8. Glade CP, Van Erp PEJ, Werner-Schlenzka H, et al A clinical flow cytometric model to study remission and relapse in psoriasis. *Acta Derm Venereol*. 1998;78:180–185
9. Herron MD, Hinckley M, Hoffman MS, et al Impact of obesity and smoking on psoriasis presentation and management. *Arch Dermatol*. 2005;141:1527–1534
10. Horn EJ, Fox KM, Patel V, et al Are patients with psoriasis undertreated? Results of National Psoriasis Foundation survey. *J Am Acad Dermatol*. 2007;57:957–962
11. James WD, Berger TG, Elston DM. *Andrews' diseases of the skin. Clinical dermatology*. Philadelphia: Saunders Elsevier; 2006
12. Jankowiak B, Krajewska-Kulak E, Van Damme-Ostapowicz K, et al The need for health education among patients with psoriasis. *Dermatol Nurs*. 2004;16:439–441
13. Javitz H, Ward M, Farber E, et al The direct cost of care for psoriasis and psoriatic arthritis in the United States. *J Am Acad Dermatol*. 2002;46:850–860
14. Kavli G, Forde O, Arnesen E, et al Psoriasis: familial predisposition and environmental factors. *Br Med J*. 1985; 291: 999–1000
15. Kimball AB, Gladman D, Gelfand JM, et al National psoriasis foundation clinical consensus on psoriasis comorbidities and recommendations for screening. *J Am Acad Dermatol*. 2008;58:1031–1042
16. Kimball AB, Robinson D Jr, Wu Y, et al Cardiovascular disease and risk factors among psoriasis patients in two US healthcare databases, 2001–2002. *Dermatology*. 2008;217: 27–37
17. Lindegard B. Diseases associated with psoriasis in a general population of 159, 200 middle-aged, urban, native Swedes. *Dermatologica*. 1986;172:298–304
18. Lumholt G. *Psoriasis: Prevalence, Spontaneous Course and Genetics- A Census study on the Prevalence of Skin Disease on the Faroer Islands*. Copenhagen: GEC, GAD; 1963
19. Najarian DJ, Gottlieb AB. Connections between psoriasis and Crohn's disease. *J Am Acad Dermatol*. 2003;48: 805–821
20. Naldi L, Patrazzini F, Peli L, et al Dietary factors and the risk of psoriasis: results of an Italian case-control study. *Br J Dermatol*. 1996;134:101–106
21. National Psoriasis Foundation, Psoriasis Overview and Treatment, November 2008. URL <http://www.psoriasis.org>
22. Rapp SR, Feldman SR, Exum ML, et al Psoriasis causes as much disability as other major medical diseases. *J Am Acad Dermatol*. 1999;41:401–407
23. Schafer T. Epidemiology of psoriasis. *Dermatology*. 2006; 212:327–337
24. Wolff K, Johnson RA, Suurmond D. *Fitzpatrick's Color Atlas and Synopsis of Clinical Dermatology*. New York: McGraw-Hill; 2005

Sports Dermatology: Prevention

Brian B. Adams

The four main categories of skin conditions that afflict the athlete include infections, trauma, inflammation, and encounters with the environment. Knowledge of the etiology of cutaneous skin problems of athletes helps the clinician best formulate a prevention plan. Most of the skin ailments that sideline athletes can be prevented through proper disqualification, appropriate use of equipment, and selective use of pharmacologic agents.

9.1 Infections

The four main types of infections that affect the athlete are bacteria, fungi, viruses, and parasites. In general, parasitic infestations play a relatively small role in sports dermatology. However, all contact athletes need screening before practice and competition to ensure that infestations with lice and scabies do not cause epidemics.

9.1.1 General Prevention Techniques

Some athletes are particularly susceptible to infections because of intense and prolonged skin-to-skin contact and trauma, inherent to athletic activity, which disturbs the normal epidermal barrier and allows for microorganism penetration. Sweating provides an ideal microenvironment (warm and moist) for microorganism growth.

B.B. Adams
Department of Dermatology,
University of Cincinnati,
Cincinnati, OH, USA
e-mail: brianadams@pol.net

Finally, athletes transmit infections among team competitors through sharing equipment (Table 9.1).

Basic prevention principles for athletes include modifying these risk factors (Table 9.2). No athlete should share towels, pads (shoulder, knee, elbow), helmets, hats, gloves, sweatbands, clothing, footwear, or razors. Athletic trainers should also be careful to ensure that they do not cross-contaminate any communal source. For example, once a trainer dips a tongue depressor into a jar of gel and applies it to an athlete, that depressor must be discarded. Any subsequent applicator that gets dipped into that container must be clean though not necessarily sterile.

Athletes should always consider placing a barrier between their skin and the athletic environment. During practice and competition (if allowed) athletes who anticipate prolonged and intense skin-to-skin contact with competitors should wear synthetic moisture-wicking clothing to cover exposed areas. Loose-fitting clothing made of this fabric keeps the athletes cool and their skin dry while creating a physical barrier between themselves and potentially infectious competitors. Athletes should also wear synthetic moisture-wicking socks at all times. The feet of athletes become warm and moist as a result of their athletic activity and experience occlusion by athletic footwear, which further exacerbates the risk of infection of tinea pedis (Table 9.3).[1]

Athletes should never go barefoot on the locker room or shower floors. Poolside is equally infectious and athletes should always wear sandals in these situations. One group of investigators cultured dermatophytes each time they examined the pool and locker room floors every other week for a year.[2] Additionally, once experiencing a traumatic break in their skin, the athlete should carefully bandage the area.

Appropriate cleansing remains a cornerstone of infection control among sports teams. Immediately after

Table 9.1 Evidence for transmission of Staphylococcus by fomites

Equipment type	Epidemic study	Level of evidence
Fencing sensor wires	MMWR, 2003	+
Whirlpools	Kazakova	+
	Begier	+++
	Bartlett	+++
	Seidenfeld	–
	Lindenmayer	–
Weights	Kazakova	+
Sharing towels	Kazakova	+
	Begier	–
	Seidenfeld	–
	Sosin	–
	Lindenmayer	–
Sharing equipment	Begier	–
	Seidenfeld	–
	Sosin	–
	Lindenmayer	–
Tape sharing	Seidenfeld	–
Elbow pad use	Sosin	+++
	Seidenfeld	++
	Bartlett	+++
Athletic tape use	Sosin	+++
	Bartlett	+++
Skin lubricants use	Bartlett	+++

From Adams.[1] With permission from Springer Science and Business Media LLC
"–" no statistical association
"+" suggested link
"++" increased risk but not statistically significant
"+++" statistically significant increased risk

Table 9.2 Prevention techniques to avoid skin infection epidemics

Frequent, if not daily, skin checks by athletes and trainers
Daily showers immediately after practices or competition
Routine antibacterial soap use in the showers
Frequent hand washing by trainers and affected athletes
Universal availability of alcohol-based, waterless, soap cleansers
Regular laundering of equipment and clothing
Mandatory no sharing policy for equipment and personal items
Required personal towels
Meticulous covering of all wounds
Use of protective gloves when using weight-lifting equipment
Universal sandal usage in the locker room and showers
Periodic formal education for the athletes, coaches, and trainers

From Adams.[1] With permission from Springer Science and Business Media LLC

Table 9.3 Preventative measures for tinea pedis and tinea ungium

Synthetic moisture-wicking socks
Immediate showers after sporting activity
Sandals or other footwear while in shower and locker room or pool deck
Thorough feet washing
Regular cleaning of shower, locker room, and pool floors
Daily application of antifungal cream to feet

From Adams.[1] With permission from Springer Science and Business Media LLC

practice or competition, athletes should shower with antibacterial soap. Athletes and trainers should liberally and frequently use soapless cleansers with moisturizers while in the training room. It is vital that athletic trainers use these cleansers between caring for separate athletes. Salient and judicious placement of these cleansers in the training room help ensures its use.

Athletes, coaches, and trainers must together ensure timely diagnosis and prompt therapy of skin infections; daily skin examinations of athletes who experience intense skin-to-skin contact are mandatory. Often, a medley of clinicians care for athletes on the high school level and coordination of care can be difficult. One study demonstrated the untoward effects of having wrestlers return to wrestling before their communicable skin disease was adequately treated.[3] This study demonstrated that a series of wrestlers were incorrectly diagnosed and treated for herpes gladiatorum when in fact they actually had impetigo (70%), tinea corporis gladiatorum (10%), and eczema (10%). Eighty percent of these sidelined wrestlers returned to wrestling without proper treatment for their bacterial and fungal eruptions and 10% (eczema) of the benched athletes had no infection at all.[3] Specific National Collegiate Athletic Association (NCAA) guidelines exist that assist clinicians in the disposition of infected athletes. Adherence to these guidelines can prevent epidemics.

9.1.2 Specific Prevention Techniques

While these general methods significantly decrease the incidence of skin infections in athletes, specific recommendations exist for each unique condition. Herpes simplex virus causes two different types of skin conditions in athletes. First, in outdoor athletes, the ultraviolet rays (both direct and reflected) can activate herpes labialis. One double-blind placebo controlled study of skiers demonstrated that 71% of those using placebo lip balm developed herpes labialis; no skiers assigned to use sunscreen on their lips developed herpes labialis.[4] Another study demonstrated that skiers that took valacyclovir 400 mg twice daily starting 12 h before skiing experienced significantly fewer outbreaks of herpes labialis.[5]

Herpes simplex virus (specifically HSV-1) also causes epidemics in wrestlers (Fig. 9.1). To address these epidemics, one research team examined the

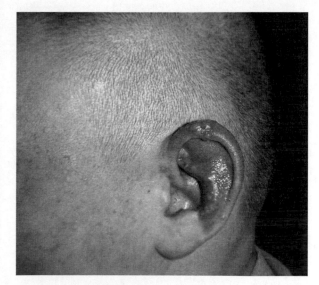

Fig. 9.1 Herpes gladiatorum of the ear (From Adams.[1] With permission from Springer Science and Business Media LLC)

effectiveness of season-long pharmacological prophylaxis.[6] This double-blind placebo controlled study had four distinct groups. The first section represented wrestlers whose initial herpes lesion occurred more than 2 years prior; half of these individuals took placebo and half took 500 mg of valacyclovir. None of the athletes who took valacyclovir in this section developed herpes while 33% of the wrestlers who took placebo developed herpes. The second section represented athletes who had first had a history of herpes less than 2 years prior to the start of the study. The athletes who took valacyclovir developed herpes 21% of the time whereas 33% of those athletes who had placebo developed herpes. Though differences among groups do not exist upon close statistical analysis, season-long prophylaxis with 1 g of valacyclovir seems prudent and allows maximal athletic participation.

Methicillin resistant *Staphylococcus aureus* (MRSA) has caused many epidemics in athletes at many ability levels. Athletes with positive skin cultures for MRSA need to also have their nares swabbed for culture. Mupirocin 2% applied twice daily to the nares for 1 week significantly decreases nasal carriage. This process should be repeated twice per year to decrease the athlete's *staphylococcal* carriage.[1] In repeated cutaneous disease, clinicians should also consider the perianal, groin, and axillae regions as possible sites of *staphylococcal* colonization. The same mupirocin 2% application process for the nares works also for the perianal, groin, and axillae areas.

As athletes spend time in the whirlpool while rehabbing an injury, they risk developing hot tub folliculitis caused by *Pseudomonas*. Whirlpools must be cleaned routinely and adequately chlorinated to prevent hot tub folliculitis. The free chlorine level should be at least 0.6 mg/L and the pH kept between 7.2 and 7.8. Unfortunately, adequate chlorination does not ensure bacteria-free water. In 16% of *Pseudomonas* folliculitis epidemics, unfortunately, the chlorination has been adequate.[7,8] Pools with *Pseudomonas* necessitate a hyperchlorination with 5 mg/L for 3 days.[9]

Other bacterial infections that occur in athletes such as erythrasma (groin and axillae) and pitted keratolysis (feet) propagate in warm and moist microenvironments (Fig. 9.2). Wearing synthetic moisture-wicking undergarments and socks prevent those infections. Some of these types of socks also possess antimicrobial properties. Athletes predisposed to pitted keratolysis may find it helpful to apply aluminum chloride (which is quite drying) to the soles and interdigitally before exercising.

Tinea corporis gladiatorum, caused by *Trichophyton tonsurans,* causes frequent epidemics among wrestling teams. Teams and their staff frequently clean the mats before and after practice, though only one study has ever documented dermatophyte presence on the mats.[10] Two studies have examined pharmacological prevention of tinea corporis gladiatorum. Itraconazole (400 mg every other week), in an open-label prospective trial, decreased the incidence from 27% to 0%.[11] A subsequent randomized placebo controlled study of 100 mg of weekly fluconazole significantly decreased the incidence of tinea corporis gladiatorum.[12]

As a complication of their skin becoming warm and sweaty, athletes also frequently develop tinea versicolor. Prevention of this condition thwarts the persistent discoloration (either hyperpigmentation or hypopigmentation) of the skin that occurs subsequently. Once per week, athletes can apply selenium sulfide 2.5% to the predisposed areas and wash off after 15 min.[1]

While no direct evidence-based medicine exists to support this specific recommendation, athletes with recurrent tinea pedis should indefinitely apply topical antifungal agents to their soles and interdigital regions on the weekends. This recommendation relates in part to one study that revealed a decrease in the prevalence of tinea pedis from 21.5% to 6.9% over 3 years after bathers used an antifungal powder upon leaving the pool.[13] Athletes, with recurrent tinea pedis, should consider obtaining new shoes; one study documented dermatophytes in 15% of shoes kept in storage for 1–4 weeks.[14]

9.2 Trauma

While skin infections can sideline athletes and disrupt team activities, trauma causes the most common cutaneous ailments in athletes. Friction between the athlete's skin and athletic equipment results in bullae and occasionally erosions. Depending on location, these physical disruptions in the skin may result in significant decrease in athletic ability secondary to pain. The primary risk factors for the development of bullae include ill-fitted equipment, moisture, heat, and prolonged activity. Athletes typically experience friction on their hands, feet, groin, shoulders, face, and nipples.

Several approaches assuage friction bullae production (Table 9.4). First and foremost, athletes need to wear properly fitted footwear. Shoes that are too small or too large can result in bullae. Special lacing techniques can ameliorate bullae on the feet by preventing slippage in shoes that are too large (Fig. 9.3). Slip-resistant shoe insoles also help prevent bullae by not allowing the toes to slam into the toe box. Brand new shoes need to be gradually included into the exercise regimen. Wearing new shoes for a prolonged period during intense activity can lead to bullae.

Athletes should also wear synthetic moisture-wicking clothing (including socks); decreasing the degree of wet clothing and equipment decreases the incidence of bullae. Before the development of frank bullae, athletes experience warmth in the skin on the affected area. Some socks have extra padding in these "hot spots" to decrease bulla formation while other socks

Table 9.4 Prevention of friction bullae

Category	Method
Equipment	Gloves
Shoes	Adequately sized toebox Nonslip insoles Supple shoes Unique lacing techniques
Socks	Double-layered Padded Synthetic moisture-wicking
Topical agents	Aluminum chloride Drying powders Micronized wax and silicone powder Petroleum jelly Tissue adhesives

From Adams.[1] With permission from Springer Science and Business Media LLC

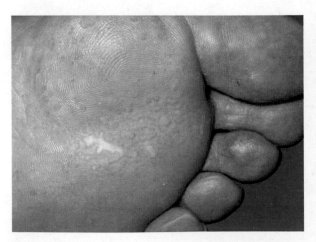

Fig. 9.2 Pitted keratolysis

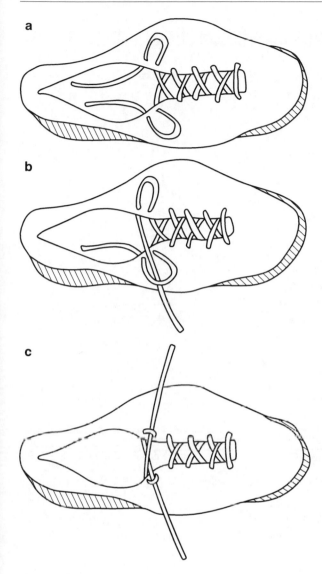

Fig. 9.3 (**a**) Rather than lacing across to the opposite hole, lace the shoestring through the hole on the same side. (**b**) Through each of the loops made by the lacing procedure in (**a**), lace across to the opposite side. (**c**) Finally pull up, out, and tight. This snuggly stabilizes the heel and ankle for athletic participation (From Adams.[1] With permission from Springer Science and Business Media LLC)

lack seams that can contribute to bulla genesis. Athletes can also decrease friction by wearing two layers of synthetic moisture-wicking clothing.

Athletes whose hands come in contact with implements also can acquire bullae on their hands; gloves serve to decrease the amount of friction.

Athletes can also apply topical antiperspirants to these "hot spots" to decrease moisture. In addition, lubricants applied to these hot spots decrease the coefficient of friction between the skin and the equipment.

These lubricants include cosmetically elegant vehicles but also cheaper alternatives such as a petroleum jelly. There remains one caveat to the use of these occlusive agents. In the short term, the coefficient of friction is reduced but after about 3 h the occlusive nature of these agents results in a decrease in transepidermal water loss and supersaturation of the epidermis. This excess local moisture thus increases the chance of bullae formation. Commercially available tissue adhesives also serve to decrease the degree of friction experienced by the epidermis.

Athletes' skin that chronically experience these frictional forces develops calluses. These callosities occur in anatomic locations that relate to specific athletic activities (Table 9.5) and help prevent future bullae. The same methods that prevent bullae acutely prevent calluses in the long term.

Other frictional forces result not in bullae but in painful erosions. Common locations for these eruptions include the nipples (runners) and thighs (cyclists). Prevention of these erosions requires a multifaceted approach. First, athletes should apply a barrier between the "hot spots" and the clothing. Petroleum jelly and multiple commercially available substances decrease the coefficient of friction thus preventing epidermal breakdown. Synthetic moisture wicking clothing (including undergarments) also decrease friction by adding a layer that will, instead of the skin, experience the shearing forces and by wicking away moisture from the skin. Without additional moisture, the epidermis is less likely to develop erosions. Runners may also purchase patches to apply over their nipples to decrease friction.

These shearing forces when experienced on the sole of the foot can cause talon noire. Black heel (or talon noire) may appear clinically similar to malignant melanoma. Heel cups may help prevent talon noire.

Surfer's and cyclist's nodules represent another sports-related traumatic skin condition (Fig. 9.4). Surfer's nodules occur on the knees and feet; protective padding on these areas prevent the nodules. Interestingly, cold-water surfers develop surfer's nodules more frequently than surfers in warm water. While paddling out to catch waves in cold water, surfers rest on their board only on their knees and feet; this intense focal pressure results in nodular formation. Warm water surfers can lie prone on their board and thus distribute their weight equally. Cold-water surfers can decrease the incidence of surfer's nodules by wearing wet suits that permit them to lie prone on the board in

Table 9.5 Sport-specific callosities

Sport	Location	Etiology
Archery	Fourth fingertip	Bowstring hand
Baseball	Palms	Batting
	First finger	Pitching
Billiards	Nondominant, palmar aspect thumb and first finger; dorsal aspect second finger	Holding the cue
Bowling (no holes)	Throwing hand, third and fourth fingers	Throwing ball
With holes	Throwing hand, second, third, and fourth lateral fingers	Throwing ball
Canoeing/crew/kayaking/rowing	Palms (depends on oar type)	Rowing
Cycling	Ischial tuberosities	Peddling
Dance	Distal toes	Dancing ballet
Equestrian	Fingers and palms	Holding on to reins
Fishing	Thumb and opposite first finger	Reeling in fish
Golf	Dominant hand, first finger and opposite palm, and opposite third finger	Swinging club
Gymnastics	Palms	Horse, parallel bar, rings
In-line skating	Leg	Pushing off while skating
Karate/judo	Lateral sides of hands and heels	Blows, chops, kicks
Tennis (badminton, racquetball, squash)	Dominant palm and thumb	Swinging racquet
Track and field (discus)	Throwing hand, all palmar aspects of fingers except thumb	Throwing discus
Shot put	Hypothenar eminence	Throwing shot
Distance runners	Heel ("runner's bump")	Running
Weightlifters	Palms, web spaces between thumb and first fingers	Lifting

From Adams.[1] With permission from Springer Science and Business Media LLC

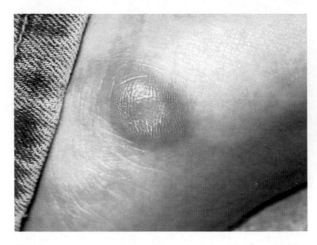

Fig. 9.4 Like cyclists and surfers, skaters wearing tight-fitting skates may develop athletes' nodules such as seen here on the medial aspect of the foot

cold water.[1] Cyclists develop morphologically similar nodules in sacrococcygeal area. Properly fitted and padded seats, along with padded biking shorts, decrease the incidence of cyclist's nodules.[1]

Athlete's toenail occurs in myriad athletes (Fig. 9.5). To prevent these nail changes, athletes need to cut their nails straight across so that the pressure of the toe box distributes equally across the nail. The shoe's toe box must allow adequate room. Unique lacing techniques ensure that the most distal toenails do not slam into the toe box.

Combined forces (heat, moisture, and friction) create acne mechanica in athletes (Fig. 9.6 and Table 9.6). The focus of prevention for acne mechanica aims to decrease all three factors on the skin. Athletes must shower immediately after practicing or competing. The use of mildly abrasive soaps may also decrease the

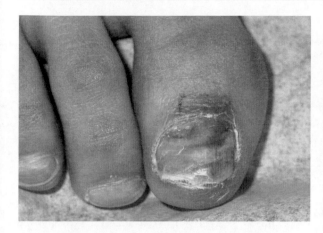

Fig. 9.5 A tight-fitting figure skate resulted in this athlete's toenail abnormality

Table 9.6 The location and cause of acne mechanica depending on sport

Sport	Acne location	Etiology
Dancers	Trunk	Beneath tight leotard
Football	Chin	Chin straps
	Shoulders	Shoulder pads
	Upper inner arm	Shoulder pad straps
	Forehead, cheeks	Helmet
Golfers	Lower lateral back	Golf bag while carrying it
Hockey	Chin	Chin straps
	Shoulders	Shoulder pads
	Upper inner arm	Shoulder pad straps
	Forehead, cheeks	Helmet
Shot putters	Neck	Shot put before launch
Tennis	Back	Heavy warm clothes
Weightlifters	Upper back	Plastic/vinyl bench cover
	Upper central chest	Weight bar
Wrestlers	Chin, neck periauricular	Headgear
	Elbows, knees	Elbow and kneepads

From Adams.[1] With permission from Springer Science and Business Media LLC

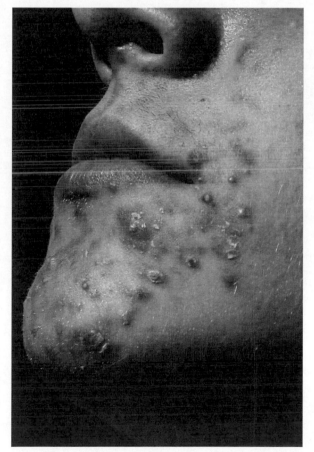

Fig. 9.6 Acne mechanica (From Adams.[1] With permission from Springer Science and Business Media LLC)

incidence of acne mechanica. Athletes can also use keratolytic agents to prevent acne mechanica. Synthetic moisture-wicking clothing keeps the skin cool and dry and decreases friction. Athletes can use fragments of this type of clothing to form a barrier beneath chin-straps, knee pads, and elbow pads.

9.3 Inflammation

Both allergic and irritant contact dermatitis occur in athletes; their equipment and environment can cause eruptions (Fig. 9.7 and Table 9.7). Topical medication and equipment alternatives allow sensitized athletes (allergic contact dermatitis) to compete and practice without incident. If no equipment alternatives exist, athletes should apply tape, coban wrap, tissue adhesive, petroleum jelly, or another barrier between the offending equipment and the skin. Athletes sensitized to poison ivy, poison oak, and poison sumac can apply bentoquatam (commercially available as IvyBlock) to their skin to prevent allergic reactions; these athletes need to apply this medication at least 15 min before going outdoors and reapply every 4 h.[1]

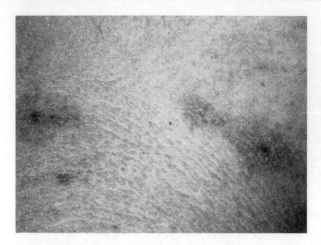

Fig. 9.7 Note the linear pattern characteristic of poison ivy. Also note the black dots in several of the lesions. These dots represent oxidized uroshiol, the protein responsible for poison ivy

Irritant contact dermatitis results from a direct toxic irritation of the skin with some agent in the environment; an athlete's own immune system plays little initial role in the pathogenesis (unlike allergic contact dermatitis). Athletes decrease their risk for irritant contact dermatitis by placing a barrier between their skin and the environmental irritant. Such barriers include waterproof gloves, wet suits, petroleum jelly, and clothing to decrease the amount of exposed skin.

Some irritants will wash away if too much time has not elapsed.

Several types of urticaria occur in athletes. Athletes can prevent cholinergic urticaria with antihistamines; also a gradual increase in athletic intensity may result in habituation that allows the athlete to participate without bouts of urticaria. Cold-urticaria-susceptible athletes should wear cold weather synthetic moisture-wicking clothing; using several layers of such clothing maximizes heat retention. Some authors have suggested that cyproheptadine hydrochloride best prevents cold urticaria.[15] Athletes with solar urticaria need to apply broadband blocking water-resistant sunscreen frequently. The use of sun-protective athletic clothing and broad-brimmed hats also helps prevent solar urticaria. Athletes with severe recalcitrant solar urticaria may require antimalarial agents or desensitization with ultraviolet radiation. Inert oily substances applied to the exposed skin in sensitized athletes, prevents the exceedingly rare condition, aquagenic urticaria.

Some athletes develop exercise-induced anaphylaxis. A study of 278 athletes reported that over three-quarters of those affected identified running as a trigger of their disease.[16] Several factors exacerbate exercise-induced anaphylaxis including extreme temperatures, eating before exercise, and ingesting NSAIDS (nonsteroidal anti-inflammatory drugs), aspirin, and B-lactam antibiotics (Table 9.8). Some of the notable foodstuffs that trigger exercise-induced anaphylaxis include barley, beans, broccoli, cheese, chicken, eggs, garlic, grapes, lettuce, peaches, peanuts, rye, shellfish, tomatoes, and wheat.[17] By avoiding these triggers, athletes can mitigate outbreaks. Ketotifen appears to prevent exercise-induced anaphylaxis-related angioedema[18] and cromolyn mitigates the exercise-induced anaphylaxis-related respiratory-related symptoms.[19] The symptoms of exercise-induced anaphylaxis do not occur consistently during each athletic activity; however, athletes with this disorder should never exercise alone.

Table 9.7 The etiologies of the various sports-related types of irritant contact dermatitis

Category	Sport	Designation	Irritant
Playing field	Mountaineering	Canyoning hands	Irritant Forces of nature (rocks, water, wind)
	Soccer	Cement burns	Calcium oxide
	Swimming	Pool dermatitis	Halogenated compounds in pool water
Athletes' implements	Basketball	Basketball pebble fingers	Pebbled nicked ball
	Hockey	Hockey dermatitis	Fiberglass
	Injured athletes	Pack dermatitis	Ammonium nitrate
	Board surfers	Surf rider's dermatitis	Mixed (board, salt, sand)
Athletes themselves	Baseball	Baseball pitcher's friction dermatitis	Questionable coarse clothing
	Swimming	Swimmer's shoulder	Hair stubble

From Adams.[1] With permission from Springer Science and Business Media LLC

Table 9.8 Critical history questions to ask the athlete with suspected exercise-induced angioedema/anaphylaxis

Do you experience EIA flares more frequently when you…
Exercise in very cold or very hot conditions?
Eat certain foods before exercising?
Take aspirin, ibuprofen (or other NSAIDS), or antibiotics before exercising?

From Adams.[1] With permission from Springer Science and Business Media LLC

Table 9.9 Sports for which studies have specifically illustrated reasons for increased ultraviolet damage

Sports	Reasons for increased ultraviolet damage
Triathalon, cycling, baseball, softball, golf	Gross exposure to severe level of UV rays
Skiing, soccer, runners	Failure to apply sunscreen
Outdoor athletes	High wind
Outdoor athletes	High temperatures
Outdoor athletes	Sweating
Skiing, snowboarding, swimming	Reflectance of UV rays

From Adams.[1] With permission from Springer Science and Business Media LLC

Table 9.10 Smart sun safety tips for athletes

Avoid, if possible the sun between 10 am and 3 pm
Apply SPF 30 sunscreen one half hour before practicing in outdoor sports
Reapply sunscreen often while sweating or swimming
Wear hats
Wear sun-protective clothing

From Adams.[1] With permission from Springer Science and Business Media LLC

Table 9.11 Factors influencing the protection factor of an athlete's clothing

Variable of fabric	Effect on protection factor
Nylon, wool, silk	Relatively increases
Cotton, rayon, linen	Relatively decreases
Dark color	Increases
UV absorbers added	Increases
Increasing wetness	Decreases
Increasing numbers of washes	Increases

From Adams.[1] With permission from Springer Science and Business Media LLC

9.4 Environmental Encounters

Environmental conditions also put athletes at risk to develop several other dermatologic conditions. Athletes practice and compete during the peak hours of ultraviolet exposure (10 AM to 4 PM). Several studies note an excessive exposure among athletes (Table 9.9). For instance, in the Tour de Suisse, the cyclists experienced up to 17 times their MED (the minimal UV dose to barely cause the skin to be pink).[20] Another study revealed that athletes' sweat reduces, by 40%, the amount of ultraviolet exposure required for sunburn.[21] Outdoor winter athletes and beach athletes must also endure significant reflectance of the ultraviolet rays.

Avoidance of ultraviolet exposure prevents not only the acute effects of the sun (sunburn, bullae, sun poisoning) but also the long-term effects (premature aging, wrinkles, sun spots) and skin cancer (Table 9.10). When possible, athletes should avoid practicing during the peak hours of ultraviolet radiation. Athletes should

wear water-resistant SPF 30+ sunscreen and reapply frequently with sweating and water exposure.

Unfortunately, athletes – despite their obvious increased risk – do not often use sunscreen. In one study, 85% of 200 collegiate athletes never used sunscreen. Only 6% of these collegiate athletes used sunscreen at least 3 of 7 days of the week.[22] This same study identified one of the major barriers to athletes' use of sunscreen as the lack of access to it. By making sunscreen readily available in the training rooms of high schools, colleges, and professional venues, medical providers can increase the likelihood of athletes' sunscreen use.

In addition to sunscreen, athletes should wear hats and sun-protective clothing. Broad-brimmed hats do not allow athletes to forego sunscreen use on their face, however, as sand and snow (two common sporting activity venues), reflect a great deal of ultraviolet radiation. Experts assign the term UPF to describe the relative ultraviolet-protective value of clothing. Several factors of athletic clothing influence ultraviolet protection (Table 9.11). Nylon, silk, and wool possess higher sun-protective factors than do other fabric types. Darker-colored clothes block more ultraviolet rays as do tighter weave fabrics (though they will be hotter). The initial launderings of athletic clothing improve its sun-protection ability. However, in general when an athlete's clothing becomes wet (either through sweating or from the environment) the sun protection ability of the clothing decreases.[1]

On the opposite spectrum from the sun and warmth, frostbite and chilblains can occur in winter sport athletes. To prevent these cold-weather-related ailments, athletes can layer synthetic moisture-wicking clothing; outerwear should be waterproof. Winter athletes should avoid wearing metal jewelry as it conducts heat. Commercially available warming packets can be placed in gloves or shoes.

As they practice and compete, athletes also must endure insect (bees, flies, wasps, yellow jackets, hornets) attacks. Several methods assuage the attack of these insects. First, athletes should avoid wearing bright colors. Scented products and shiny jewelry also attract insects. Second, most arthropod pests have a specific time of day that they prevail; avoidance of this time helps prevent arthropod stings. Products containing 20% (or greater) DEET deter insect bites. Long-sleeved synthetic moisture-wicking clothing keeps the athlete cool but also protected from insect bites. Athletes should also wear sandals in grass to prevent stepping on one of these insects. Some insects are social insects and release a pheromone if destroyed; this pheromone incites all nearby yellow jackets, for instance, to swarm around the destroyed insect. All sporting venues should remove trash receptacles from areas of athlete congregation to prevent stings.[1]

Insults from insects are not all that athletes must endure; aquatic athletes who frequent areas where sea urchins and starfish are prevalent should wear protective boots. Swimmers who use chlorinated pools, instead of the ocean may develop a condition termed green hair. Green hair occurs in light haired aquatic athletes exposed to water rich in copper. To prevent green hair, these athletes should shampoo immediately after water exposure; shampooing with copper chelating shampoos also deters the production of green hair.[1]

9.5 Summary

Knowledge of the etiology of cutaneous skin problems of athletes reviewed here helps the clinician best formulate a prevention plan. Most of the skin ailments that sideline athletes can be prevented by following the guidelines included in this chapter.

References

1. Adams BB. *Sports Dermatology*. New York: Springer; 2006
2. Detandt M, Nolard N. Dermatophytes and swimming pools: seasonal fluctuations. *Mycoses*. 1988;31:495–500
3. Dworkin MS, Shoemaker PC, Spitters C, et al Endemic spread of herpes simplex virus type I among adolescent wrestlers and their coaches. *Pediatr Infect Dis J*. 1999;18:1108–1109
4. Rooney JF, Bryson Y, Mannix ML, et al Prevention of ultraviolet-light induced herpes labialis by sunscreen. *Lancet*. 1991;338:1419–1422
5. Spruance SL, Hamill ML, Hoge WS, et al Valacyclovir prevents reactivation of herpes simplex labialis in skiers. *JAMA*. 1988;269:1597–1599
6. Anderson BJ. The effectiveness of valacyclovir in preventing reactivation of herpes gladiatorum in wrestlers. *Clin J Sport Med*. 1999;9:86–90
7. Fox AB, Hambrick GW. Recreationally associated Pseudomonas aeruginosa folliculitis. *Arch Dermatol*. 1984;120:1304–1307
8. Spitalny KC, Voot RL, Witherell LE. National survey on outbreaks associated with whirlpool spas. *Am J Public Health*. 1984;74:725–726
9. Thomas P, Moore M, Bell E, et al Pseudomonas dermatitis associated with a swimming pool. *JAMA*. 1985; 253:1156–1159
10. El Fari M, Graser Y, Presber W, et al An epidemic of tinea corporis caused by Trichophyton tonsurans among children (wrestlers) in Germany. *Mycoses*. 2000;43:191–196
11. Hazen PG, Weil ML. Itraconazole in the prevention and management of dermatophytosis in competitive wrestlers. *J Am Acad Dermatol*. 1997;36:481–482
12. Kohl TD, Martin DC, Nemeth R, et al Fluconazole for the prevention and treatment of tinea gladiatorum. *Pediatr Infect Dis J*. 2000;19:717–722
13. Gentles JC, Evans EGV, Jones GR. Control of tinea pedis in a swimming bath. *Br Med J*. 1974;2:577–580
14. Jello L, Getz ME. Recovery of dermatophytes from shoes and shower stalls. *J Invest Dermatol*. 1954;22:17–24
15. Briner WW. Physical allergies and exercise. *Sport Med*. 1993;15:365–373
16. Shaddick NA, Liang MH, Partridge AJ, et al The natural history of exercise induced anaphylaxis: survey results from a

10-year follow-up study. *J Allergy Clin Immunol*. 1999; 104:123–127

17. Adams ES. Identifying and controlling metabolic skin disorders. *Phys Sportsmed*. 2004;32:29–40
18. Nichols AW. Exercise-induced anaphylaxis and urticaria. *Clin Sports Med*. 1992;11:303–312
19. Adams BB. Exercise-induced anaphylaxis in a marathon runner. *Int J Dermatol*. 2002;41:394–396
20. Moehrle M, Heinrich L, Schmid A, et al Extreme UV exposure of professional cyclists during selected outdoor activities. *Photodermatol Photoimmunol Photomed*. 2000;201: 44–45
21. Moehrle M, Koehle W, Dietz K, et al Reduction of minimal erythema dose by sweating. *Photodermatol Photoimmunol Photomed*. 2000;16:260–262
22. Hamant E, Adams BB. Sunscreen use among collegiate athletes. *J Am Acad Dermatol*. 2005;53:237–241

Prevention of Cosmetic Problems

10

Zoe Diana Draelos

Cosmetic problems can be prevented through proper diagnosis and the use of carefully selected products. These products typically fall in the over-the-counter (OTC) realm and can be classified as true cosmetics or OTC drugs. Products that are considered cosmetics include moisturizers, lip balms, and shaving preparations while OTC drugs include sunscreens and antiperspirants. This chapter examines the use of these products in the prevention of cosmetic-related skin disease including facial eczema, eyelid dermatitis, cheilitis, postinflammatory hyperpigmentation, hyperhidrosis, and acne. These are common cosmetic problems that can be exacerbated or alleviated based on the dermatologist's ability to correctly recommend prescription and complimentary nonprescription therapies.

10.1 Facial Eczema

The face is the most complex area of the entire body because more products are designed for facial use than any other. The face contains sebaceous, eccrine, and apocrine glands, as well as keratinized and transitional skin. The face is also characterized by numerous follicular structures in the form of pigmented terminal hairs in the eyebrows, eyelashes, and male beard combined with white fine downy vellus hairs over the rest of the face. These follicular structures are the transition between the skin on the surface of the face and the follicular ostia associated with the follicle and sebaceous glands. This skin cannot be reached by traditional cosmetics and skin care products, but irritant or allergic reactions that occur at the skin surface can impact this follicular lining. Thus, moisturizer and cleanser formulations for the face must be hypoallergenic, non-comedogenic, and non-acnegenic, since the face is capable of all these reaction patterns.

10.1.1 Facial Moisturizers

Facial moisturizers are the most important cosmetic in the prevention of facial eczema. These moisturizers attempt to mimic the effect of sebum and the intercellular lipids composed of sphingolipids, free sterols, and free fatty acids. They intend to provide an environment allowing healing of the stratum corneum barrier by replacement of the corneocytes and the intercellular lipids. Yet, the moisturizing substances must not occlude the sweat ducts, or miliaria will result; must not produce irritation at the follicular ostia, or an acneiform eruption will result; and must not initiate comedonal formation.

Moisturizers are used to heal barrier-damaged skin by minimizing transepidermal water loss (TEWL) and creating an environment optimal for healing. There are three categories of substances that can be combined to enhance the water content of the skin, which include occlusives, humectants, and hydrocolloids (Table 10.1). Occlusives are oily substances that retard TEWL by placing an oil slick over the skin surface, while humectants are substances that attract water to the skin, not from the environment, unless the ambient humidity is 70%, but rather from the inner layers of the skin. Humectants draw water from the viable dermis into the

10

Z.D. Draelos
Department of Dermatology,
Duke University School of Medicine,
Durham, NC, USA
e-mail: zdraelos@northstate.net

R.A. Norman (ed.), *Preventive Dermatology in Infectious Diseases*,
DOI 10.1007/978-0-85729-847-8_10, © Springer-Verlag London Limited 2012

Table 10.1 Facial moisturizer categories

Moisturizer category	Ingredients	Skin effect
Occlusive	Petrolatum, mineral oil, cetyl alcohol, dimethicone, cyclomethicone, soybean oil, lanolin, shea butter, cocoa butter, sesame oil, borage oil, all vegetable oils	Prevent water evaporation from skin, smooth desquamating corneocytes, place protective film over nerve endings to alleviate itch, add skin shine
Humectant	Glycerin, hyaluronic acid, sodium PCA, sorbitol, propylene glycol, vitamins, gelatin	Act as a sponge to hold water within the skin enabling hydration
Hydrocolloid	Proteins, hyaluronic acid, colloidal oatmeal	Create a physical barrier to water evaporation from the skin

viable epidermis and then from the nonviable epidermis into the stratum corneum. Lastly, hydrocolloids are physically large substances, which cover the skin, thus retarding TEWL.

The best moisturizers to prevent facial eczema combine occlusive and humectant ingredients to combine the benefit of both categories. For example, a well-formulated moisturizer might contain petrolatum, mineral oil, and dimethicone as occlusive agents. Petrolatum is the synthetic substance most like the natural intercellular lipids, but too high a concentration will yield a sticky, greasy ointment. The aesthetics of petrolatum can be improved by adding dimethicone, also able to occlude water loss, but allowing a reduction in the petrolatum concentration and a thinner, more acceptable formulation. Mineral oil is not quite as greasy as petrolatum, but still an excellent barrier repair agent that further improves the ability of the moisturizer to spread, yielding enhanced aesthetics. The addition of glycerin to the formulation will allow water attraction to the xerotic facial skin from the dermis, speeding hydration. It is through the careful combination of these ingredients that facial moisturizers can be constructed to prevent and heal facial eczema.

10.1.2 Facial Cleansers

The second most important cosmetics for the prevention of facial eczema are cleansers. Facial hygiene is an important concern; however, the cleanser must normalize the biofilm without damaging the stratum corneum skin barrier. The biofilm is the thin layer of sebum, eccrine sweat, apocrine sweat, skin care products, cosmetics, medications, environmental dirt, bacteria, and fungus that is present on the facial skin surface. Thus,

a cleanser must remove sebum, p. acnes, other bacteria, Malassezia, other fungi, and Demodex to maintain the health of the facial skin. Good facial hygiene is a careful balance between maintaining a healthy biofilm while preserving the integrity of the barrier by leaving the intercellular lipids intact and preventing facial eczema. This can be challenging because cleansers cannot accurately differentiate between sebum and intercellular lipids. It is further challenged by the ever-changing sebum production of the facial glands, which varies by both age and climate, and the different bacteria with which the body comes in contact.

Cleansers for the face must be selected to maintain hygiene while preserving the intercellular lipids, which form the skin barrier. The three major chemical categories of cleansers are soaps, syndets, and combars, which can be placed on a variety of cleansing implements from the hands to a washcloth to a disposable face cloth (Table 10.2). True soap is a specific type of cleanser with an alkaline pH of 9–10 created by chemically reacting a fat and an alkali to create a fatty acid salt with detergent properties. Soap efficiently removes both sebum and intercellular lipids making it an excellent general facial cleanser, but a poor choice for dry, sensitive facial skin. Milder cleansing for normal to dry facial skin is found in the syndet cleansers, which contain sodium cocoyl isethionate formulated at a neutral pH of 5.5–7. This more neutral pH removes fewer intercellular lipids, making it a cleanser suitable for the prevention of facial xerotic eczema. If the patient has extremely dry facial skin or tendencies toward eczematous skin conditions, a moisturizing liquid cleanser that leaves behind a thin layer of petrolatum, dimethicone, or vegetable oils should be selected for prevention of disease recurrence. Finally, extremely dry sensitive skin should be cleansed with a lipid-free cleanser, based on sodium laurel lauryl sulfate, for facial eczema prevention.

Table 10.2 Cleanser categories

Cleanser category	Formulation	Appropriate patient selection
Soap (Ivory, P &G; pure and natural, Jergens)	Fatty acid salt, pH 9–10	Normal-to-oily skin, general cleansing
Syndet (Dove, Unilever; Olay Bar, P & G)	Synthetic detergent (sodium cocoyl isethionate), pH 5.5–7	Normal-to-dry skin, general cleansing
Combar (Dial, Dial Corporation; Irish Spring, Coast, Colgate-Palmolive)	Soap and syndet combined, pH 7–9	Triclosan antibacterial useful in patient with wound infection, bacterial colonization, or body odor
Moisturizing body wash (Olay Ribbons, P & G; Dove Nutrium, Unilever)	Synthetic detergent combined with petrolatum, dimethicone, and/or vegetable oils	Extremely dry skin, similar to conditioning shampoo, leaves behind a thin film of occlusive moisturizers to minimize skin scaling and roughness
Lipid-free cleanser (Cetaphil, Galderma; Aquanil, Person and Covey; CeraVe Cleanser, Coria)	Sodium laurel sulfate with cetyl alcohol and stearyl alcohol	Dry, sensitive skin

10.2 Eyelid Dermatitis

The most sensitive skin on the entire body is located on the eyelids. The eyelid skin moves constantly as the eyes open and close, thus it must possess unique mechanical properties. It must be thin enough for rapid movement yet strong enough to protect the tender eye tissues. Eyelid tissue shows the state of health and age of an individual more rapidly than any other skin of the body. When others comment on a tired appearance, they are usually assessing the appearance of the eyes and the eyelid tissue. When others comment on a sickly appearance, they are also assessing the appearance of the eyes and the eyelid tissue. The eyelid skin appears to age quickly resulting in the presence of redundant upper eyelid tissue and lower eyelid bags. The redundant upper eyelid tissue is due to loss of facial fat, cumulative collagen loss in the eyelid skin from UV exposure, and the effect of gravity pulling down the upper eyelid skin. Lower eyelid bags are also due to the effect UV damage and gravity, but edema or swelling may also contribute. This edema may be due to retained body fluids or the release of histamine from inhaled allergens. All of these factors contribute to the complexity of the eyelid skin.

The eyelids are the thinnest skin on the body; hence the eyelids are the most common site for irritant contact dermatitis and allergic contact dermatitis, either from products that are directly applied to the eyelids or from products transferred to the eyelids by the hands. The eyelid skin also has a paucity of sebaceous glands, making it a common area of skin dryness. While there are no hairs on the eyelids themselves, the eyelashes form an interesting transition between the keratinized eyelid skin and the cartilage of the tarsal plate giving structure to the edge of the eyelid. Tearing from the eye impacts the skin of the eyelid, since wetting and drying of the eyelid tissues can predispose to dermatitis.

The eyelids are also a common source of symptoms induced by allergies. These symptoms can be itching, stinging, and/or burning. Most persons with these symptoms respond by vigorously rubbing the eyelids. This can cause mechanical damage to the eyelid skin from minor trauma resulting in sloughing of portions of the protective stratum corneum to major trauma resulting in small tears in the skin. Most of the skin on the body responds by thickening when rubbed. Eyelid skin will also thicken, but this predisposes to decreased functioning and worsening of the symptoms.

10.2.1 Eyelid Cosmetics

Eyelids are also a common site for cosmetic adornment. There are more individual colored cosmetics for the eyelid area than any other body area to include mascara, eyeliner, eye shadow, and eyebrow pencil.

These cosmetics and the products used to remove them can be a source of both allergic and irritant contact dermatitis. The most common cause of cosmetic eyelid dermatitis is the use of light-reflective pigments in eye shadow powders or creams. Mica, bismuth oxychloride, fish scale, and ground minerals are used to create the iridescent appearance of the cosmetic when applied to the eyelid skin. These small particles can create irritation when placed on sensitive eyelid skin, resulting in an irritant contact dermatitis. Cosmetic-induced eyelid dermatitis can be prevented by selecting matte finish eyelid cosmetics without the light-reflective particles.

10.2.2 Eyelid Moisturizers

The most common cause of eyelid dermatitis is barrier disruption from xerotic eczema. Since the eyelid is relatively poor in oil glands, dry eyelid skin is frequently seen due to overly aggressive removal of lipids. This may be due to the use of a strong cleanser or products designed to solubilize oil-based waterproof cosmetics, such as mascara and eyeliner. Anything that damages the intercellular lipids or the corneocytes will result in eyelid eczema. Thus, eyelid hygiene must achieve a careful balance between the removal of excess sebum and old cosmetics to prevent eyelash infections and seborrheic blepharitis, while preventing damage to the intercellular lipids and ensuing eyelid eczema. Moisturizers for the eye area should be composed of occlusive substances that have minimal chance for allergic or irritant reactions, reduced ability to enter the eye, and excellent moisturizing properties (CeraVe, Coria).

10.2.3 Eyelid Cleansers

The use of eyelid moisturizers should be complemented by the formulation of cleansers designed to maintain the biofilm around the eye area. Cleansing of the eyelid tissue is indeed a delicate task. Typically, the skin should be handled very gently, due to its thin nature, and cleansing should remove excess sebum while preserving the intercellular lipids. Lipid-free cleansers (Table 10.2) are excellent to prevent eyelid dermatitis. If more aggressive cleansing is required, such as provided by a foaming face wash (Olay Foaming Face Wash, P & G) an appropriate moisturizer must be selected that will provide an environment for healing while the intercellular lipids are resynthesized (Cetaphil Cream, Galderma).

10.3 Cheilitis

Inflammation of the lip tissues, known as cheilitis, can be related to a variety of causes including lip-licking, irritant contact dermatitis, allergic contact dermatitis, actinic damage, and eczema. Cheilitis is a condition that combines both medical and cosmetic treatments, since lip balms and lipsticks may be an important part of disease prevention, or in some cases, the cause of the cheilitis.

Cheilitis is basically an inflammation of the lips. This inflammation may be due to defective cellular repair from actinic damage, which leads to leukoplakia and chronic lip peeling. This is perhaps the most common cause of cheilitis in men. Alternatively, cheilitis may be due to an allergic reaction to cosmetics. The most common culprit is castor oil, which is found in the majority of lipsticks. Irritation from medications or lip-licking may also contribute. The irritation may be due to retinoids applied elsewhere on the face migrating to the lips or maceration from repeated wetting and drying of the lips. Lastly, there may be individuals who have defective oil production from the tiny oil glands found on the periphery of the lip where the transitional mucosa meets the keratinized skin. These sebaceous glands, also known as Fordyce spots, appear as yellow dots within the red vermillion. These individuals could be viewed as having a type of lip eczema.

10.3.1 Xerotic Cheilitis

In the female patient, lipsticks can be used to prevent and treat xerotic cheilitis. Lipsticks are mixtures of waxes, oils, and pigments in varying concentration to yield the characteristics of the final product. A moisturizing lipstick designed to prevent cheilitis should contain a high concentration of waxes combined with some oils to create an environment optimal for maintenance of the transitional lip barrier. The waxes commonly incorporated into lipstick formulations are white beeswax, candelilla wax, carnauba wax, ozokerite wax, lanolin wax, ceresin wax, and other synthetic waxes. Usually, lipsticks contain a combination of these waxes carefully selected and blended to achieve the desired melting point. Oils are then selected (i.e., castor oil, white mineral oil, lanolin oil, hydrogenated vegetable oils) to form a film suitable for application to the lips. The oils provide emolliency in the lipstick, making the lips feel smooth and soft.

Lip balms can also be used in the treatment and prevention of cheilitis. They can be viewed as moisturizers for the lips without the pigments contained in the previously discussed lipsticks. Lip balms are designed to reduce TEWL creating an environment optimal for lip healing. The best prevention for xerotic cheilitis is the use of lip balm at night prior to bed (Lip Moisture SPF15, Neutrogena). The lips are at rest at night and the lip balm the greatest effect when applied at this time.

10.3.2 Allergic Contact Cheilitis

Allergic contact dermatitis is also a cause of cheilitis, which can be difficult to diagnose. Several ingredients unique to lipstick formulation can cause allergic contact dermatitis in the sensitized patient.[1] Castor oil, found in almost all lipsticks due to its excellent ability to dissolve bromo acid dyes, is a cause of allergic contact lip cheilitis.[2-4] Another common lipstick sensitizer is the bromo acid dyes, one of which is eosin (D and C Red No. 21).[5] Eosin is used in the indelible red lipsticks designed to stain the lips and extend the amount of time color remains on the lips. Many long-wearing lip products contain this allergen. In addition to causing allergic contact dermatitis, the bromo acid dyes may also cause irritant contact dermatitis and worsen lip dryness. Other ingredients in

lipstick that may cause allergic contact dermatitis include: ricinoleic acid,[6] benzoic acid,[7] lithol rubine BCA (Pigment Red 57–1),[8] microcrystalline wax,[9] oxybenzone,[10] propyl gallate,[11] and C18 aliphatic compounds.[12]

10.4 Postinflammatory Hyperpigmentation

Postinflammatory hyperpigmentation is a common cosmetic problem of the entire body that is best prevented rather than treated. The prevention of postinflammatory hyperpigmentation may be difficult, especially in Fitzpatrick skin types III and higher. This unsightly pigmentation can occur after casual or deliberate sun exposure, unintended injury to the skin, or following skin surgery. A successful treatment must remove existing pigment from the skin, shut down the manufacture of melanin, and prevent the transfer of existing melanin to the melanosomes. Currently, there is no topical prescription or OTC product that achieves these three goals. The following discussion divides the prevention and treatment of postinflammatory hyperpigmentation into the prescription pigment-lightening agents such as hydroquinone mequinol, tretinoin, and azelaic acid (Table 10.3); and the botanical OTC agents such as ascorbic acid, licorice extract, alpha lipoic acid, kojic acid, aleosin, and arbutin. There is no doubt that the prescription products are more effective than the botanical derivatives, but both are discussed for completeness.

Table 10.3 Skin-lightening ingredients for postinflammatory hyperpigmentation

Skin-lightening ingredient	Effect on melanogenesis	Relative efficacy
Hydroquinone	Inhibits tyrosinase by interfering with copper binding reducing conversion of dihydroxyphenylanlanine (DOPA) to melanin	Highest
Azelaic acid	Inhibits tyrosinase by interfering with copper binding reducing conversion of DOPA to melanin	Moderate
Kojic acid	Inhibits tyrosinase by interfering with copper binding reducing conversion of DOPA to melanin	Moderate
Arbutin	Decreases tyrosinase activity without affecting messenger RNA expression	Moderate
Liquirtin	Increases melanin granule dispersion	Low
Vitamin C	Interacts with copper ions to reduce dopaquinone and blocks dihydrochinindol-2-carboxyl acid oxidation	Low

10.4.1 Prescription Hyperpigmentation Topical Agents

10.4.1.1 Hydroquinone

The gold standard for hyperpigmentation therapy in the United States remains hydroquinone. This substance is actually quite controversial, having been removed from the OTC markets in Europe and Asia. Concern arose because oral hydroquinone has been reported to cause cancer in mice fed large amounts of the substance. While oral consumption probably is not related to topical application, hydroquinone remains controversial because it actually is toxic to melanocytes. Hydroquinone, a phenolic compound chemically known as 1,4 dihydroxybenzene, functions by inhibiting the enzymatic oxidation of tyrosine and phenol oxidases. It covalently binds to histidine or interacts with copper at the active site of tyrosinase. It also inhibits RNA and DNA synthesis and may alter melanosome formation, thus selectively damaging melanocytes. These activities suppress the melanocyte metabolic processes inducing gradual decrease of melanin pigment production.[13]

Hydroquinone is available in both the OTC and prescription markets in the US. The maximum concentration in OTC formulations is 2% while most prescription formulations are 4%. It is possible to compound hydroquinone creams as high as 8%, but the formulations are unstable with rapid oxidation represented by browning of the product. In all formulations, hydroquinone is unstable, turning brown upon contact with air. Once the hydroquinone has oxidized, it is no longer active and should be discarded.

Prescription hydroquinone formulations have tried to increase the potency of formulations by adding penetration enhancers such as glycolic acid, sunscreens, and tretinoin as a supplemental pigment lightening agent. Other prescription formulations have added microsponges to create time delivery of hydroquinone to the skin while others have placed the hydroquinone in a special canister dispenser.

The initiation of hydroquinone prior to elective cosmetic surgery is the best preventative for minimizing and possibly eliminating postinflammatory hyperpigmentation. Hydroquinone can be used to decrease pigment production prior to the skin surgery that will ultimately drive pigment production.

10.4.1.2 Mequinol

Mequinol is the newest prescription skin-lightening agent approved in the US. It has also received approval in Europe. It is chemically known as 4-hydroxyanisole. Other names include methoxyphenol, hydroquinone monomethyl ether, and p-hydroxyanisole. Mequinol is available in the US in a 2% concentration and is commercially marketed as a prescription skin lightener in combination with 0.01% tretinoin as a penetration enhancer and vitamin C, in the form of ascorbic acid and ascorbyl palmitate, to enhance skin lightening. These active agents are dissolved in an ethyl alcohol vehicle. The exact mechanism of action accounting for the skin-lightening properties of mequinol is unknown; however, it is a substrate for tyrosinase, thereby acting as a competitive inhibitor in the formation of melanin precursors. It does not damage the melanocyte as does hydroquinone.

Mequinol can be irritating to the skin and cause hyperpigmentation in persons with sensitive skin. Prior to picking this ingredient for the prevention of postinflammatory hyperpigmentation, a small test site should be selected to daily application for 2 weeks. If no skin darkening occurs, the mequinol may be suitable for the prevention of postinflammatory hyperpigmentation. It may actually be the 0.01% tretinoin that is the irritant in the presently available commercial mequinol formulation, rather than the mequinol itself (Solage, barrier therapeutics).

10.4.1.3 Tretinoin

Topical tretinoin is used alone and in combination with hydroquinone as prescription pigment lightening treatment. Tretinoin has an effect on skin pigmentation as seen by a decrease in cutaneous freckling and lentigenes.[14] It is the irregular grouping and activation of melanocytes that accounts for the dyspigmentation associated with photoaging,[15] but normalization of this change has been histologically demonstrated with retinoids.[16] While this effect is more dramatic with topical tretinoin, topical retinol has been thought to provide similar effects as a cosmeceutical. For persons with difficult-to-manage postinflammatory hyperpigmentation, tretinoin can be combined with hydroquinone and a topical corticosteroid, to reduce inflammation, in a presently marketed combination formulation (TriLuma, Galderma).

10.4.1.4 Azelaic Acid

Azelaic acid is available currently as a 15% gel approved in the US for the treatment of rosacea (Finacea, Intendis). It is a 9-carbon dicarboxylic acid obtained from cultures of Pityrosporum ovale that may be a treatment alternative for individuals allergic to hydroquinone. Although its lightening effects are mild, several large studies done with a diverse ethnic background population have compared its efficacy to that of hydroquinone.[17,18] It too interferes with tyrosinase activity, but may also interfere with DNA synthesis. It appears to have a specificity for abnormal melanocytes and for this reason has been used to suppress the progression of lentigo maligna to lentigo maligna melanoma. Azelaic acid may be an alternative to the previously mentioned prescription formulations in persons with sensitive skin or an allergy to other pigment lightening ingredients for the prevention of postinflammatory hyperpigmentation.

10.4.2 Nonprescription Hyperpigmentation Topical Agents

There are a variety of nonprescription topical agents that are available in cosmeceuticals and cosmetics to prevent postinflammatory hyperpigmentation. None of these ingredients are as efficacious as hydroquinone; however, they are considered safe for use both in the US and worldwide.

10.4.2.1 Ascorbic Acid

Ascorbic acid, also known as vitamin C, is used in the treatment and prevention of postinflammatory hyperpigmentation. It interrupts the production of melanogenesis by interacting with copper ions to reduce dopaquinone and blocking dihydrochinindol-2-carboxyl acid oxidation.[19] Ascorbic acid, an antioxidant, is rapidly oxidized when exposed to air and is of limited stability. High concentrations of ascorbic acid must be used with caution as the low pH can be irritating to the skin actually precipitating postinflammatory hyperpigmentation.

10.4.2.2 Licorice Extract

Licorice extracts are being used as topical anti-inflammatories to decrease skin hyperpigmentation. The active agents are known as liquiritin and isoliquertin, which are glycosides containing flavenoids.[20] Liquiritin induces skin lightening by dispersing melanin. It is typically applied to the skin in a dose of 1 g/day for 4 weeks to see a clinical result. Irritation is fortunately not a side effect.

10.4.2.3 Alpha Lipoic Acid

Alpha lipoic acid is found in a variety of antiaging cosmeceuticals to function as an antioxidant, but it may also have very limited value in postinflammatory hyperpigmentation. It is a disulfide derivative of octanoic acid that is able to inhibit tyrosinase. However, it is a large molecule and cutaneous penetration to the level of the melanocyte is challenging.

10.4.2.4 Kojic Acid

Kojic acid, chemically known as 5-hydroxymethyl-4H-pyrane-4-one, is one of the most popular cosmeceutical skin-lightening agents found in cosmetic counter skin-lightening creams distributed worldwide. It is a hydrophilic fungal derivative obtained from Aspergillus and Penicillium species. It is the most popular agent employed in the Orient for the treatment of melasma.[21] Some studies indicate that kojic acid is equivalent to hydroquinone in pigment-lightening ability.[22] The activity of kojic acid is attributed to its ability to prevent tyrosinase activity by binding to copper. It may be useful in postinflammatory hyperpigmentation.

10.4.2.5 Aleosin

Aleosin is a low-molecular-weight glycoprotein obtained from the aloe vera plant. It is a natural hydroxymethyl-chromone functioning to inhibit tyrosinase by competitive inhibition at the dihydroxyphenylanlanine (DOPA) oxidation site.[23,24] In contrast to hydroquinone, it shows no cell cytotoxicity; however, it has a limited ability to penetrate the skin due to its hydrophilic nature. It is sometimes mixed with arbutin to enhance its skin-lightening abilities.

10.4.2.6 Arbutin

Arbutin is obtained from the leaves of the vaccinicum vitis-idaca and other related plants. It is a naturally occurring gluconopyranoside that causes decreased tyrosinase activity without affecting messenger RNA expression.[25] It also inhibits melanosome maturation. Arbutin is not toxic to melanocytes and is used in a variety of pigment-lightening preparations in Japan at concentrations of 3%. Higher concentrations are more efficacious than lower concentrations, but a paradoxical pigment darkening and postinflammatory hyperpigmentation may occur.

10.4.3 Sunscreens

Sunscreens are another product category that can be used to prevent postinflammatory hyperpigmentation by minimizing the pigmenting effect of ultraviolet (UV) radiation. Sunscreens are designed to absorb UVA radiation (320–360 nm), accounting for pigmentation, and UVB radiation (290–320 nm), accounting for sunburn. Table 10.4 summarizes the more commonly used UVA and UVB filters. The primary UVA absorbers on this list are the benzophenones, anthralinates, and avobenzone. The primary UVB absorbers are the PABA derivatives, salicylates, and cinnamates; substances that absorb both UVB and UVA are titanium dioxide and

Table 10.4 Cosmeceutical sunscreens

Sunscreen categories	Spectrum of protection	Ingredients
Organic UVB filters	290–320 nm	Octyl methoxycinnamate, ocytocrylene, octyl salicylate
Organic UVA filters	320–360 nm	Ecamsule, avobenzone, oxybenzone, menthyl anthranilate
Inorganic UVB/UVA filters	Total reflection of all radiation	Zinc oxide, titanium dioxide

zinc oxide. Most quality sunscreens to prevent postinflammatory hyperpigmentation combine these ingredients to yield a product with excellent photoprotection that is cosmetically elegant.

10.4.3.1 UVA Filters and Prevention of Tanning Response

The UVA absorbers are most important in the prevention of postinflammatory hyperpigmentation. UVA absorbers can be divided into organic and inorganic subgroups. The organic subgroup undergoes a chemical reaction, known as resonance delocalization, to transform the UVA energy into heat. The main organic UVA absorber in sunscreens that prevent postinflammatory hyperpigmentation is avobenzone. Avobenzone must be combined with other organic filters because it is rapidly degraded by UV exposure. Almost 36% of the avobenzone in a sunscreen formulation becomes chemically inactive on initial exposure. Thus, avobenzone is combined with oxybenzone and octocrylene to enhance its photostability. Other UVA organic filters, such as the anthranilates (menthyl anthranilate), can be added as secondary agents.

However, some of the most effective UVA photoprotectants are the organic filters zinc oxide and titanium dioxide. These white powders primarily reflect UVA radiation, but may also absorb a small amount. They also reflect UVB radiation. Zinc oxide is available as a microfine powder, but it cannot be used in high concentration due to the white-skin appearance created. Typically, zinc oxide is only used in concentrations of 2% or less for this reason. The newer nanoparticle zinc oxide is transparent, but very controversial. The controversy revolves around the ability of nanoparticle zinc oxide to penetrate the skin and create a permanent nonreactive dermal reservoir. The safety of this reservoir is unknown at this writing, leading the cosmetics industry to voluntarily refrain from use of this material until a better understanding of its skin effects can be obtained.

Titanium dioxide is typically used in a larger particle size than zinc oxide. The term micronized is used to describe these particles because they are of many different sizes as compared to the even size of microfine particles. The microfine formulations produce less skin whitening than the micronized formulations. Both particulates are often silicone-coated to decrease the generation of secondary oxygen radicals when struck by UV radiation. Thus, the most effective inorganic sunscreens for preventing postinflammatory hyperpigmentation are zinc oxide and titanium dioxide while the most effective organic sunscreen is stabilized avobenzone. However, the sunscreen filter is just as important as the ability of the sunscreen to stay on the skin preventing postinflammatory hyperpigmentation.

10.4.3.2 Sunscreen Longevity

Providing superior longevity of the sunscreen film on the skin surface and preventing postinflammatory hyperpigmentation can be accomplished by imparting water-resistant characteristics, since sweat, humidity, and a moist environment are the three most common factors that result in sunscreen failure (Table 10.5).

Water resistance is predicated on the fact that water soluble and oil-soluble substances do not mix. Thus, if a sunscreen is predominantly oil, with minimal water, it will not dissolve in the presence of water or perspiration. However, oil-dominant sunscreens are greasy and sticky, imparting poor aesthetics. This has led to

development of silicone-based sunscreens, since silicone is an oil that is not greasy or sticky and has excellent water-resistant properties.

Another method of imparting water resistance to a sunscreen is to alter or eliminate the emulsifier. The emulsifier allows water and oil-soluble ingredients to coexist as one continuous phase. Unfortunately, the sunscreen emulsifier will also allow perspiration or swimming pool water to mix with the oily ingredients, facilitating removal. This has led to the development of acrylate cross polymers and liquid crystal gels as the vehicle without an emulsifier. This increases the longevity of the sunscreen, an important consideration on areas such as the face that are prone to pigmentation following surgery.

The last method used to confer sunscreen longevity in a moist environment is predicated on creating a film resistant to water removal. This can be accomplished with phospholipids, structurally similar to natural sebum, that create a thin oily film on the skin. Polymers can also be used to create a thin water-resistant film on the skin surface.

10.4.3.3 SPF and Sunscreen Efficacy

Another important consideration in sunscreen efficacy is the amount of photoprotection afforded by the product. It has been traditionally thought that a sunscreen with an SPF of 15 was sufficient. Recently, newer sunscreen formulations have been introduced with higher SPF ratings, providing added benefits. While an SPF of 15 was thought to be sufficient for the prevention of sunburn, it is not optimal for protection against postinflammatory hyperpigmentation. A higher SPF cannot be achieved without providing additional UVA photoprotection. At present, no rating system exists for the UVA qualities of a sunscreen.

In summary, a sunscreen to prevent postinflammatory hyperpigmentation should contain broad-spectrum UVA photoprotective ingredients, water-resistant qualities, and a high SPF.

10.5 Hyperhidrosis

Another common cosmetic problem is unwanted axillary perspiration. Clearly, the biggest advance in the treatment of this condition is the injection of

Table 10.5 Water-resistant sunscreens

Chemical technology	Mechanism of efficacy
Water-in-oil emulsions	Oil is the main ingredient and resists removal by water
Silicones	Hydrophobic oily liquid that resists removal by water and forms film over skin surface
Acrylate crosspolymer	No emulsifier required which prevents water from dissolving the sunscreen, used in titanium dioxide preparations
Liquid crystal gels	Hydrophobic emulsifiers used that resist water, used in titanium dioxide preparations
Phospholipid emulsifiers	Substances engineered to mimic natural sebum (potassium cetyl phosphate) with water-resistant properties
Film forming polymers	Thin polymer film formed over the skin with inherent water resistance

botulinum toxin, which produces dramatic long-term sweat reduction. Yet antiperspirants remain a viable effective alternative in some patients. Antiperspirants can even be combined with botulinum toxin to prolong or increase the effect.

Antiperspirants function to reduce both apocrine and eccrine sweat. Eccrine sweat is a clear, odorless fluid of pH 4–6.8 composed of 98–99% water, sodium chloride, lower fatty acids, lactic acid, citric acid, ascorbic acid, urea, and uric acid. Apocrine sweat is a turbid, viscous, odorless fluid of pH 6–7.5 that has high content water, in addition to protein, carbohydrate waste materials, and sodium chloride. The amount of eccrine perspiration is much greater than the amount of apocrine perspiration. An effective antiperspirant must reduce both types of perspiration.

10.5.1 Antiperspirant Mechanism of Action

To reduce axillary hyperhidrosis, the antiperspirant must reach some 25,000 eccrine glands and coagulate the sweat duct protein. Antiperspirants contain metal salts that alter intraductal keratin fibrils to cause eccrine duct closure and formation of a horny plug, which obstructs sweat flow to the skin surface.[26] The plug is formed by aluminum and zirconium metal salts.[27] The original antiperspirant formulation was a 25% solution of aluminum chloride hexahydrate in distilled water, but it was extremely irritating.[28] More modern antiperspirant formulations contain aluminum chloride, aluminum chlorohydrate, aluminum zirconium chlorohydrate, and buffered aluminum sulfate.[29] These metals provide a better balance between efficacy and skin irritation.

An effective antiperspirant must reduce sweat by at least 20% as mandated by the FDA, since antiperspirants are regulated as OTC drugs. Antiperspirants labeled as highly effective must reduce sweat by at least 30%. The antiperspirant must create a long-lasting plug in the sweat duct ostia quickly. This is best accomplished by evenly spreading the antiperspirant in the axillary vault. If the antiperspirant does not touch the sweat duct, it will not work. The active agent in the newer antiperspirants is aluminum-zirconium tetrachlorohydrexgly complex. This complex can reduce axillary perspiration by 40–60%. These aluminum salts have an acidic pH of 3.0–4.2.[30] Irritation is reduced

by incorporating skin conditioning agents, such as dimethicone or cyclomethicone, into the formulation. The silicone imparts skin soothing properties to the skin irritated by the antiperspirant ingredients.

10.5.2 Optimizing Antiperspirant Efficacy

Antiperspirants can fail to control hyperhidrosis for many reasons. The most common reason is use of a poor formulation that does not contain an optimal active ingredient mix and appropriate vehicle construction to deliver results. Antiperspirants also fail because an even film cannot be obtained that covers the entire armpit. The antiperspirant must be in contact with each and every eccrine and apocrine duct in the armpit to work. Thus, the applicator should be domed to fit into the axilla and dispense a thick even film of product. The film must be somewhat water-resistant or it will be rinsed away by perspiration before the plug can be formed in the ducts. For this reason, the armpit should be dry when the product is applied. Many dermatologists recommend that patients apply an OTC or prescription antiperspirant and then occlude the armpit with plastic wrap. If the patient sweats profusely under the occlusion, the perspiration may wash away the active ingredients before a plug can be formed. Thus, the occlusion may decrease the efficacy of the antiperspirant rather than increase efficacy due to enhanced penetration.

Another possible cause for antiperspirant failure is inconsistent application. Compliance is important to achieve optimal results. It takes about 10 days of antiperspirant application for the complete plug to be formed in the sweat duct. If the patient decides after 3 days of application that the antiperspirant has not worked sufficiently, they have not given the product an adequate trial. Furthermore, the plug is completely gone 14 days after the last application. Continuous daily application is necessary to achieve and maintain the sweat reduction effect.

Another consideration is the depth of the plug within the sweat duct. Plugs that are more deeply placed in the sweat gland will provide better sweat reduction than those that are superficially situated. If the plug is very close to the surface, it is possible that it can be removed by the rubbing of clothing or shaving. Patients who complain that antiperspirants do not work may wish to wear loose fitting clothing around the armpits and use only light razor pressure when shaving the armpits. The deepest plugs are created by prescription aluminum chloride solutions, but these formulations must be used carefully as they can irritate skin and ruin natural fabrics, such as rayon, cotton, and silk. More superficial plugs are created by OTC antiperspirants containing aluminum chlorohydrate. Intermediate depth plugs are created by OTC antiperspirants containing aluminum zirconium chlorohydrate.

Optimizing antiperspirant efficacy requires the use of a well-formulated product that is consistently applied to the entire armpit as a thin film. One of the newer formulations uses aluminum-zirconium tetrachlorohydrexgly complex, which has good efficacy with minimal skin irritation (Secret Platinum, P & G). This irritation is further reduced by the presence of dimethicone in the vehicle, which also provides for easy spreadability of a thin water-resistant film. Efficacy can be further enhanced by applying the antiperspirant twice daily. The bedtime application is actually more important than the morning application because the body is at rest and sweating reduced. The reduced sweating decreases the removal of the antiperspirant from the armpit and allows the active ingredient to remain in contact with the skin longer creating a stronger plug. Thus, antiperspirants can be optimized to provide prevention for the cosmetic problem of hyperhidrosis.

10.6 Acne

Perhaps the most bothersome cosmetic problem to prevent is acne. Many skin care products have been accused of causing or worsening acne. Is there a true cause-and-effect relationship between skin care or cosmetic product use and the onset of acne? Sometimes this is difficult to ascertain. The final topic of discussion in this chapter addresses the issue of acne cosmetica, a term used to describe acne caused by the application of topical products.

10.6.1 Acne Cosmetica

Acne cosmetica is a concept that was developed many years ago when there was concern that cosmetics could indeed cause comedones formation. The issue of come-

dogenicity in relation to cosmetics arose in 1972 when Kligman and Mills described a low-grade acne characterized by closed comedones on the cheeks of women ages 20–25.[31] Many of these women had not experienced adolescent acne. The authors proposed that substances present in cosmetic products induced the formation of closed comedones and, in some cases, a papulopustular eruption. Presently, personal conversations with Dr. Kligman indicate that he no longer believes currently marketed cosmetics cause comedones formation, yet acne related to cosmetics remains a problem.

Lists remain in the literature of ingredients that supposedly cause acne, yet it is practically impossible to find formulations devoid of these substances. The list contains some of the most effective emollients (octyl stearate, isocetyl stearate), detergents (sodium lauryl sulfate), occlusive moisturizers (mineral oil, petrolatum, sesame oil, cocoa butter), and emulsifiers found in the cosmetic industry.[32] A product line that excluded all these ingredients would exhibit poor efficacy and aesthetics.

The skin care industry has developed the nomenclature of noncomedogenic and nonacnegenic to assure the consumer that the product does not cause acne; however, these claims carry no scientific validity as they are strictly for marketing purposes. The claims were developed to create a new consumer image for cosmetic lines designed to minimize acne. While testing is not required to make these claims, most large companies voluntarily will use established industry tests to ensure product safety and substantiate their claims.

Many manufacturers, however, make noncomedogenic and nonacnegenic claims based on the safety profiles of the individual ingredients in the formulation. This is inaccurate. Noncomedogenic and nonacnegenic claims should be made based on clinical testing of the finished formulation. There are several established methods of testing cosmetic products.

10.6.2 Comedogenicity Testing

Comedogeniticity testing is typically carried out on either the rabbit ear or the human upper back. Rabbit ear testing is forbidden in the European Union and has been largely abandoned in the US as most companies wish to advertise that their products do not involve animal testing. Human testing is conducted on the upper back of individuals who have demonstrated the ability to form comedones. This is confirmed by performing a cyanoacrylate biopsy on the upper back of volunteers. The biopsy is obtained by placing cyanoacrylate glue on a microscope slide and allowing the acrylate to polymerize, adhering the stratum corneum to the glass slide. The slide is then peeled from the upper back and a thin layer of stratum corneum along with follicular contents is removed. The number of comedonal plugs removed is counted and should be at least ten to provide an adequate sample size. The cosmetic for comedogenicity testing is applied to the upper back under occlusion Monday through Friday for 2 weeks.

At the end of the testing period, the cyanoacrylate biopsy is repeated. One negative control patch is applied with no cosmetic and one positive control patch is applied with coal tar. The final counts are obtained by viewing the slide upside down with a low magnification microscope and counting in a 1 cm squared field. If the number of comedonal plugs increases as compared to baseline, the cosmetic is considered comedogenic. If the number of comedonal plugs remains the same or decreases, the cosmetic can be labeled noncomedogenic. This type of human testing is safe and appears to accurately predict the comedogenic potential of a cosmetic.

10.6.3 Comedogenic Ingredients

There are many frequently used cosmetic ingredients that have been associated with comedones formation. Perhaps mineral oil is the most common. Several cosmetic lines have been founded on the premise that mineral oil is a "bad" ingredient and avoidance of this material creates a "good" facial cosmetic. Mineral oil is a lightweight, inexpensive oil that is odorless and tasteless. Mineral oil may have been comedogenic in the past, but in current forms used in cosmetic formulations it is not comedogenic. Mineral oil is available for purchase in industrial and cosmetic grades. Industrial grade mineral is used as a machine lubricant and may be contaminated with tar by-products, which are comedogenic. However, cosmetic grade mineral oil is certified pure by the supplier and is noncomedogenic. No quality cosmetic company would use industrial grade mineral oil in their products.

Most of the ingredients of old that were considered comedogenic were derived from petroleum distillates. It is well-known in dermatology that tar is comedogenic. If a raw material is contaminated with tar, it may cause comedones formation. With new mass spectroscopy and better control on the manufacture of cosmetic materials, by-product contamination is rare. Most cosmetic companies require purity testing from their suppliers and then retest shipments of raw materials for purity in their own laboratories. The risk of ruining a good reputation based on a poor-quality raw material is too great in today's competitive market. The old lists of comedogenic substances probably need to be retired in the modern marketplace.

10.6.4 Acneiform Eruptions and Cosmetics

Acnegenicity must be distinguished from comedogenicity. While comedogenicity is rare, acnegenicity is much more common from skin care products. Comedogenicity results in the formation of comedones while acnegenicity results in the formation of inflammatory perifollicular papules. These papules may represent true acne with the involvement of the sebaceous gland or may simply represent a perifollicular acneiform eruption, which is undoubtedly more common.

Many patients note the occurrence of "breakouts" following the use of moisturizers, facial foundations, sunscreens, etc. These patients typically present with perifollicular papules and pustules in a random distribution over the face. This eruption appears within 24–48 h after wearing the facial product. This is insufficient time for true acne to develop as evidenced by follicular rupture. However, it is sufficient time for an irritant contact dermatitis to develop. Most liquid formulations contain an emulsifier that allows the oily and water-soluble ingredients to coexist in one continuous phase. These emulsifiers can also emulsify sebum and create perifollicular irritation. Most companies test their product for acnegenicity for this reason. The tests usually involve an in-use test where volunteers use the product for 12 weeks with every 4-week evaluation by a dermatologist. All adverse reactions are recorded. If these perifollicular eruptions do not occur, the product can then accurately claim the formulation to be nonacnegenic.

Persons who are prone to acneiform eruptions should prevent cosmetic problems by use-testing a new cosmetic or skin care product inside the elbow for five consecutive nights. If no problems arise, the product can then be applied to an area lateral to the eye for five consecutive nights. If no problems present, the product can be applied to the entire face. This type of testing can best prevent a total facial eruption.

10.7 Summary

This chapter has discussed prevention of the common cosmetic problems including facial eczema, eyelid dermatitis, cheilitis, postinflammatory hyperpigmentation, hyperhidrosis, and acne. The proper selection of skin care products can aid in prevention. Adequate treatment of these conditions is best addressed through the use of pharmaceuticals in conjunction with OTC drugs, such as sunscreens and antiperspirants, along with the use of skin care products, such as moisturizers, skin-lightening agents, and cleansers. A complete understanding of cosmetic problems involves understanding all the product categories available for therapeutic intervention.

References

1. Sulzgerger MD, Boodman J, Byrne LA, Mallozzi ED. Acquired specific hypersensitivity to simple chemicals. Cheilitis with special reference to sensitivity to lipsticks. *Arch Dermatol.* 1938;37:597–615
2. Sai S. Lipstick dermatitis caused by castor oil. *Contact Derm.* 1983;9:75
3. Brandle I, Boujnah-Khouadja A, Foussereau J. Allergy to castor oil. *Contact Derm.* 1983;9:424–425
4. Andersen KE, Neilsen R. Lipstick dermatitis related to castor oil. *Contact Derm.* 1984;11:253–254
5. Calan CD. Allergic sensitivity to eosin. *Acta Allergol.* 1959;13:493–499
6. Sai S. Lipstick dermatitis caused by ricinoleic acid. *Contact Derm.* 1983;9:524
7. Calnan CD. Amyldimethylamino benzoic acid causing lipstick dermatitis. *Contact Derm.* 1980;6:233
8. Hayakawa R, Fujimoto Y, Kaniwa M. Allergic pigmented lip dermatitis from lithol rubine BCA. *Am J Contact Derm.* 1994;5:34–37
9. Darko E, Osmundsen PE. Allergic contact dermatitis to lipcare lipstick. *Contact Derm.* 1984;11:46
10. Aguirre A, Izu R, Gardeazabal J, et al. Allergic contact cheilitis from a lipstick containing oxybenzone. *Contact Derm.* 1992;27:267–268
11. Cronin E. Lipstick dermatitis due to propyl gallate. *Contact Derm.* 1980;6:213–214
12. Hayakawa R, Matsunaga K, Suzuki M, et al. Lipstick dermatitis due to C18 aliphatic compounds. *Contact Derm.* 1987;16:215–219
13. Halder RM, Richards GM. Management of dischromias in ethnic skin. *Dermatol Ther.* 2004;17:151–157
14. Weinstein GD, Nigra TP, Pochi PE, et al. Topical tretinoin for treatment of photodamaged skin. *Arch Dermatol.* 1991;127:659–665
15. Gilchrest BA, Blog FB, Szabo G. Effects of aging and chronic sun exposure on melanocytes in human skin. *J Invest Dermatol.* 1979;73:141–143
16. Bhawan J, Serva AG, Nehal K, et al. Effects of tretinoin on photodamaged skin a histologic study. *Arch Dermatol.* 1991;127:666–672
17. Fitton A, Goa KL. Azelaic acid. a review of its pharmacological properties and therapeutic efficacy in acne and hyperpigmentary skin disorders. *Drugs.* 1991;5:780–798
18. Balina LM, Graupe K. treatment of melasma. 20% azelaic acid versus 4% hydroquinone cream. *Int J Dermatol.* 1991;30(12):893–895
19. Espinal-Perez LE, Moncada B, Castanedo-Cazares JP. A double blind randomized trial of 5% ascorbic acid vs. 4% hydroquinone in melasma. *Int J Dermatol.* 2004; 43(8):604–607
20. Amer M, Metwalli M. Topical Liquiritin improves melasma. *Int J Dermatol.* 2000;39(4):299–301
21. Lim JT. Treatment of melasma using kojic acid in a gel containing hydroquinone and glycolic acid. *Derm Surg.* 1999;25:282–284
22. Garcia A, Fulton JE Jr. The combination of glycolic acid and hydroquinone or kojic acid for the treatment of melasma and related conditions. *Dermatol Surg.* 1996;22(5):443–447
23. Choi S, Lee SK, Kim JE, et al. Aloesin inhibits hyperpigmentation induced by UV radiation. *Clin Exp Dermatol.* 2002;27:513–515
24. Jones K, Hughes J, Hong M, et al. Modulation of melanogenesis by aloesin: a competitive inhibitor of tyrosinase. *Pigment Cell Res.* 2002;15:335–340
25. Hori I, Nihei K, Kubo I. Structural criteria for depigmenting mechanism of arbutin. *Phytother Res.* 2004;18:475–469
26. Shelley WB, Hurley HJ Jr. Studies on topical antiperspirant control of axillary hyperhidrosis. *Acta Derm Venereol.* 1975;55:241–260
27. Jass HE. Rationale of formulations of deodorants and antiperspirants. In: Frost P, Horwitz SN, eds. *Principles of Cosmetics for the Dermatologist.* St. Louis: CV Mosby; 1982:98–104
28. Emery IK. Antiperspirants and deodorants. *Cutis.* 1987; 39:531–532
29. Morton JJP, Palazzolo MJ. Antiperspirants. In: Whittam JH, ed. *Cosmetic Safety: A Primer for Cosmetic Scientists.* New York: Marcel Dekker; 1987:221–263
30. Calogero AV. Antiperspirant and deodorant formulation. *Cosmet Toilet.* 1992;107:63–69
31. Kligman AM, Mills OH. Acne cosmetica. *Arch Dermatol.* 1972;106:843
32. Fulton JE, Pay SR, Fulton JE. Comedogenicity of current therapeutic products, cosmetics, and ingredients in the rabbit ear. *J Am Acad Dermatol.* 1984;10:96–105

Nutrition, Vitamins, and Supplements

11

Evangeline B. Handog and Trisha C. Crisostomo

Everyone has the right to a standard of living adequate for the health and well-being of himself and his family, including food.

Universal Declaration of Human Rights

Adequate nutrition is essential for health and for the management of disease. From the earliest stages of life until old age, proper food and good nutrition is fundamental for survival, physical growth, mental development, performance and productivity, health and well-being.

The right to food and nutrition, and the right to be free from hunger and malnutrition are international human rights being promoted by the World Health Organization (WHO) and other intergovernmental organizations since 1948. In the Rome Declaration on World Food Security (World Food Summit, 1996), heads of state and governments reaffirmed "the right of everyone to have access to safe and nutritious food, consistent with the right to adequate food and the fundamental right of everyone to be free from hunger."[1]

The various nutrients, vitamins, and minerals can be acquired through a balanced diet, but more often than not, supplements are needed to maintain this equilibrium and prevent malnutrition. In 2000, WHO reported 150 million children less than 5 years old having protein–energy malnutrition, but this figure is slowly decreasing. It is distressing to note that WHO also reported 49% of the 10.7 million deaths among children less than 5 years old each year in the developing world are associated with malnutrition.[1]

Malnutrition is most commonly caused by a deficiency in nutrients. It may be caused by insufficient ingestion, abnormal absorption or inadequate utilization of nutrients. However, it may also be caused by an intake excess. WHO reports an emerging epidemic of obesity. Three hundred million adults are diagnosed with obesity, 17.6 million of which are children in developing countries.[1]

Nutritional diseases may present initially or eventually with cutaneous signs and symptoms. This chapter aims to describe the common nutritional disorders encountered by dermatologists and how to prevent them.

11.1 Definition

11.1.1 Nutrition

Nutrition is the process by which a living being takes in substances such as food and nutrients and uses them for life, growth, and the preservation of health.[2] Nutrients are substances not synthesized by the body in enough amounts and thus must be supplemented by the diet. These include proteins, fats, carbohydrates, vitamins, minerals, and water. The required amounts of each essential nutrient differ according to the age and physiologic state of the individual.[3]

E.B. Handog (✉)
Department of Dermatology, Asian Hospital
and Medical Center, Filinvest Corporate City,
Muntinlupa, Alabang, Philippines
e-mail: handogmd@pacific.net.ph

R.A. Norman (ed.), *Preventive Dermatology in Infectious Diseases*,
DOI 10.1007/978-0-85729-847-8_11, © Springer-Verlag London Limited 2012

Table 11.1 Body mass index (BMI) classification

BMI (kg/m^2)	Classification
<18.5	Underweight
18.5–24.9	Normal
25.0–29.9	Overweight
30.0–39.9	Obese
>40	Morbidly obese

BMI = weight (kilograms)/[height(meters)]^2

11.1.2 Body Mass Index

Body mass index (BMI) is computed by dividing the person's weight in kilograms by the square of his height in meters. A BMI within the range of 18.5–24.9 kg/m^2 is normal, a BMI of 25.0–29.9 kg/m^2 is categorized as overweight, a BMI of 30.0–39.9 kg/m^2 is considered obesity and a BMI of >40 kg/m^2 is morbid obesity. WHO suggests that a BMI over 25 is responsible for 64% of male and 77% of female cases of noninsulin-dependent diabetes mellitus (NIDDM). A BMI below 18.5 is considered underweight. BMI measurement is a very quick and simple way of assessing malnutrition, but it does not reflect differences in frame size.[4] Table 11.1 summarizes the BMI value and its corresponding classification.

11.1.3 Degrees of Malnutrition and Treatment

11.1.3.1 Protein–Energy Malnutrition

A lack of intake of protein and energy causes loss of both body mass and adipose tissue, although both may not be necessarily found in a given individual. This disorder is found in conditions wherein the socioeconomic factors limit the quantity and quality of food. The problem is heightened when energy intake is insufficient so that the dietary proteins are utilized as fuel rather than for the synthesis of body protein.[5]

Protein–energy malnutrition may occur in adults. The most observable change is the loss of subcutaneous fat from prominent deposits. The skin turns dry and rough and loses its elasticity. Follicles become more prominent. Follicular hyperkeratosis ensues, giving the skin texture similar to a nutmeg grater. Brown pigmentation develops around the oral, orbital, and malar areas. Patients with acne observe that this condition disappears, yet lesions resume when nutrition is restored. Hair growth is slow. It falls out prematurely and turns gray. Nail growth is impeded. Bacterial infections such as furunculosis, impetigo, skin ulcers, and sores are common due to associated unsanitary environment.[2]

Malnourished children from developing countries may present with either of two conditions. The first is *marasmus*, which in Greek means "wasting." It is a prolonged deficiency of protein and calories, and is a major contributing factor to mortality in infancy and early childhood. It is usually caused by weaning problems due to disease, poor hygiene, poverty, and cultural factors. Symptoms include dry, wrinkled loose skin due to a marked loss of subcutaneous fat. The loss of fat pads in the buccal area brings about the "monkey facies." Hair is thin, grows slowly, and easily falls out or breaks. Nails may be fissured and nail growth is retarded. There is no edema or dermatosis in this condition.[2]

The second condition is *kwashiorkor*, which in Ghana language literally means "the first child gets when the second is on the way." It is a severe deficiency in protein, usually occurring when the child is weaned onto a starchy diet. Changes in pigmentation may be found around the perioral area, the lower extremities, and around previous wounds, ulcerations, and other injuries. In children with fair skin, depigmentation starts with blanchable erythema evolving into small, dusky purple patches that do not blanch. In children with dark-skinned complexion, depigmentation is more obvious, evolving into waxy "enamel paint" spots on the trunk, diaper area, trochanters, knees, and ankles. The lesions have sharp edges and are elevated. Large areas of erosions that resemble "flaky paint" or "crazy paving" are seen in severe cases. Linear fissures can be found around the pinna, popliteal, antecubital and axillary areas, interdigits, in the center of the lips, and at the edge of the foreskin of the penile shaft. These lesions are brought about by intermittent tension. The skin is easily damaged; therefore, care must be taken to avoid acute trauma and chronic pressure injuries in bedridden children. Hair findings show the "flag sign," wherein there are alternating bands of dark and pale hair. These bands reflect the alternating periods of adequate and inadequate nutrition.[2]

Protein–energy malnutrition rarely occurs alone. Concomitant nutritional deficiencies commonly seen include deficits in folic acid, thiamine, riboflavin, nicotinic acid, pyridoxine, and vitamin A.

11.1.3.2 Obesity

Malnutrition may also be due to excess in nutrients. Obesity may be seen as an interplay of environmental and genetic factors. It is a condition wherein there is an excess of adipose tissue. This term is not analogous to being overweight, for the reason that muscular individuals may exceed their ideal weight for height without having an excess of adipose tissue. Aside from the BMI, we may measure adiposity by skin-fold thickness (anthropometry), underwater weighing (densitometry), or getting the waist-to-hip ratio, wherein abnormal values would be >0.9 for women and >1.0 in men.[6]

Body fat and fat distribution are affected by gender, age, degree of physical activity, and a number of drugs such as phenothiazines, antidepressants, antiepileptics, and steroids. Body fat increases with age in both men and women.[6]

The WHO reports that obesity in school children is estimated at 10% in industrialized countries such as Japan, US, and some countries in the European continent. Overweight and obesity during childhood lead to an increased risk of becoming overweight and obese in adulthood, as well as an increased prevalence of obesity-related disorders.[1]

In adults, the prevalence of obesity is 10–25% in most countries of Western Europe, 20–25% in some countries in the Americas, up to 40% in some countries in Eastern Europe, and more than 50% in some countries in the Western Pacific.[1]

With obesity, there is an increased risk of hypertension, cardiovascular disease, diabetes, gall bladder disease, sleep apnea, and osteoarthritis. Cutaneous man infestations associated with obesity include intertrigo due to friction between excessive fat folds, striae, and acrochordons. Acanthosis nigricans is characterized by a gray–brown velvety plaque found on the face, inner thighs, antecubital and popliteal fossae, umbilicus, and perianal area.[2]

11.2 Vitamins

11.2.1 Definition

Vitamins are organic compounds that cannot be synthesized by humans and therefore must be ingested to prevent metabolic disorders. The term "*vitamine*" was coined by Funk in the early 1900s which came from two words: "*amine*," which was the chemical that he was able to isolate from rice polishings, which he believed to preserve life, "*vita*." He further went on to define avitaminosis and deficiency disorders.[7]

11.2.2 Recommended Dietary Allowance

The recommended dietary allowances or recommended daily allowances (RDA) are based on the evaluation of the Food and Nutrition Board of the National Research Council on the correct amount of essential nutrients sufficient to meet the needs of a healthy individual. It is defined as the average daily dietary intake level that is sufficient to meet the nutrient requirements of nearly all healthy individuals of a specific sex, age, life stage, or physiologic condition (pregnancy or lactation).[3] RDAs are based on many types of evidence on nutrients, including replacement studies in persons with deficiency, biochemical assessments of function in relation to intake, epidemiologic studies, and extrapolation of data from animal experiments. The objective of these recommendations is to provide a safety factor appropriate to each nutrient by exceeding the actual requirements of most individuals.[8]

Water-soluble vitamins include the vitamin B-complex and vitamin C (Tables 11.2 and 11.3). Fat-soluble vitamins include vitamins A, D, E, and K (Tables 11.4 and 11.5). A balanced diet will ensure an individual of both water-soluble and fat-soluble vitamins (Tables 11.6 and 11.7).

11.2.3 Hypervitaminosis/ Hypovitaminosis

11.2.3.1 Vitamin A

Vitamin A consists of all naturally occurring active forms, which include retinol and retinylesters, and the carotenoids. This fat-soluble vitamin is essential for normal epithelial proliferation, keratinization, and the transduction of visual images by the retina.[9]

The major causes of vitamin A deficiency are inadequate diet, malabsorption of fat and liver disease. It can be assessed by taking the serum retinol level.[2]

Table 11.2 Recommended dietary allowances (RDA) of water-soluble vitamins for children (modified from dietary reference intakes of the Food and Nutrition Board of the National Research Council)

Life-stage group	VitaminB1 (thiamin) mg/day	Vitamin B2 (riboflavin) mg/day	Vitamin B3 (niacin) mg/day	Vitamin B5 (pantothenic acid) mg/day	VitaminB6 (pyridoxine) mg/day	Vitamin B12 (cyanocobalamin) µg/day	Folate µg/day	Vitamin C (ascorbic acid) mg/day	Vitamin H (biotin) µg/day
Infants									
0–6 months	0.2	0.3	2	1.7	0.1	0.4	65	40	5
7–12 months	0.3	0.4	4	1.8	0.3	0.5	80	50	6
Children									
1–3 years	0.5	0.5	6	2	0.5	0.9	150	15	8
4–6 years	0.6	0.6	8	3	0.6	1.2	200	25	12
Males									
9–13 years	0.9	0.9	12	4	1.0	1.8	300	45	20
14–18 years	1.2	1.3	16	5	1.3	2.4	400	75	25
Females									
9–13 years	0.9	0.9	12	4	1.0	1.8	300	45	20
14–18 years	1.0	1.0	14	5	1.2	2.4	400	65	25

Table 11.3 RDA of water-soluble vitamins for adults (modified from dietary reference intakes of the Food and Nutrition Board of the National Research Council)

Life-stage group	Vitamin B1 (thiamin) mg/day	Vitamin B2 (riboflavin) mg/day	Vitamin B3 (niacin) mg/day	Vitamin B5 (pantothenic acid) mg/day	Vitamin B6 (pyridoxine) mg/day	Vitamin B12 (cyanocobalamin) µg/day	Folate µg/day	Vitamin C (ascorbic acid) mg/day	Vitamin H (biotin) µg/day
Males									
19–30 years	1.2	1.3	16	5	1.3	2.4	400	90	30
31–50 years	1.2	1.3	16	5	1.3	2.4	400	90	30
50–70 years	1.2	1.3	16	5	1.7	2.4	400	90	30
>70 years	1.2	1.3	16	5	1.7	2.4	400	90	30
Females									
19–30 years	1.1	1.1	14	5	1.3	2.4	400	75	30
31–50 years	1.1	1.1	14	5	1.3	2.4	400	75	30
50–70 years	1.1	1.1	14	5	1.5	2.4	400	75	30
>70 years	1.1	1.1	14	5	1.5	2.4	400	75	30
Pregnancy									
<18 years	1.4	1.4	18	6	1.9	2.6	600	80	30
19–30 years	1.4	1.4	18	6	1.9	2.6	600	85	30
31–50 years	1.4	1.4	18	6	1.9	2.6	600	85	30
Lactation									
<18 years	1.4	1.4	17	7	2.0	2.8	500	115	35
19–30 years	1.4	1.4	17	7	2.0	2.8	500	120	35
31–50 years	1.4	1.4	17	7	2.0	2.8	500	120	35

Vitamin A deficiency may have ocular manifestations such as night blindness and diseases of the conjunctiva, sclera and cornea, such as xerosis conjunctivae, Bitot spots, xerosis corneae, and keratomalacia. Cutaneous manifestations include dermomalacia where in the large areas of the body have dry, wrinkled skin covered with fine scales. Phrynoderma or "toad skin" is a type of follicular hyperkeratosis which is also seen in vitamin A deficiency. Lesions may present as flesh-colored or hyperpigmented filiform, conical or large papules with large horny centers usually seen on the elbows and knees.[2]

WHO has strategies for controlling vitamin A deficiency which aim to provide an adequate intake through a combination of dietary improvement including breast-feeding, supplementation, and food fortification.[1]

Acute vitamin A intoxication may occur after ingestion of 500,000 IU or greater by adults or proportional

Table 11.4 RDA of fat-soluble vitamins for children (modified from dietary reference intakes of the Food and Nutrition Board of the National Research Council)

Life-stage group	Vitamin A (µg/day)	Vitamin D (µg/day)	Vitamin E (mg/day)	Vitamin K (µg/day)
Infants				
0–6 months	400	5	4	2.0
7–12 months	500	5	5	2.5
Children				
1–3 years	300	5	6	30
4–6 years	400	5	7	55
Males				
9–13 years	600	5	11	60
14–18 years	900	5	15	75
Females				
9–13 years	600	5	11	60
14–18 years	700	5	15	75

Table 11.5 RDA of fat-soluble vitamins for adults (modified from dietary reference intakes of the Food and Nutrition Board of the National Research Council)

Life-stage group	Vitamin A (µg/day)	Vitamin D (µg/day)	Vitamin E (mg/day)	Vitamin K (µg/day)
Males				
19–30 years	900	5	15	120
31–50 years	900	5	15	120
50–70 years	900	10	15	120
>70 years	900	15	15	120
Females				
19–30 years	700	5	15	90
31–50 years	700	5	15	90
50–70 years	700	10	15	90
>70 years	700	15	15	90
Pregnancy				
<18 years	750	5	15	75
19–30 years	770	5	15	90
31–50 years	770	5	15	90
Lactation				
<18 years	1,200	5	19	75
19–30 years	1,300	5	19	90
31–50 years	1,300	5	19	90

amounts by children (over 100 times the RDA). Symptoms include skin desquamation, abdominal pain, nausea, vomiting, and muscle weakness. Chronic intoxication occurs after intake of 50,000 IU/day for several months. Symptoms include desquamation, pruritus, facial dermatitis, dryness of the mucous membranes, erythema, brittle nails, cheilitis, and alopecia, which are reversible upon cessation of overdosing.[2]

Table 11.6 Common food sources of water-soluble vitamins (modified from dietary reference intakes of the Food and Nutrition Board of the National Research Council)

Vitamin	Food source
Vitamin B1 (thiamin)	Enriched, fortified, or whole-grain products; bread and bread products, mixed foods whose main ingredient is grain, and ready-to-eat cereals
Vitamin B2 (riboflavin)	Organ meats, milk, bread products, and fortified cereals
Vitamin B3 (niacin)	Meat, fish, poultry, enriched and whole-grain breads and bread products, fortified ready-to-eat cereals
Vitamin B5 (pantothenic acid)	Chicken, beef, potatoes, oats, cereals, tomato products, liver, kidney, yeast, egg yolk, broccoli, whole grains
Vitamin B6 (pyridoxine)	Fortified cereals, organ meats, fortified soy-based meat substitutes
Vitamin B12 (cyanocobalamin)	Fortified cereals, meat, fish, poultry
Folate	Enriched cereal grains, dark leafy vegetables, enriched and whole-grain breads and bread products, fortified ready-to-eat cereals
Vitamin C (ascorbic acid)	Citrus fruits, tomatoes, tomato juice, potatoes, brussels sprouts, cauliflower, broccoli, strawberries, cabbage, and spinach
Vitamin H (biotin)	Liver and smaller amounts in fruits and meats

Table 11.7 Common food sources of fat-soluble vitamins (modified from dietary reference intakes of the Food and Nutrition Board of the National Research Council)

Vitamin	Food source
Vitamin A	Liver, dairy products, fish, darkly colored fruits, and leafy vegetables
Vitamin D	Fish liver oils, flesh of fatty fish, liver and fat from seals and polar bears, eggs from hens that have been fed vitamin D, fortified milk products, and fortified cereals
Vitamin E	Vegetable oils, unprocessed cereal grains, nuts, fruits, vegetables, meats
Vitamin K	Green vegetables (collards, spinach, salad greens, broccoli), brussels sprouts, cabbage, plant oils, and margarine

11.2.3.2 B Vitamins

Vitamin B_1 (thiamine) deficiency may present as either of two conditions. Beriberi is commonly found in Asians and presents with symptoms of fatigue, peripheral neuropathy, polyneuritis, heart failure, edema, angular stomatitis, and glossitis. Wernicke-Korsakoff syndrome presents as thiamine deficiency with symptoms of apathy, loss of memory, and confabulations. A deficiency in this vitamin may be associated with other B-complex vitamin and folate deficiency.[2]

A deficiency in riboflavin or vitamin B_2 may result in glossitis, angular stomatitis or perlèche, cheilosis of vertical fissures of the lip, and lesions resembling seborrheic dermatitis distributed along the nasolabial folds, cheeks, forehead, and postauricular area.[2]

Pellagra is the deficiency in vitamin B_3 or niacin and is characterized by the triad of dermatitis, diarrhea, and dementia. Cutaneous symptoms are found on areas that are exposed to the sun or localized pressure. It begins as erythema of the dorsal aspect of both hands with associated pruritius, burning, and edema. Vesicles may appear, coalesce to form bullae then burst. Dry brown scales may form. These scales are thicker and larger on the face, and may evolve into pustules. These lesions may become hard, rough, cracked, blackish, and brittle. Painful fissures develop in the palms and digits. In severe cases, the skin is covered with scales and blackish crusts due to hemorrhages. Lesions on the upper extremities may follow a "glove" or "gauntlet" distribution, while lesions on the lower extremities do not exceed the proximal malleoli, giving a "boot" distribution. On the face, lesions are usually found on the nose, forehead, cheeks, and chin giving a "butterfly" appearance. Lesions on the neck seen as a broad band encircling the neck are known as the Casal's necklace.[2]

There have been no reported cutaneous changes in humans deficient in vitamin B_5 or pantothenic acid.[2]

Vitamin B_6 (Pyridoxine) deficiency reveals seborrhea-like lesions on the face, scalp, neck, shoulders, buttocks, and perineum. Similar to riboflavin deficiency, one may also find angular stomatitis, cheilosis, and glossitis. Other symptoms include anorexia, nausea, vomiting, and neurologic findings such as hyperesthesia, ascending paresthesia, altered vibration and position sense, and hypoactive deep tendon reflexes.[2]

Cutaneous findings of a deficiency in cyanocobalamin or vitamin B_{12} include generalized hyperpigmented macules and patches found on flexural areas, palmar creases, soles, knuckles, and oral mucosa. Nail plates may also develop longitudinal, hyperpigmented streaks. Individuals with this deficiency may also present with graying of hair and a beefy red tongue.[2]

Cutaneous changes due to a deficiency in folic acid are rare but it has been reported to cause scaly papules and plaques on the face, trunk and extensor aspects of the extremities, stomatitis, and glossitis. Megaloblastic anemia is found in individuals deficient in folic acid. When treating this deficiency, it is important to check for a concomitant deficiency in vitamin B_{12}. If this is overlooked, treatment with folate supplements will improve the anemia, but can progress to neurologic damage due to the cyanocobalamin deficiency.[2]

Biotin, also known as vitamin H, is found in the diet, but is also synthesized by bacteria found in the human intestines. A deficiency in this vitamin may either be acquired or inborn. An acquired deficiency is commonly caused by an excessive intake of the avidin-containing egg whites, which blocks the absorption of biotin. Symptoms include fine desquamation on the extremities, periorificial eczema, alopecia, pallor and atrophy of the tongue. Inborn deficiencies of the enzymes holocarboxylase synthetase or biotinidase may cause biotin deficiency due to malabsorption and ineffective metabolism. Symptoms include a generalized erythematous scaly rash similar to ichthyosis or seborrheic dermatitis, alopecia of the scalp, eyebrows and eyelashes, absence of lanugo hair. Corneal ulcers and keratoconjunctivitis may develop.[2]

11.2.3.3 Vitamin C

Ascorbic acid, ascorbate, or vitamin C is a water-soluble vitamin most commonly found in citrus fruits and green vegetables. It is critical in wound healing due to its important role in collagen synthesis. It also has a role in regenerating active vitamin E and increases cholesterol excretion.[10]

Scurvy or the deficiency in the intake of vitamin C begins with symptoms of follicular hyperkeratosis and the appearance of corkscrew hairs. Perifollicular purpura then ensues, seen commonly on the lower extremities. There is poor wound healing and old scars may break down. Other associated symptoms include edema of the lower extremities and gingival necrosis.

Marginal deficiencies increase the risk of cancer, cardiovascular disease, hypertension, decreased immunity, diabetes and cataracts.[2]

An increased intake of vitamin C may cause dose-dependent symptoms. An intake of greater than 1 g/day may cause an increase in oxalate excretion. Those taking 2 g/day may produce kidney stones in some cases. Doses greater than 2 g/day may cause diarrhea, nausea, stomach cramping, excess urination, and skin rashes.[11]

11.2.3.4 Vitamin D

Vitamin D is a steroid hormone which is important in calcium regulation and tissue growth and differentiation, including the skin. It comprises a number of related molecules, wherein only a few can be ingested, namely, vitamin D_2 (ergocalciferol) and vitamin D_3 (cholecalciferol). A deficiency of this vitamin may cause an abnormality in the absorption and transport of calcium into the bone. An acquired deficiency of this vitamin is caused by inadequate diet, malabsorption, or a decreased exposure to ultraviolet B (UVB) radiation. Symptoms include osteomalacia, muscle weakness, and alopecia. Chronic ingestion of excessive amounts of vitamin D (50,000–100,000 U/day) may produce hypervitaminosis D with symptoms such as weakness, lethargy, headache, nausea and polyuria, and metastatic calcification.[12]

11.2.3.5 Vitamin E

Vitamin E is a group of eight fat-soluble compounds, with α-tocopherol as the only active form found in humans. Deficiency of this vitamin is rare and occurs in individuals with chronic liver disease and fat malabsorption syndromes such as celiac disease and cystic fibrosis. Symptoms include nerve damage, lethargy, apathy, inability to concentrate, staggering gait, low thyroid hormone levels, decrease immune response, and anemia. Marginal deficiency in vitamin E is more common and is associated with an increased risk of cardiovascular disease and cancer. Vitamin E toxicity will cause adverse effects such as increased risk of bleeding, diarrhea, abdominal pain, fatigue, reduced immunity, and transiently raised blood pressure.[13]

11.2.3.6 Vitamin K

Vitamin K deficiency causes hemorrhage due to an abnormal coagulation. This may occur in any part of the body, but this may manifest cutaneously as purpura. The confirmatory test that can be requested is a prothrombin time measurement.[2]

11.3 Supplements

11.3.1 Antioxidants

Two types of chemical reactions occur widely in nature, namely oxidation and reduction. Oxidation involves the loss of electrons, while reduction is the gain of electrons. Oxidation and reduction reactions always occur together. Highly reactive molecules can oxidize molecules that were formerly stable causing them to become unstable species, such as free radicals. A free radical is defined as a chemical with an unpaired electron that can be neutral, positively charged, or negatively charged. Therefore, without antioxidants, a single free radical can cause damage to numerous molecules. However, despite the actions of antioxidant nutrients, some oxidative damage will still occur, and accumulation of this damage throughout life is believed to be a major factor in aging and disease.[13]

An antioxidant is any substance that significantly decreases the adverse effects of reactive species, such as reactive oxygen and nitrogen species, on the normal physiological function in humans.[14]

Human cells, most especially those found in the epidermis, possess an efficient antioxidant system, including enzymatic and nonenzymatic reductants, that deactivate reactive oxygen species (ROS) and reduce oxidized molecules such as lipid peroxides.[14]

11.3.1.1 Endogenous Antioxidants

Endogenous antioxidants are those found inherently in the epidermis, using either enzymatic and nonenzymatic reductants deactivating the ROS and reducing oxidized molecules. These include tocopherols (vitamin E) and ascorbic acid (vitamin C).[14]

Fig. 11.1 Interacting network of nonenzymatic endogenous antioxidants

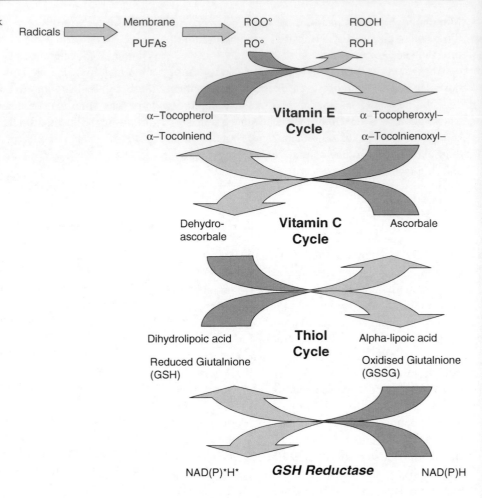

The main advantage of endogenous antioxidants is their low toxicity potential since they are innate components of the organism (Fig. 11.1).[14]

Alpha-Lipoic Acid

Lipoic acid is a very powerful antioxidant due to its being both aqueous and lipid-soluble, its anti-inflammatory activity, and its easy penetrability in the skin when topically applied due to it being a small, stable molecule.[15] Its mechanism of action of preventing UV-induced photo-oxidative damage is due to the down-modulation of NF-B activation and inhibition of tyrosinase activity by chelating the copper ions.

Coenzyme Q10

Coenzyme Q10 (CoQ10) is a powerful free radical inhibitor that acts on hindering lipid peroxidases from forming plasma membranes. It also has a very important role in cellular energy production and works in the mitochondrial adenosine triphosphate (ATP) energy-producing pathway of the cell. It may also play a role in preventing oxidative stress-induced cellular apoptosis since it is in the mitochondria where the final apoptotic signal is dispatched. It is reported that oral CoQ10 improves cellular energy production while topical CoQ10 is shown to inhibit collagenase expression in UV-irradiated human fibroblasts.[15] It can regenerate reduced tocopherol 3–30 times greater than tocopherol within membranes.

Glutathione

The glutathione system, also called the "master antioxidant," is our first line of defense against peroxidation in the body. The liver contains the greatest amount while the heart and muscles show lower quantities. It is found both in the epidermis and the dermis, particularly within the fibroblasts. Glutathione peroxidase is a major detoxifier of hydrogen peroxide in the cytoplasm, along with catalase.[10]

11.3.1.2 Exogenous Antioxidants

An immense inflammation can overpower the antioxidant defense system of the skin and lead to tissue destruction, thus the use of exogenous antioxidants, both topical and systemic. These include α-hydroxy acids (AHAs) and the various plant antioxidants such as anapsos, silymarin, soybeans, and tea. They are naturally occurring organic acids that are often referred to as fruit acids because they are found mostly in citrus fruits, apples, and grapes (Table 11.8).

Anapsos

Anapsos comes from the tropical fern *P. leucotomos*, which has in vitro antioxidant and immunomodulating

Table 11.8 Common food sources of exogenous antioxidants

Antioxidant	Food source
Carotenoids	
Beta-carotene	Carrots, various fruits
Lutein, zeaxanthin	Kale, collards, spinach, corn, eggs, citrus
Lycopene	Tomatoes and processed tomato products
Flavonoids	
Anthocyanidins	Berries, cherries, red grapes
Flavanols (catechins, epicatechins, procyanidins)	Tea, cocoa, chocolate, apples, grapes
Flavanones	Citrus foods
Flavonols	Onions, apples, tea, broccoli
Proanthocyanidins	Cranberries, cocoa, apples, strawberries, grapes, wine, peanuts, cinnamon
Isothiocyanates	
Sulforaphane	Cauliflower, broccoli, broccoli sprouts, cabbage, kale, horseradish
Phenols	
Caffeic acid, ferulic acid	Apples, pears, citrus fruits, some vegetables
Sulfides/thiols	
Diallyl sulfide, allyl methyl trisulfide	Garlic, onions, leeks, scallions
Dithiolthiones	Cruciferous vegetables (broccoli, cabbage, bok choy, collards)
Whole grains	Cereal grains

properties. It has been used in the treatment of psoriasis and vitiligo. It is shown to inhibit lipid peroxidation, ROS formation, phototoxicity, and acute sunburn in humans in vivo following acute ultraviolet (UV) light exposure.[14]

Isoflavone Genistein

Genistein is a soy derivative which has been reported to have antioxidant, anticarcinogenesis, particularly breast and prostate cancers, and estrogen-like properties, thus improving the skin condition of postmenopausal women. Its action is in the protection of oxidative and photodynamically damaged DNA and downregulation of UVB-activated signal transduction cascade.[16]

Procyanidins

The seeds of red grapes are the richest source of procyanidins. Similar to polyphenols, it has antioxidant properties and is shown to inhibit lipid peroxidation.[15]

11.3.1.3 Botanical Antioxidants

All plants protect themselves from oxidation following UV exposure in the outdoor environment. They work by quenching singlet oxygen and ROS. Most of these botanical antioxidants can be classified as flavonoids, carotenoids, and polyphenols.[17]

Chamomile

Chamomile or *Matricaria recutita* inhibits UVB-induced pigmentation by avoiding ET-1-induced DNA synthesis. Its main ingredient is α-bisabolol. It has antiallergic, antineoplastic, and analgesic properties. Studies have shown that it has antimicrobial effects against *Staphylococcus sp.* and *Candida sp.* It has also been shown to promote wound healing and exhibit anti-inflammatory activity.[18]

Curcumin

Curcumin is a polyphenol antioxidant extracted from the tumeric root. Its effect has been shown to be greater than that of vitamin E. Tetrahydrocurcumin is added to cosmetic products and functions as an antioxidant. It prevents the lipids from the moisturizer from becoming rancid.[17]

Echinacea

Echinacea contains polysaccharides and glycoproteins, flavonoids, caffeic and ferulic acid derivatives, volatile oils, alkamides, polyenes, and pyrrolizine alkaloids which stimulate immunity and protect collagen.[18]

Garlic

Garlic has potent antimicrobial and antioxidant activity primarily due to alkylcysteine sulfoxides, specifically alliin. Other components include polysaccharides, saponins, and vitamins A, B_2, and C. It also stimulates immunity and has anti-yeast activity.[18]

Gingko Biloba

Gingko biloba contains unique polyphenols such as terpenoids, flavonoids, and fl avonol glycosides that have anti-inflammatory effects that have been linked to anti-radical and anti-lipoperoxidant effects in experimental fibroblast models. There is increased collagen and extracellular fibronectin as demonstrated by radio-isotope assay.[17]

Green Tea

Polyphenols can be found in tea (*Camellia sinensis*) and is produced during the tea leaf processing. Green tea contains predominantly monomeric polyphenol catechins, whereas black tea contains polymeric polyphenols. In humans, polyphenols has been shown to inhibit UV-induced erythema and inflammation.[14]

Licorice

The roots of the licorice plant contain saponosides (glycyrrhizine) which serve as an emollient, flavonoids which are antioxidants, and glycyrrhetinic and glycyrrhizinic acids which have anti-inflammatory and wound healing effects. Glabridin is the main ingredient of licorice extract. It inhibits tyrosinase activity in vitro without affecting DNA synthesis.

Pycnogenol

Pycnogenol is derived from the bark of the French maritime pine (*Pinus pinaster*). It is several times more powerful than vitamins C and E. It recycles vitamin C, regenerates vitamin E, and increases the endogenous antioxidant enzyme system. Its active ingredient is proanthocyanidin.[17]

Resveratrol

Resveratrol is a phytoalexin found in grape seeds and Mulberry tree (*Morus alba*). It has anti-inflammatory effects and inhibits cyclooxygenase and hydroperoxidase functions.[19]

Silymarin

Silymarin comes from the extract of the thistle *Silybum marianum* and has been used in the treatment of liver diseases due to its powerful antioxidant properties. It has been reported to inhibit the actions of UV radiation on living cells, and thus is a potential topical reagent in preventing and treating photodamage.[14]

Soybean

Soybean milk extracts has been shown to reduce the melanin deposition within the swine epidermis. It prevents UVB-induced pigmentation in vivo, similar to soybean trypsin inhibitor STI.[20]

11.3.2 Minerals

11.3.2.1 Recommended Dietary Allowances

The RDA of minerals differ according to life-stage group (Tables 11.9 and 11.10). These mineral nutrients can be acquired through a balanced intake of the following common food sources (Table 11.11).

Table 11.9 RDA of minerals for children (modified from dietary reference intakes of the Food and Nutrition Board of the National Research Council)

Life-stage group	Calcium (mg/day)	Chromium (μ g/day)	Copper (μ g/day)	Fluoride (mg/day)	Iodine (μ g/day)	Iron (mg/day)	Magnesium (mg/day)	Manganese (mg/day)	Molybdenum (μ g/day)	Phosphorus (mg/day)	Selenium (μ g/day)	Zinc (mg/day)
Infants												
0–6 months	210	0.2	200	0.01	110	0.27	30	0.003	2	100	15	2
7–12 months	270	5.5	220	0.5	130	11	75	0.6	3	275	20	3
Children												
1–3 years	500	11	340	0.7	90	7	80	1.2	17	460	20	3
4–8 years	800	15	440	1	90	10	130	1.5	22	500	30	5
Males												
9–13 years	1,300	25	700	2	120	8	240	1.9	34	1,250	40	8
14–18 years	1,300	35	890	3	150	11	410	2.2	43	1,250	55	11
Females												
9–13 years	1,300	21	700	2	120	8	240	1.6	34	1,250	40	8
14–18 years	1,300	24	890	3	150	15	360	1.6	43	1,250	55	9

Table 11.10 RDA of minerals for adults (modified from dietary reference intakes of the Food and Nutrition Board of the National Research Council)

Life-stage group	Calcium (mg/day)	Chromium (µg/day)	Copper (µg/day)	Fluoride (mg/day)	Iodine (µg/day)	Iron (mg/day)	Magnesium (mg/day)	Manganese (mg/day)	Molybdenum (µg/day)	Phosphorus (mg/day)	Selenium (µg/day)	Zinc (mg/day)
Males												
19–30 years	1,000	35	900	4	150	8	400	2.3	45	700	55	11
31–50 years	1,000	35	900	4	150	8	420	2.3	45	700	55	11
50–70 years	1,200	30	900	4	150	8	420	2.3	45	700	55	11
>70 years	1,200	30	900	4	150	8	420	2.3	45	700	55	11
Females												
19–30 years	1,000	25	900	3	150	18	310	1.8	45	700	55	8
31–50 years	1,000	25	900	3	150	18	320	1.8	45	700	55	8
50–70 years	1,200	20	900	3	150	8	320	1.8	45	700	55	8
>70 years	1,200	20	900	3	150	8	320	1.8	45	700	55	8
Pregnancy												
<18 years	1,300	29	1,000	3	220	27	400	2.0	50	1,250	60	12
19–30 years	1,000	30	1,000	3	220	27	350	2.0	50	700	60	11
31–50 years	1,000	30	1,000	3	220	27	360	2.0	50	700	60	11
Lactation												
<18 years	1,300	44	1,300	3	290	10	360	2.6	50	1,250	70	13
19–30 years	1,000	45	1,300	3	290	9	310	2.6	50	700	70	12
31–50 years	1,000	45	1,300	3	290	9	320	2.6	50	700	70	12

Table 11.11 Common food sources of minerals

Mineral	Food source
Calcium	Almonds, figs, beans, carrots, pecans, raisins, brown rice, apricots, garlic, dates, spinach, sesame seeds, brazil nuts, cashews, papaya, avocados, celery
Chromium	Brewer's yeast, clams, cheese, corn oil, whole grains
Copper	Soy beans, brazil nuts, bone meal, raisins, legumes, seafoods, black strap molasses
Iodine	Kelp, dulse, beets, celery, lettuce, irish moss, grapes, mushrooms, oranges
Iron	Kelp, raisins, figs, beets, soy beans, bananas, asparagus, carrots, cucumbers, sunflower seeds, parsley, grapes, watercress
Magnesium	Honey, almonds, tuna, kelp, pineapple, pecans, green vegetables
Manganese	Celery, bananas, beets, egg yolks, bran, walnuts, pineapples, asparagus, whole grains, leafy green vegetables
Phosphorus	Mushrooms, cashews, oats, beans, squash, pecans, carrots, almonds
Potassium	Spinach, apples, tomatoes, strawberries, bananas, lemons, figs, celery, mushrooms, oranges, papaya, pecans, raisins, pineapple, rice, cucumbers, brussels sprouts
Selenium	Brazil nuts, meats, tuna, plant foods
Sodium	Turnips, raw milk, cheese, wheat germ, cucumbers, beets, string beans, seafoods, lima beans, okra, pumpkins
Sulfur	Bran, cheese, eggs, cauliflower, nuts, onions, broccoli, fish, wheat germ, cucumbers, turnips, corn
Zinc	Mushrooms, liver, seafoods, soy beans, sunflower seeds, brewer's yeast

11.3.2.2 Calcium

In an adult, there is approximately 1–2 kg of calcium present in the body, 99% of which is found in the skeletal system. RDA ranges from 1,000 to 1,200 mg/day. However, some individuals increase their oral supplementation to 1,500–2,000 mg/day to prevent osteoporosis. A feedback mechanism exists to regulate hormonal regulation of intestinal absorption of calcium, resulting in an almost constant daily net calcium absorption of approximately 200–400 mg/day.[12]

An inadequate intake of calcium during growth may increase the risk of osteoporosis later in life. Osteoporosis is defined as a reduction of bone mass or density, characterized by a decrease in bone strength. In taking calcium supplements, it should be taken in doses <600 mg at a time, as the calcium absorption fraction decreases at higher doses. Calcium supplements should be computed based on the elemental calcium content, and not the weight of the calcium salt. Calcium carbonate is best taken with food since it requires acid for solubility. Calcium citrate can be taken at any time. Although side effects from calcium supplements are rare, individuals with a history of kidney stones should have a 24-h urine calcium determination before starting calcium to avoid hypercalciuria.[12]

11.3.2.3 Copper

Copper plays an integral role in iron metabolism, melanin synthesis, and central nervous system function. Deficiency of this mineral is rare, although it may be found in premature infants who are fed mild diets and in infants with malabsorption. Patients with malabsorptive diseases and nephritic syndrome and in patients treated for Wilson's disease with chronic high doses of oral zinc, which can interfere with copper absorption, may acquire copper deficiency anemia. Menkes kinky hair syndrome, a cross-linked metabolic disease of copper metabolism presents with symptoms such as mental retardation, hypocupremia, and decreased circulating ceruloplasmin. Children diagnosed with this disease often die within 5 years due to dissecting aneurysms or cardiac rupture.[11]

Copper deficiency is diagnosed by a finding of low serum levels of copper (<65 m g/dL) and low ceruloplasmin levels (<18 mg/dL).[11]

Copper toxicity can, in severe cases, cause kidney failure, liver failure, and coma. In Wilson's disease, mutations in the copper-transporting *ATP7B* gene lead to accumulation of copper in the liver and brain. However, low blood levels of copper are detected due to decreased ceruloplasmin.[11]

11.3.2.4 Iron

Chronic iron deficiency may manifest as anemia, glossitis, cheilosis, koilonychia, and hair loss. Hemosiderosis or chronic excess intake of iron would cause a bronze pigmentation of the skin, cirrhosis of the liver, diabetes mellitus, cardiomyopathy, and an increased risk in porphyria cutanea tarda.[2]

11.3.2.5 Selenium

The mineral selenium is necessary for the function of glutathione peroxidase, an antioxidant enzyme. A deficiency in selenium causes cardiomyopathy, muscle pain and weakness, nail changes similar to Terry's nails (found in patients with hepatic cirrhosis), dyschromotrichia, and macrocytosis. Selenium poisoning can occur after ingestion of water containing large amounts of the metal. Acute selenium intoxication may cause cutaneous findings such as alopecia, paronychia, possible nail loss, and reddish pigmentation of the nails, hair, and teeth.[2]

11.3.2.6 Zinc

Zinc is essential for the formation and function of the immune system. It plays a role in the sense of taste and in wound healing.

Acrodermatitis enterohepatica is an autosomal recessive disease that may cause zinc deficiency due to a defect in zinc absorption. The initial manifestations are usually seen when an infant is weaned from human to cow's milk. Hallmark features include dermatitis, diarrhea, and alopecia.[21]

Toxicity may be caused by inhalation, oral ingestion, or intravenous administration. Inhalation of zinc oxide fumes by welders leads to a condition called metal-fume fever or brass chills, with symptoms such as fever, chills, excessive salivation, headaches, cough, and leukocytosis. Contamination of dialysis fluids with zinc from the adhesive on the dialysis coils or from galvanized pipes may also cause zinc toxicity with symptoms such as anemia, fever, and central nervous system disturbances.[22]

11.4 Conclusion

An excess or deficiency in certain vitamins and minerals may manifest characteristically in the skin. The "toad skin" appearance found in hypovitaminosis A, the Casal's necklace in hypovitaminosis B3, and the

perifollicular purpura found in scurvy are just a few examples of distinctive dermatologic manifestations. Armed with the knowledge of this chapter, if one is to be presented with a patient with these symptoms, a diagnosis is very hard to miss.

The WHO, together with the different health sectors and their national programs, has come up with a global strategy to fight malnutrition. However, prevention is always superior to cure. A well-balanced diet, along with the various supplements available in the market, will ensure a healthy individual.

Our vision is of *a world where people everywhere, at every age, enjoy a high level of nutritional well-being, free from all forms of hunger and malnutrition.*

World Health Organization

References

1. World Health Organization. Nutrition for Health and Development: A global agenda for combating malnutrition. World Health Organization; 2000. http://whqlibdoc.who.int/hq/2000/WHO_NHD_00.6.pdf; 2007 Accessed 11.12.07
2. Nieves D, Goldsmith L. Cutaneous changes in nutritional disease. In: Freedberg I, Eisen A, Wolff K, et al, eds. *Fitzpatrick's Dermatology in General Medicine*. 6th ed. New York: McGraw-Hill; 2003
3. Dwyer J. Nutritional requirements and dietary assessment. In: Kasper D, Braunwald E, Fauci A, et al, eds. *Harrison's Principles of Internal Medicine*. 16th ed. New York: McGraw-Hill; 2005
4. Denke M, Wilson J. Assessment of nutritional status. In: Fauci A, Braunwald E, Isselbacher K, et al, eds. *Harrison's Principles of Internal Medicine*. 14th ed. New York: McGraw-Hill; 1998
5. Denke M, Wilson J. Protein and energy malnutrition. In: Fauci A, Braunwald E, Isselbacher K, et al, eds. *Harrison's Principles of Internal Medicine*. 14th ed. New York: McGraw-Hill; 1998
6. Flier J, Maratos-Flier E. Obesity. In: Kasper D, Braunwald E, Fauci A, et al, eds. *Harrison's Principles of Internal Medicine*. 16th ed. New York: McGraw-Hill; 2005
7. Bereston E. Vitamins in dermatology. A J Clin Nutr. 1954;2(2):133–139
8. Denke M, Wilson J. Nutrition and nutritional requirements. In: Fauci A, Braunwald E, Isselbacher K, et al, eds. *Harrison's Principles of Internal Medicine*. 14th ed. New York: McGraw-Hill; 1998
9. Meyers D, Maloley P, Weeks D. Safety of antioxidant vitamins. *Arch Int Med*. 1996;156(9):925–935
10. Pugliese P. The skin's antioxidant systems. *Dermatol Nurs*. 1998;10(6):401–416
11. Russell R. Vitamin and trace mineral deficiency and excess. In: Kasper D, Braunwald E, Fauci A, et al, eds. *Harrison's*

Principles of Internal Medicine. 16th ed. New York: McGraw-Hill; 2005

12. Bringhurst FR, Demay M, Krane S. Bone and mineral metabolism in health and disease. In: Kasper D, Braunwald E, Fauci A, et al, eds. *Harrison's Principles of Internal Medicine.* 16th ed. New York: McGraw-Hill; 2005

13. Quiroga R. Anti-aging medicine as it relates to dermatology. In: Burgess C, ed. *Cosmetic Dermatology.* Berlin: Springer; 2005

14. Sorg O, Antille C, Saurat J. Retinoids, other topical vitamins, and antioxidants. In: Rigel D, Weiss R, Lim H, et al, eds. *Photoaging.* New York: Marcel Dekker; 2004

15. Graf J. Anti-aging skin care ingredient technologies. In: Burgess C, ed. *Cosmetic Dermatology.* Berlin: Springer; 2005

16. Wei H, Saladi R, Yuhun L, et al Isoflavone genistein: photoprotection and clinical implications in dermatology. *J Nutr.* 2003;133:3811 S–3819 S

17. Draelos ZD. Cosmeceutical botanicals: part 1. In: Draelos ZD, ed. *Cosmeceuticals.* Philadelphia: Elsevier Saunders; 2005

18. Thornfeldt C. Cosmeceutical botanicals: part 2. In: Draelos ZD, ed. *Cosmeceuticals.* Philadelphia: Elsevier Saunders; 2005

19. Jang M, et al Cancer chemopreventive activity of resveratrol, a natural product derived from grapes. *Science.* 1997; 275(5297): 218–220

20. Paine C, et al An alternative approach to depigmentation by soybean extracts via inhibition of the PAR-2 pathway. *J Invest Dermatol.* 2001;116(4):587–595

21. Neldner K. Acrodermatitis enterohepathica and other zinc-deficiency disorders. In: Freedberg I, Eisen A, Wolff K, et al, eds. *Fitzpatrick's Dermatology in General Medicine.* 6th ed. New York: McGraw-Hill; 2003

22. Falchuk K. Disturbances in trace elements. In: Fauci A, Braunwald E, Isselbacher K, et al, eds. *Harrison's Principles of Internal Medicine.* 14th ed. New York: McGraw-Hill; 1998

Vaccines for Viral Diseases

12

Ivan D. Camacho and Brian Berman

Vaccination against viral agents has considerably alleviated the burden associated with viral diseases and has saved millions of lives worldwide. Global vaccination eradicated diseases like polio and other vaccines have led to a significant decline in infection rates and related complications of viral diseases. Important criteria for a disease to be susceptible of global elimination are that the disease is specific to humans and that there are no animal reservoirs for the infection.

Three types or viral vaccines are currently available:

- Attenuated live viral vaccines: these vaccines contain viruses that have been modified to produce an immune response without causing the disease. A risk of mutation to a pathogenic form is possible. These include measles, mumps, oral polio, rubella, varicella, and yellow fever.
- Killed viral vaccines: these vaccines contain viral particles that have been deactivated, causing an immune reaction but not an infection. These include influenza, rabies, Japanese encephalitis, etc.
- Recombinant antigens: specific immunogenic viral proteins are subtracted to induce antibody formation against that virus. The hepatitis B vaccine is one example of this kind of vaccine.

The efficacy of a vaccine is measured by the length of immunity and the percentage of vaccinated individuals displaying immunity. Vaccines stimulate the production of IgG and IgA secretory antibodies by B-cell lymphocytes and the elimination of human leukocyte antigen-matched infected cells by CD8+ T lymphocytes. CD4+ T lymphocytes present antigens to B-cells resulting in long-lasting immunity, even without antibody test results.[1]

12.1 Paramyxoviruses

Paramyxoviruses encompass a heterogeneous family of RNA viruses including measles virus, mumps virus, parainfluenza virus, and respiratory syncytial virus.

Vaccination for measles, mumps, and rubella is typically given in combination in the MMR vaccine, providing efficacious immunity with fewer immunizations and to a large target population. MMR is part of the US centers for disease control and prevention (CDC) Recommended Immunization Schedule. MMR is a live attenuated virus vaccine that is provided as a first dose for children 12–18 months of age and a second dose for children 4–6 years of age. Second doses may be given to adolescents ages 11–18 (if not received before) and adults that were either recently exposed to measles, previously vaccinated with killed measles vaccine, healthcare workers, or international travelers. MMR should not be administered to immunocompromised patients, patients with allergy to neomycin, and pregnant women. Pregnancy should be avoided in the following 4 weeks to an immunization.[2]

12.1.1 Measles (Rubeola)

Measles virus is a highly contagious airborne virus that causes the typical prodrome of fever, malaise, conjunctivitis, photophobia and cough, followed 48 h later

I.D. Camacho (✉)
Department of Dermatology and Cutaneous Surgery,
University of Miami Miller School of Medicine,
Miami, FL, USA
e-mail: icamacho2@med.miami.edu

R.A. Norman (ed.), *Preventive Dermatology in Infectious Diseases*,
DOI 10.1007/978-0-85729-847-8_12, © Springer-Verlag London Limited 2012

by a characteristic maculopapular rash. About 75% of household contacts to infected patients will develop the disease. Measles virus is related to orthomyxoviruses, which cause mumps and influenza, but is not related to togaviruses, which cause German measles or rubella. Since humans are the only reservoir to the infection, global eradication of measles is feasible, with a goal date of 2010.

The measles vaccine is produced by culturing the Moraten virus strain in chick embryo cells. Vaccination produces 95–99% serologic evidence of immunity after two doses of vaccine and life-long immunity.[3] The vaccination produces a mild noncontagious infection, with occasional fever (15%) and a transient viral exanthem. Encephalitis and subacute sclerosing panencephalitis are rare adverse effects.[4] In the last decade, an aerosolized measles vaccine has been administered, providing superior immunogenicity and fewer side effects.[5]

12.1.2 Mumps

Live attenuated mumps vaccine produces a mild, non-communicable infection, providing 93–97% of serological evidence of immunity after one vaccination. However, the duration of the immunity is not clear, with efficacy rates ranging from 75% to 95% as demonstrated during outbreaks. Low-grade fever, mild parotitis, and a viral exanthema are the most common side effects.[6, 7]

12.1.3 Rubella (German Measles)

The rubella vaccine is grown in human diploid fibroblast cell cultures, producing high antibody titers in 97% of immunized individuals and lifelong protection.[8] Arthritis is a common side effect in adults (40%), followed by fever, lymphadenopathy, and a viral exanthema (15%).

12.2 Human Herpes Viruses

Herpesviruses comprise eight types of viruses that are known to be pathogenic in humans.

Herpes simplex virus type 1 (HSV-1) is one of the most prevalent viruses, causing oral and perioral gingivostomatitis, and the most common type of herpesvirus infections. Although several topical and systemic antiviral medications are routinely used for treatment and prophylaxis of HSV-1 infections, no successful vaccines have been developed. Herpes simplex virus 2 (HSV-2) is generally a cause of herpetic genital lesions, although oral lesions have been reported. Epstein–Barr virus (HSV-4) is associated with multiple presentations, including infectious mononucleosis, Burkitt's lymphoma in African children, nasopharyngeal carcinoma in Asian populations, and oral hairy leukoplakia. Cytomegalovirus (HSV-5) may present as sialadenopathy in immunocompetent individuals, birth defects in infected fetuses, and stomatitis in immunosuppressed patients. Human herpesvirus type 6 (HSV-6) is the cause of exanthema subitum (roseola infantum). Herpes virus type 8 (HSV-8 or Kaposi's sarcoma-related herpes virus [KSHV]) is the etiologic agent for Kaposi's sarcoma in patients with AIDS. HSV-8 has also been associated with primary effusion lymphoma and multicentric Castelman's disease, both encountered in HIV-positive patients, as well as myeloma multiple and lymphoproliferative disorders. From this group of viruses, only the varicella zoster virus (VZV) (HSV-3) has an approved vaccine available.

12.2.1 Varicella Zoster Virus (HSV-3)

VZV is an enveloped double-stranded DNA virus that causes varicella (chicken pox) as a primary infection and presents in the form of herpes zoster (shingles) as a reactivation of a latent VZV in the sensory ganglia of previously infected individuals. VZV is an airborne pathogen and the virus also sheds from infected vesicles.

The varicella vaccine was developed using a live-attenuated Oka strain varicella virus, and was approved for use in 1995, proving to be safe, effective, and reducing the rate of infection by 60–90%.[9] Varicella vaccination is currently recommended for all people at high risk for exposure who do not have a reliable history of varicella infection or serological evidence of VZV infection, including healthcare workers, those who live or work in environments where transmission is likely (corrections, military bases, daycare centers, colleges, etc.), women wanting to become pregnant, and international travelers. Susceptible children may be vaccinated after 12 months of age; susceptible individuals over 13 years of age should receive two doses, at least 4 weeks apart. The varicella vaccine is contraindicated in pregnant women and pregnancy should be avoided for 4 weeks after immunization. The live attenuated Oka strain varicella vaccine does not effectively prevent herpes zoster or postherpetic neuralgia because it does not provide enough antigenic load to enhance the cell-mediated immune response to VZV.

A herpes zoster live vaccine (Zostavax, Merck) developed to reduce the manifestation of shingles and its complications was approved by the FDA in 2006, for use in patients over 60 years of age. The zoster vaccine contains 18,700–60,000 plaque-forming units of virus and is estimated to be 14 times more potent than the varicella vaccine. The vaccine proved to be safe and efficacious in reducing the morbidity in immunocompetent elderly patients. The vaccine reduced the incidence of herpes zoster by more than 50% and reduced pain and discomfort of affected individuals by 61.1%, compared to the placebo group. The incidence of postherpetic neuralgia decreased by 66.5%, and the severity and duration of pain in those who develop the disease was 61% less than the control group.[10] Erythema, swelling, and pain at the injection site are the most common side effects. Varicella-like rashes may also develop. The live attenuated vaccine is contraindicated in immunocompromised patients and is given as a single subcutaneous dose. Further studies on long-term effectiveness and cost-effectiveness will provide important information for the extended use of this vaccine.

Although the effect of the zoster vaccine on the incidence of herpes zoster was less among individuals over 70 years old compared to individuals with ages ranging from 60 to 69 years (65.5% vs. 55.4%) the effect of the vaccine on the severity of illness and the development of postherpetic neuralgia was greater among the older age group (66.8% vs. 65.7%).[11]

12.3 Human Papillomavirus

Human papillomavirus (HPV) is a nonencapsulated, double-stranded DNA virus that affects the skin and mucoses, and is the cause of common diseases such as cervical neoplasia and anogenital warts. In the US,

over six million cases of HPV infection are documented each year, and approximately 50% of people will carry HPV at some point in their life. Two distinct groups have been identified: oncogenic stains and non-oncogenic strains. Fifteen HPV types are considered high risk for cervical cancer, types 16 and 18 being the most common, accounting for about 70% of cervical cancers in women. HPV types 6 and 11 cause more than 90% of anogenital warts. Vaccination prevention with a vaccine could be 90%.[12]

A HPV quadrivalent vaccine (Gardasil, Merck) against the most prevalent high-risk HPV types was approved by the FDA to reduce the incidence of cervical, vaginal and vulvar cancer, and anogenital warts. This vaccine contains recombinant HPV type-specific virus-like particles made of L1 capsid protein of types 6, 11, 16, and 18. The vaccine has proven to be successful in the prevention of cervical cancer and genital warts by 90% in the vaccine group when compared with placebo.[13]

This vaccine is FDA-approved for use in females 9–26 years of age, and a priority review was announced to extend the potential use to women aged 27 through 45. The vaccine should be given to patients in the approved ages even if they are already carries of other HPV types or have suffered HPV disease. The vaccine is given intramuscularly, at days 1, 60, and 180, covered by most health insurance plans or may be provided through a patient assistance program. Pain, swelling, and local erythema at the site of injection are the most common adverse reactions.

Many experts believe that boys and young men as well as immunosuppressed organ transplant recipients and HIV-positive individuals may benefit from HPV vaccination, protecting themselves against anogenital warts, penile, and anal carcinomas. The European Commission approved the use of this vaccine in males ages 9–15 in an effort to decrease the incidence of genital warts, penile and anal cancers, and reduce cervical cancer in sexual contacts of these individuals. The effectiveness of vaccination in males still needs further investigation.

A bivalent prophylactic vaccine containing virus-like particles of HPV 16 and 18 was also investigated, showing good efficacy against HPV infection (91.6%), but requires further investigation regarding its duration of protective effects and administration standards.[14] However, virus-like particle HPV vaccines failed to improve the rate of viral clearance in women already infected with HPV types 16 and 18, and should not be used to treat the infection.[15]

Therapeutic vaccines in which induced enhanced cell-mediated immunity produces lesion regression have been studied, showing lack of efficacy in human trials for the treatment of genital warts but some promising results in a patient with metastatic cervical cancer.[16, 17] Further trials will explore other therapeutic vaccination strategies to include multiple HPV types and using different antigens.[18]

12.4 Poxviruses

Poxviruses are an extensive family of viruses that include molluscipoxvirus (molluscum contagiosum virus), orthopoxvirus (vaccinia), parapoxvirus (orf), pseudocowpox, yatapoxvirus (tanapox), and cowpox virus, the causing agent of smallpox (variola) and the only virus in this group with an approved vaccine.

12.4.1 Cowpox (Smallpox: Variola)

The smallpox vaccine was the first human vaccine, created by Edward Jenner in 1796, becoming the model for success of viral vaccines. Smallpox was finally eradicated worldwide in 1977 and just over the past years became a concern that it could be used for bioterrorist purposes since it is highly contagious and has a high mortality rate. Smallpox is an airborne and fomite transmitted virus from active skin lesions, and characteristically presents with a febrile prodrome followed by a deep-seated papulo-vesicular rash with subsequent pustule and scab formation.

The smallpox vaccine is a suspended live vaccine derived from the vaccinia virus, similar to the cowpox virus. Although this vaccine is not routinely administered, it is provided to US military personnel and reserves are maintained in case of a bioterrorist outbreak. Pustule formation, local erythema, and pain are common adverse effects, but in the new era of smallpox vaccination other side effects such as erythema multiforme-like rashes and urticarial hypersensitivity reactions have been seen.[19] Postvaccinal encephalomyelitis and death have occurred. Generalized vaccinia is also rare reported complication of smallpox vaccination.[20]

Some physicians are not familiar with the estimated rate of death related to smallpox vaccination (1 in 1,000,000), and vaccination contraindications such as myocardial infarction, angina, congestive heart failure, steroid eye drop use, and the nonemergency vaccination of those younger than age 18.[21] Coadministration of smallpox vaccine with vaccine immune-globulin (VIG) decreases the severity of smallpox in exposed individuals, if administered within 4 days of known exposure.

The development of recombinant vaccines will result in good immunity with fewer complications. A second-generation smallpox vaccine (ACAM2000) was approved in 2007 by the FDA for the inoculation of people at high risk of exposure to smallpox and could be used to protect individuals and populations during a bioterrorist attack.

References

1. Plotkin SA. Immunologic correlates of protection induced by vaccination. *Pediatr Infect Dis J*. 2001;20(1):63–75
2. Watson JC, Hadler SC, Dykewicz CA, et al Measles, mumps, and rubella – vaccine use and strategies for elimination of measles, rubella, and congenital rubella syndrome and control of mumps: recommendations of the Advisory Committee on Immunization Practices (ACIP). *MMWR Recomm Rep*. 1998;47(RR-8):1–57
3. Watson JC, Pearson JA, Markowitz LE, et al An evaluation of measles revaccination among school-entry-aged children. *Pediatrics*. 1996;97(5):613–618
4. Peltola H, Heinonen OP. Frequency of true adverse reactions to measles-mumps-rubella vaccine. A double-blind placebo-controlled trial in twins. *Lancet*. 1986;1(8487):939–942
5. Bennett JV, Fernandez de Castro J, Valdespino-Gomez JL, et al Aerosolized measles and measles-rubella vaccines induce better measles antibody booster responses than injected vaccines: randomized trials in Mexican schoolchildren. *Bull World Health Organ*. 2002;80(10):806–812
6. Kim-Farley R, Bart S, Stetler H, et al Clinical mumps vaccine efficacy. *Am J Epidemiol*. 1985;121(4):593–597
7. Hersh BS, Fine PE, Kent WK, et al Mumps outbreak in a highly vaccinated population. *J Pediatr*. 1991;119(2):187–193
8. Chu S Y, Bernier RH, Stewart JA, et al Rubella antibody persistence after immunization. Sixteen-year follow-up in the Hawaiian Islands. *JAMA*. 1988;259(21):3133–3136
9. Vázquez M, LaRussa PS, Gershon AA, et al Effectiveness over time of varicella vaccine. *JAMA*. 2004;291(7):851–855
10. Kimberlin DW, Whitley RJ. Varicella-zoster vaccine for the prevention of herpes zoster. *N Engl J Med*. 2007;356(13):1338–1343
11. Oxman MN, Levin MJ, Johnson GR, et al Shingles Prevention Study Group. A vaccine to prevent herpes zoster and postherpetic neuralgia in older adults. *N Engl J Med*. 2005;352(22):2271–2284

12. Muñoz N, Bosch FX, de Sanjosé S, et al International Agency for Research on Cancer Multicenter Cervical Cancer Study Group. Epidemiologic classification of human papillomavirus types associated with cervical cancer. *N Engl J Med.* 2003;348(6):518–527

13. Villa LL, Costa RL, Petta CA, et al Prophylactic quadrivalent human papillomavirus (types 6, 11, 16, and 18) L1 virus-like particle vaccine in young women: a randomised double-blind placebo-controlled multicentre phase II efficacy trial. *Lancet Oncol.* 2005;6(5):271–278

14. Harper DM, Franco EL, Wheeler C, et al GlaxoSmithKline HPV Vaccine Study Group. Efficacy of a bivalent L1 viruslike particle vaccine in prevention of infection with human papillomavirus types 16 and 18 in young women: a randomised controlled trial. *Lancet.* 2004;364(9447):1757–1765

15. Hildesheim A, Herrero R, Wacholder S, et al Effect of human papillomavirus 16/18L1 virus-like particle vaccine among young women with preexisting infection: a randomized trial. *JAMA.* 2007;298(7):743–753

16. Santin AD, Bellone S, Gokden M, et al Vaccination with HPV-18 E7-pulsed dendritic cells in a patient with metastatic cervical cancer. *N Engl J Med.* 2002;346(22):1752–1753

17. Vandepapeliere P, Barrasso R, Meijer CJ, et al Randomized controlled trial of an adjuvanted human papillomavirus (HPV) type 6 L2E7 vaccine: infection of external anogenital warts with multiple HPV types and failure of therapeutic vaccination. *J Infect Dis.* 2005;192(12):2099–2107

18. Urman CO, Gottlieb AB. New viral vaccines for dermatologic disease. *J Am Acad Dermatol.* 2008;58(3):361–370

19. Bessinger GT, Smith SB, Olivere JW, James BL. Benign hypersensitivity reactions to smallpox vaccine. *Int J Dermatol.* 2007;46(5):460–465

20. Lewis FS, Norton SA, Bradshaw RD, et al Analysis of cases reported as generalized vaccinia during the US military smallpox vaccination program, December 2002 to December 2004. *J Am Acad Dermatol.* 2006;55(1):23–31

21. Dellavalle RP, Heilig LF, Francis SO, et al What dermatologists do not know about smallpox vaccination: results from a worldwide electronic survey. *J Invest Dermatol.* 2006;126(5):986–989

Prevention of Sexually Transmitted Diseases from Office to Globe

13

Kim K. Dernovsek

13.1 Introduction

My interest in prevention of sexually transmitted diseases (STDs) was borne out of my own frustration in managing the maladies of my dermatologic patients over the last 25 years. As they suffered the consequences of what they had understood would be "safe" sex, via condom use, I began to contemplate that strategy. "Safe sex" originated in the early 1980s as the "buzz-word" for promotion of condom use to high-risk population groups to prevent sexual transmission of HIV/AIDS. Since condoms doubled as barrier contraceptive devices, it was not long before "safe sex" became the prevention strategy of the era. With the use of a simple "prophylactic" device, the condom, adults and teens alike could, in theory, prevent both HIV transmission and pregnancy. They could be "safe" in their sexual practices. In the 1980s and 1990s, it became customary for physicians to caution patients to "practice safe sex." Then, during the late 1990s, as rising rates of chronic, viral, skin-to-skin transmitted STDs became an increasingly widespread public health problem, the medical literature quietly transitioned to the more accurate description, "safer" sex. Yet "safe sex," long written into classroom curricula and medical pamphlets, was in its second-generation as the prevention strategy for the general public. It was not until one of those people got a sexually transmitted disease (STD) and ended up as a patient that the idea that "sex" was not really "safe" had become a reality for that

K.K. Dernovsek
Departments of Dermatology and Family Medicine,
University of Colorado Health Sciences Center,
Pueblo, CO, USA
e-mail: kdernovsek@gmail.com

patient and doctor. I began to feel the havoc wreaked in the lives of my patients by diseases that could have been prevented by different choices. Ultimately, I came full circle in my own thinking, from my early venereal-disease–clinic years of "see'em and treat'em," to becoming an advocate for primary prevention via behavior change.

Certainly there are few physicians who *want* to manage STDs and the complexities of coinfections, reportability, contact tracking, and the coincidental emotional overlay. It follows that the dermatologist who is *least* interested in managing STDs would be *most* interested in encouraging prevention, lest a patient with an STD show up for a clinic appointment. Surely, practicing physicians everywhere would unanimously concur that prevention of STDs would be a goal worth achieving for patients and doctors alike.

How to *really* prevent the now-myriad STDs has become increasingly complex with vaccines, palliative treatment, condoms, etc. Is it any wonder that there is a grassroots movement toward a holistic approach of utter simplicity? Yet the generations since the 1960s are quick to dismiss the concept of true primary prevention, via behavior change, labeling it as religious or political ideology or simply calling it "unrealistic." What *is* realistic is that the patients of this millennium are concerned about their health. They want healthy skin, healthy genitalia, healthy reproductive tracts, and they want to live. They don't want to die of an STD.

The scientific evidence establishes the failure of the condom "risk reduction" approach used over the last 25 years and the data support that people can change their sexual behavior to healthy lifestyles, i.e., primary prevention via "risk avoidance." In this chapter I present the magnitude of the problem, the failure of the past paradigm, the current trends in sexual behavior, a directive counseling approach to patients in the office, and a low-cost vision for health based on the world's best success against HIV to date. There is no other area of public health where we as physicians might, with such a simple approach, have a positive impact and save lives. Whether in the office caring for individual patients, or whether in implementing a new public health paradigm in our local community or around the globe, the opportunity exists for all physicians and healthcare providers to play a role. The vision is to put an end to the suffering and death from STDs the world over by motivating patients to choose healthy sexual lifestyles.

13.2 The Magnitude of the Problem of STDs

The possible adverse consequences of sexual intercourse are varied and well-documented in the literature and include in excess of 25 sexually transmitted infections.[1] More than 65 million people in the United States alone are living with an incurable STD[2] and the financial burden of management of STDs is at an estimated cost to our healthcare system of 17 billion dollars annually.[1]

Dermatologists diagnose and treat lice, molluscum contagiosum, and scabies, all of which can be transmitted by sexual activity and yet are so readily transmitted that nonsexual skin-to-skin contact is their most common presentation. Such skin-to-skin transmission is well-understood by dermatologists who are likewise the experts for diagnosing the manifestations of lymphogranuloma venereum (LGV), syphilis, granuloma inquinale, chancroid, herpes simplex virus (HSV), and genital warts from human papilloma virus (HPV). Physicians may be called upon to manage long-term sequelae such as pelvic inflammatory disease and infertility caused by gonorrhea or chronic asymptomatic chlamydia infection. Sexually acquired hepatitis (A, B, or C) can induce serious morbidity via chronic active hepatitis leading to cirrhosis or resulting in liver transplantation. Patients can die from HIV/AIDS or HPV-induced cervical or penile cancer and will at the least require ongoing medical care.

Due to the chronicity, pathology, and impairment of function caused by most sexually transmitted infections, the intentional use of the traditional terminology,

STDs is warranted. Euphemistic deviation from this descriptive nomenclature is misleading to patient and doctor alike. A sexually transmitted *infection* can be treated and sometimes cured; such that the anatomical area involved can be returned to normalcy. However, a return to normal is certainly not possible for those suffering from venereal infections which are either chronic, intermittently recurring, or cause permanent pathologic damage to the involved tissues and hence by definition, are *diseases*, which are transmitted sexually, i.e., STDs.

At particular risk are current and future generations of youth since 48% of the 18.9 million new cases occurring annually are in sexually active young people aged 15–24 years.[3] It is known that young women are biologically more susceptible to chlamydia, gonorrhea, and HIV infections.[2] This is due to the ectropion of the adolescent cervix, in which there is exposed columnar epithelium for which chlamydia and gonorrhea have a predilection.[4] The squamous-columnar cell junction is likewise more exposed in the adolescent cervix, making this metaplastic transformation zone more susceptible to HPV infection.[5] Unequivocally, STDs pose a more serious health threats to our adolescent patients, whom we diagnose and treat, yet in the case of the viral STDs, cannot cure. Two of these, HSV II (progenitalis) and HPV (genital warts) are seen so regularly in dermatologic office practice so as to warrant more detailed discussion.

13.3 Dermatologic Perspective on Herpes Simplex Virus

Genital herpes (HSV I or HSV II) is most commonly caused by HSV II, which is also known to be a potent facilitator of sexual transmission of HIV infection.[6] Genital herpes is a recurrent, lifelong viral infection[7] affecting at least 50 million Americans age 12 years and older.[7] Ninety percent of these patients are unaware of their status[8] due to asymptomatic intervals between herpes outbreaks and/or undetected signs of lesions especially when hidden on mucosal surfaces of the vagina, cervix, or anus. The virus can be detected in genital secretions of most HSV-II seropositive patients who give no history of having genital herpes[9]; such asymptomatic cutaneous viral shedding likely contributes to the ease with which HSV-II is transmitted. No effective vaccine exits, intermittent or suppressive antiviral treatment does not eradicate the organism from secretions or lesions, nor does condom use fully protect. This is because both HSV-1 and HSV-2 are transmitted through direct contact: kissing, sexual contact (vaginal, oral, or anal sex), or skin-to-skin contact and can be transmitted with or without the presence of sores or other symptoms.[6]

While our nondermatologic colleagues may be baffled by herpes gladiatorum or herpetic whitlow, dermatologists understand the ease of skin-to-skin transmission where pressure, rubbing, or even simple contact is involved. This is true especially with direct droplet transmission of the infectious agent and enhanced where skin barrier alteration via erosion or microscopic fissure from xerosis exists. In the simplest of terms, there is no dermatologist who would with ungloved finger knowingly touch a herpetic vesicle, a syphilitic chancre, the rash of secondary syphilis, or the sore or drainage of chancroid or lymphogranuloma venereum (LGV). Indeed, most dermatologists would likely glove-up to do diagnostic scrapings of scabies or to curette lesions of molluscum contagiosum, even in the years predating "universal precautions."

According to the National Health and Nutrition Examinations Survey (NHANES), which is the key American ongoing population-based study, the HSV II seroprevalence rates rose 30% from 1976 to 1994.[8] It is during this same period of time that a societal liberalization of sexual mores and wide promotion of the "safe" sex condom strategy in clinics and schools was ongoing. In more recent times, alternative sexual practices are changing the natural history of genital herpes infections which had traditionally been HSV II in type. Up to 50% of first-episode genital herpes is HSV-1[10] with oral sex the most likely source, from shedding in the mouth. [11]A review of Herpes genital isolates showed that HSV I increased from 31% in 1993 to 78% in 2001, with HSV I having become the most common cause of new genital herpes on a Midwestern college campus.[10]

On a positive note, from 1999 to 2004, there has been a downward trend in HSV II seroprevalence rate toward 17%.[12] Interestingly, this correlates time-wise with implementation of the Sect. 510 Title V abstinence education initiative in 1999 when abstinence was increasingly emphasized in character-based, sex education school curriculae.[13] Simultaneously during these same years there has been a counter-cultural backlash toward "virginity" among the youth themselves.[14]

Condom use had also gone up during this period of time however this is of uncertain significance due to the theoretical offset of "risk compensation." Risk compensation is the increase in the actual risky behavior (i.e., sexual intercourse) due to the perception of being at reduced risk (i.e., via condom use), which thereby paradoxically increases the frequency of the risky behavior (i.e., sexual intercourse).

What is known with certainty is that HSV II seroprevalence rates are higher if intercourse is initiated under 18 years of age at 21.1% compared to 18 years of age and older at 14.3%.[12] HSV II seroprevalence rates are also higher if there is a greater number of lifetime partners. For example, HSV II seroprevalence is 39.9% if more than 50 partners, 20.8% if 5–9 partners, and 3.8% with only one lifetime partner.[12] Therefore, delay of sexual debut and limitation of lifetime partners is paramount to a successful genital herpes prevention strategy.

13.4 Dermatologic Perspective on Human Papilloma Virus

The second STD that dermatologists frequently manage is HPV infection, in particular, genital warts, which can be found in 1.5–13% of sexually active adults, dependent on the population group studied.[2] Any clinician has experienced the time-consuming agony of the patient newly diagnosed with either Herpes II or HPV (genital warts). It is not unusual for those newly diagnosed with genital warts to experience disclosure anxiety, relationship breakdown, depression, and fears about recurrence and transmission,[15,16] and to reduce numbers of partners (14%), use a condom (41%), or abstain from sexual intercourse (26%).[15] Fortunately our patients can be reassured that 90% of genital warts are caused by non-carcinogenic HPV types 6 and 11, although carcinogenic HPV types 16, 18, 31, 33, and 35 are found occasionally and have been associated with cervical neoplasia in females and squamous cell carcinoma in situ, bowenoid papulosis, erythroplasia of Queyrat and Bowen's disease, and squamous cell carcinoma of the anogenital and head and neck region in males and females.[17]

13.5 Gynecologic Perspective on Human Papilloma Virus

Our gynecology and primary care colleagues regularly encounter subclinical genital HPV infection since 5.5 million such new cases occur annually and it is estimated that 20 million people are currently infected, with the prevalence ranging from 28 to 46% in women under age 26.[2] Due to the ubiquitous nature of HPV genital infection in our sexually active patients, it behooves us as dermatologists to fully understand its natural history so as to correctly counsel patients in prevention. Regarding the natural history of subclinical genital HPV infection, it is reported that among sexually active college women, 26% of 608 studied were already infected at outset. Forty-three percent became infected over 3 years with 9% of them remaining infected at 2 years.[18] In another investigation, 19.7% of 553 enrolled were already infected at outset and 38.8% of the remaining 444 became infected over 2 years.[19] It is from these studies that we understand that at least 90% of subclinical HPV infections spontaneously clear. Nevertheless, persistent infection with a high-risk HPV type for at least 6 months is associated with the risk of developing a squamous intraepithelial lesion.[18] It is known that 95% of cervical cancer is associated with 8 types of HPV,[16,18] and that HPV 16 alone accounts for over 50% of cervical cancers and high-grade dysplasias.[20]

From a public health concern, it is the potential carcinogenicity of subclinical genital HPV infection that sets it apart from genital herpes infection. Unfortunately, just as treatment for visible herpetic blisters does not prevent future viral shedding, likewise treatment of visible genital warts possibly reduces, but does not eradicate HPV infectivity. Our dermatologic aim is always to remove the visible genital warts, destructively, surgically, or via a topical immune modulator. Yet it remains unclear whether reduction of HPV DNA in genital tissue impacts future transmission.[17]

Both HSV II and HPV have been generally rising in prevalence over the last 30 years despite widespread and increasing condom use by adolescents documented over the 14 years from 1991 to 2005.[21] While this may be due to "risk compensation," (above), the inadequacy of condoms to protect uncovered skin during skin-to-skin transmission is the most likely explanation. The herpes lesion may occur on skin that is not covered by the condom or may be transmitted either when visibly present or during asymptomatic periods of viral shedding. In 2001 a panel of 28 experts reviewed 138 papers and concluded that there was no epidemiologic evidence that condom use reduced the risk of HPV transmission although they "might afford some protection."[22] The center for disease control and prevention (CDCP) reported that prevention of genital HPV infection involved (1) refraining from any genital contact with another, (2) long-term mutual monogamy, (3) reduction in the number of partners and careful partner selection, and (4) that the available scientific evidence was not sufficient to recommend condoms as a primary prevention strategy.[23] In a recent study of newly sexually active college women, when partners used condoms consistently and correctly, there was a 70% reduction in HPV infection.[24] The discerning reader will recognize the terms *consistently and correctly* as significant detractors from these results (see Sect. 13.8). A CDCP publication for clinicians, in discussion of the use of condoms for decreasing efficiency of transmission of HPV, states that infections can happen in the scrotum, vulva, or perianus areas unprotected by a condom.[25]

13.6 The HPV Vaccine

An HPV vaccine that targets HPV 16, 18, 6, and 11 was developed and licensed by the Food and Drug Administration (FDA) in 2006. HPV 16 and 18 cause up to 70% of CIN II/III and anogenital cancer and HPV 6 and 11 cause up to 90% genital warts.[26] The vaccine, made from noninfectious HPV-like particles, was tested in thousands of 9–26 year-olds and found to be safe with no serious side effects.[27] Pain at the injection site occurs in 80%, site redness or swelling in 20%, fever (100°F) in 10%, site itching in 3%, and fever (102°F) in 2%.[28] These side effects and fainting comprise most of the adverse events reports on the vaccine. The serious reports (7%) have included Guillain-Barre Syndrome, blood clots, and 39 deaths, although careful analysis by experts has not found a pattern suggestive of causation by the vaccine.[29] The vaccine has nearly 100% efficacy against HPV 16, 18, 6, and 11 of at least 5 years duration with no waning immunity.[27] It is recommended for 11–26 year-old non-pregnant females and contraindicated in yeast-allergic patients.[27] Administered in a series of three injections, the total cost is $375.[30] The cost-effectiveness for HPV 16 and 18 vaccination of 12 year-old girls is estimated at $43,600 per quality adjusted life year (QALY) and cost of extension of vaccination to older girls and women is not cost-effective.[31] Since the vaccine is effective only against carcinogenic HPV types 16 and 18, women remain unprotected against 30% of cervical cancer and pre-immunization counseling is to include a recommendation for continued Pap testing after vaccine administration. Additionally, vaccine providers should notify vaccinated females that "they should continue to practice abstinence or protective sexual behaviors (i.e., condom use), since the vaccine will not prevent other sexually transmitted infections."[27]

Less than a year after FDA approval of the HPV vaccine, the governor of Texas made it mandatory, provoking widespread public concern that later resulted in overturn of this decision. The state of Virginia has made the vaccine mandatory, but with very generous opt-out provisions. Salmon et al., in a Lancet publication expressed concern that generous religious and conscientious exemptions to the HPV vaccine could cause legislators to extend the same to other childhood vaccinations, which would then be detrimental to the public's health.[32] A 2007 Journal of the American Medical Association (AMA) editorial stated: "Given that the overall prevalence of HPV types (16 and 18) associated with cervical cancer is relatively low (2.3%)[33] and that the long-term effects are unknown, it is unwise to require a young girl with a very low lifetime risk of cervical cancer to be vaccinated without her assent and her parent's consent."[34] A *New England Journal of Medicine* editorial,[35] in commenting on a large study of the quadrivalent HPV vaccine in preventing high-grade cervical lesions,[36] raised concerns that evidence was insufficient to infer the effectiveness of vaccination in prevention of CIN III or adenocarcinoma in situ and "... a cautious approach may be warranted in light of important unanswered questions about overall vaccine effectiveness, duration of protection, and adverse effects that may emerge over time." A more recent NEJM editorial raised further reasons for caution, including whether vaccinated women will be less likely to pursue cervical cancer screening and whether other HPV strains will emerge as significant oncogenic serotypes.[37] The American Cancer Society, citing probable diminished vaccine efficacy as the number of lifetime sexual partners increases, does not recommend universal vaccination among women

between 18 and 26 years of age.[38] Lastly, general questions have been raised about the applicability of the traditional compulsory vaccination paradigm to vaccination against HPV. HPV is not a highly infectious airborne disease. There is a cost to society at a loss of something else.[34] Finally, does the patient (parent) retain the right to decline a prevention modality that by one's own behavior and by regular cervical cancer screening can be prevented?

13.7 Prevention of Cervical Cancer Here and Abroad

In the United States it is estimated that there were 11,270 cases and 4,070 deaths from cervical cancer during 2009.[39] Since 95% of cervical cancer is caused by asymptomatic carcinogenic HPV present on the cervix longer than 6 months, it seems to follow that primary prevention of genital HPV infection be the method of preventing cervical cancer. "However, in populations that are screened regularly, as is typical in the U.S., cervical cancer develops rarely in women, even with persistent HPV infection. This is because women with high-grade precursor lesions are usually identified through cytologic screening, and the development of cancer can be prevented through early detection and treatment."[25] Since most cervical precancers develop slowly, nearly all cases can be prevented if a woman is screened regularly.[39] Four separate studies of women who were diagnosed with cervical cancer showed that 28.5%[40] and 30.1%[41] had never had a Pap test and 53%[42] and 56%[43] had not had a Pap test within the 3 years prior to diagnosis. The CDCP summarizes that "The single most important factor associated with invasive cervical cancer is the factor of never or rarely being screened for cervical cancer."[25]

Underscoring the role of preventive cervical screening it is noted that prior to PAP testing programs in the USA, the cervical cancer incidence per 100,000 was 38.0 whereas current rates in developed countries are less than 14.5.[44] Globally, cervical cancer killed 274,000 women in 2002 and age-standardized incidence rates per 100,000 were highest in Southern Africa at 38.2 and Eastern Africa at 42.7.[44] These sobering statistics emphasize the role of cervical Pap testing in prevention of cervical cancer and the effect of the asymptomatic progression of a long-term infection with a carcinogenic HPV subtype in settings where screening is unavailable. It is unlikely that the HPV vaccine will ever be a feasible prevention modality in the developing world countries that need it most due to high cost ($375)[30] and required administration as a series of three injections widely separated over time. Fortunately for countries where vaccines and Pap testing are unlikely to ever reach the masses, there remains a low-cost strategy, one in fact recommended by the CDCP, which states: "The surest way to prevent HPV infection is to abstain from any genital contact, including nonpenetrative intimate contact of the genital area."[25]

13.8 The Failure of the Condom Strategy

To interpret the literature on condoms and determine their role in prevention of STDs from office (individual) to globe (public health), the first step is to review the mechanism of action of the condom. The condom is a latex sheath that covers the penile shaft and glans penis with a receptacle at the tip to contain ejaculate and which must be applied by a human being, during a state of sexual arousal, to the erect penis. By design, a condom is a barrier to transmission of ejaculate containing sperm, i.e., a contraceptive device. The condom therefore is mechanically suited for protection against those pathogens known to be delivered via ejaculate: HIV, gonorrhea, and syphilis. The condom in theory provides at least some protection against those organisms that could be present in ejaculate, on the penile shaft/glans, or against any infectious organisms that might present in the recipient. Therefore condoms theoretically have the potential to be useful protecting against HSV I and II, Herpes, HPV, chlamydia, and any infectious lesion or organism covered by the condom. However, numerous STDs are or can be transmitted by skin-to-skin contact and the condom does not cover all of the potentially infected skin. So even at very best, "perfect and always" use of the condom, the condom by design will never protect against all STDs in real life.

How are condoms assessed as prophylactic devices? The FDA regulates manufacturer's pre- and postmarket compliance with industry standards of testing condom lots via the "water leak" and "air-burst" tests prior to sale. The air-burst test examines strength to resist

breakage during use and the water leak test specifies that the average defect rate should not exceed four leaking condoms per 1,000, although industry standards are more stringent at 1 per 400, with the FDA draft regulations now recommending the same.[45]

The water leak test, "under ideal conditions, is able to detect a hole 3 mm in diameter, but, in practice, the sensitivity (diameter of the smallest hole reliably detectable) is approximately 15 mm."[46] The normal human sperm has a width range of 2.5–3.5 mm (microns, i.e., 2,500 nm) and a length range of 4–5 mm.[47] Since sexually transmitted viruses vary in diameter from 0.04 to 0.15 mm,[48] a conservative, sensitive test of condoms was developed to further evaluate condoms already purchased through retail distributors (and thereby presumably having passed the water leak test).[48] This virus penetration assay was used to evaluate a broad range of condom types and brands and found that 2.6% of latex condoms allowed some virus penetration of particle size 0.032 mm.[48] By comparison, the size of HPV is 0.060 mm.[49] Hepatitis B is 0.040 mm, HIV is 0.10 mm, Herpes simplex is 0.14 mm.[42] However, the relative importance of holes is related to the volume of semen that contains an "infectious dose" of the given STD and it has been concluded that "for infectious agents with low titer and low infectivity (such as HIV), leakage through pores too small to be detected by the water leak test is not the primary public health risk of condom use."[50]

In addition to virus titer, it is known that transmission through a small hole also depends upon transcondom pressure, time for passage, viscosity of the carrier fluid, and condom thickness.[48] Fluid flow is the most important determinant of viral passage through a hole.[22] It has been demonstrated that (1) there is a "strong dependence of virus penetration on hole diameter," such that virus penetrations varied over 4–5 orders of magnitude, whereas the hole size varied over one (from 2 to 21.5 mm), i.e., roughly correlating with the Poiseuille equation of fluid flow through a cylindrical hole varying as the hole diameter to the forth power and that (2) most virus penetration is complete or nearly complete by 2 min.[51] Results from the laboratory tests were applied to determine the hypothetical relative risk of exposure to semen as a function of semen volume attributable to various independent condom use events and it was concluded that the data showed condoms to be a highly effective barrier to transmission of particles of similar size to those of the smallest STD viruses; with a strong probability of condom effectiveness when used correctly, where the etiology of STD transmission is linked to containment of preejaculate and seminal fluids or barrier coverage of lesions of the penis and there is no slippage or breakage. It was additionally noted however that for many STDs the risk of infection might not be proportional to exposure to a volume of semen and that estimation of risk requires further extrapolation because it depends also on the concentration, infectivity, and mode of transmission of the specific STD.[22] Thus it can be summarized that even if minute leakage of viral-sized particles occurs,[48] condoms do protect against STDs and in a controlled laboratory setting, transmission of infection is highly unlikely.[19,42]

Such laboratory testing is for efficacy, i.e., the improvement, achieved in a desired health outcome in a research setting in expert hands under ideal conditions. To achieve something close to efficacious use of the condom in actual life, "perfect use" must be achieved: i.e., use of the condom 100% of the time and 100% correctly each time of use. Unfortunately, in "real life," the condom often fails to protect.[52-56] That is because in actuality the best that can be achieved is "typical" use of the condom, which includes using the condom "some," "most," or "all" of the time and using it both correctly and incorrectly. Hence it is *effectiveness*, i.e., the amount of improvement in the health outcome in actual life with typical implementation, which is clinically applicable.

Condoms are known to fail in protection against pregnancy at a rate of 14%[52] and in protection at variable rates against ejaculate-delivered pathogens, the specific purpose for which they were designed.[45,46,48] Failure can occur due to "method" or "user" failure or both. "Method" failure occurs when the condom itself, as a device, fails. Types of "method" failure would result from defects incurred during manufacture or improper storage, and could include leakage or breakage during intercourse or withdrawal, or slippage during intercourse, either partially or completely.[53,55,57-60]

"User" failure refers to the condom being *used* incorrectly and represents the human component, i.e., one's (in) ability to comply with proper use during arousal and sexual intercourse. Examples of "user" failure include genital contact before condom application[61] (preejaculatory secretions can contain both infectious pathogens and sperm), flipping condom over after initial application (noting the condom to be applied "upside-down" so that when turned over contact with preejaculatory secretions on the now-exposed condom surface occurs), holes poked in condom (fingernails or jewelry from piercings), use of oil-based lubricants (known to weaken condom strength), improper positioning of condom, not holding on to condom during withdrawal resulting in ejaculate spillage and not withdrawing while penis erect (falling asleep after intercourse).[53,62]

To approach laboratory-setting efficacy of condoms in real life, "perfect condom use" (i.e., "always" (consistently) and "correctly" with each use), would need to be achieved. What scientific evidence exists for one's ability to achieve perfect use in real life? In one study of college-educated males with an average of more than 5 years of condom experience who were "consistent, 100%" condom users, it was found that altogether at least 13% of condom uses had resulted in exposure to risks of unprotected intercourse due to breakage, slippage, or failure to use condoms throughout intercourse. This calculated to 33% of the consistent condom users having been exposed to risks of disease or pregnancy in the prior month.[62] Similarly, of 186 females aged 15–21, who had reported vaginal sex in the past 14 days and who were self-described consistent (100%) condom users, 34% were found to have sperm present in vaginal fluid via Y-chromosome polymerase chain reaction assay.[63] In a study of the value of consistent condom use in adolescent females, 17.8% acquired at least one STD (chlamydia trichomoniasis, gonorrhea) despite consistent (100%) condom use.[64] Lastly, in a study of HIV serodiscordant heterosexual couples, in which 171 always used condoms, three seroconversions occurred over 24 months (1.1% incidence rate).[65] Therefore, either method (device) or user failure (incorrect use) must have occurred in order for seroconversion to HIV positivity to have taken place for any of them.

On a lighter note, a personal observation of an academically embarrassing demonstration of the complexities of correct condom use is recalled from the AIDS and STD Symposium of the 2002 American Academy of Dermatology meeting. The speaker was explaining how teens are taught in school programs to correctly use condoms by ordering steps known to be necessary for correct condom usage. To press the point he ordered dermatologists from the audience to the front, divided them into two groups and gave them each a card with a "step" in the condom use process, to put in proper order. In competition against their colleagues, the dermatologists, presumably both intelligent and manually adroit, appeared to have a great deal of difficulty ordering the steps. Ultimately each group came up with a different order of steps. In the comedy that ensued, it was never confirmed whether either group had correctly ordered the steps involved in using a condom. Since each group came up with a different order of steps, what can be concluded is that one of the groups of physicians was wrong.

The fact remains that despite years of condom public education, people still fail to use condoms correctly. What does the evidence show about whether people are able to use condoms "always," i.e., "consistently?" Three studies are concerning that, for whatever reason, people don't or won't or can't use condoms consistently. First, among a nationally representative sample of unmarried sexually experienced females aged 15–44 years who stated they "used condoms" for disease prevention, only 18.5% *always* used condoms.[66] Second, we know that among Herpes discordant couples, despite counseling to always use a condom (11 visits during 18 months), and in a vaccine trial where it was not known whether the seronegative partner had received the HSV subunit vaccine or a placebo, that only 8% "always used" a condom and 15.5% used a condom for 51–99% of sex acts.[67] In a parallel clinical trial of an HSV-2 vaccine subsequently found to be ineffective, 13% "always used" a condom and 16% used a condom for 76–99% of sexual acts, despite the counseling protocol described above and provision of free condoms at the 11 study visits.[68] Lastly is a prospective study, done prior to the development of effective antiretroviral therapy, of HIV-negative subjects whose only risk of HIV infection was a stable heterosexual relationship with an HIV-infected partner. Every 6 months the subjects were interviewed, tested for HIV, and counseled about safe sexual practices and despite the knowledge that they were at risk for a fatal disease, only 48.4% of these HIV discordant couples "always" used a condom.[69]

In addition to the problems of correct and consistent use of condoms outlined above, there are additional factors influencing condom failure in the real-life setting. The adequacy of protection against STDs will depend on the degree of infectivity of the particular STD, the prevalence of the STD in the community, the number of acts of intercourse, the user's prior experience with condoms, the age and sex of the individual, the natural

immunity of the individual, and whether lesions of other STDs are present.[70] Earlier in the chapter was described the discouraging conclusions reported by three government agencies on the existing scientific evidence for condom effectiveness in preventing HPV. Equally discouraging are the experts' conclusions regarding prevention of other STDs. Regarding chlamydia gonorrhea in women, and trichomoniasis they concluded that the available epidemiologic literature does not allow an accurate assessment of the degree of potential protection.[22] Regarding genital herpes, syphilis, and chancroid they stated that the data were insufficient to draw meaningful conclusions about the effectiveness of the latex male condom to reduce the risk of transmission.[22] The data were clear regarding the "strong evidence" for the effectiveness of condoms for reducing sexually transmitted gonorrhea for men and HIV/AIDS: that with HIV/AIDS, consistent condom use decreased the risk of HIV/AIDS transmission by approximately 85%.[22] In the more recent *Sexually Transmitted Diseases Treatment Guidelines 2006*, the CDCP states that "HIV-negative partners in heterosexual serodiscordant relationships in which condoms were consistently used were 80% less likely to become HIV-infected compared with persons in similar relationships in which condoms were not used."[71]

The scientific evidence has supported cautions offered during the early years of AIDS prevention strategy development. For example, Judson, et al. who in 1989 stated after describing the factors related to condom effectiveness: "Thus it would seem prudent not to place excessive reliance on latex condoms alone for prevention of sexually transmitted infections."[55] In 1994, d'Oro et al. reviewed barrier methods in prevention of STDs and concluded, "A consistent and strong protection may well be acceptable for treatable diseases and rare exposures, but a similar protection is clearly not satisfactory for frequent exposures and, particularly, serious or severe diseases."[56] Certainly there is no other fatal disease where it is acceptable public health policy to widely and primarily promote, around the globe, to young and old alike, a risk reduction modality in which the chance of becoming infected still remains 20%, at the universal exclusion of a risk avoidance strategy in which the chance of infection is 0%.

We have assumed that our patients cannot abstain from sex even though we understand that sex is not a mandatory biologic reflex like micturation, defecation, or sleep. We must consider the possibility that our own bias based on personal life experience has skewed our medical approach. Perhaps when we do not or have not modeled the proposed sexual behavior change, it becomes more uncomfortable for us to endorse and/or recommend it. Nevertheless we are ethically obligated to give our patients the best medical recommendation for health preservation. Therefore, for the health of our patients, is it time to rethink our STD prevention strategy from office to globe?

13.9 Defining Terminology: Safe Sex, Sex, and Abstinence

Although the medical literature currently refers to the condom method as "safer" sex, confusion over what people understand to be "safe" has prevailed. This is exemplified by varied verbiage describing condom effectiveness on packaging, such as, "safer sex, give protection, protect, are highly effective, effective, may help, will help, can reduce the risk, will reduce the risk and significantly reduce the risk."[72] As a result, directed by Public Law 106–554, the FDA proposed rules in 2005 to designate a special controls guidance document with labeling recommendations for latex condoms. The FDA concluded that condoms reduce the overall risk of STD transmission although the degree of risk reduction for different types of STDs varies with their routes of transmission. The FDA now proposes that labeling consistently utilize the terminology, "sexually transmitted diseases" and address incorrect and inconsistent use which "undermines" condom effectiveness. The FDA also proposes that labeling address the limited benefits and risks presented by N-9 spermicidal lubricant since frequent use can cause mucosal irritation, which may increase the risk of transmission of HIV.[73]

Twenty-plus years of the "safe sex" paradigm have resulted in terminology confusion for youth. In a 2000 survey of 12–17 year olds, 88% reported having heard the expression "safe sex," yet when asked to specify which behavior(s) they considered safe, 86% said not having sex/abstinence was "safe sex," 72% said "safe sex" was using a condom, 46% said birth control pills were "safe sex" and 21% said oral sex was "safe sex."[74] Regarding the practice of oral sex, specifically, a 2003 survey of 15–17 year olds revealed that 46% thought oral sex was "not as big of a deal" as sexual intercourse.

Thirty-nine percent considered oral sex "safer sex" and 19% did not know you could get an STD through oral sex.[75] These misconceptions exist despite clearly listing as "can be transmitted by oral sex" in a 2000 CDCP fact sheet: HIV, herpes, syphilis, gonorrhea, HPV, intestinal parasites (amebiasis), and hepatitis A.[76] It is not clear to teens that oral sex is a form of sexual intercourse. In the youth surveys, 63% said they had "never had sex" but 13% of those had had oral sex.[75] It is therefore paramount that we retain a precise definition: Sexual intercourse is the stimulation of a partner to orgasm via vaginal, oral, anal, nongenital activity, i.e., mutual masturbation.[77] As we communicate with clarity the correct definition of sexual intercourse, then our patients (who are themselves, community members, teachers, parents and teens) can correctly counsel that it follows that abstinence is by definition, abstinence from *all* forms of sexual intercourse. Adding an appropriate endpoint to abstinence makes it clear that "abstinence" is not just until the next Saturday night date, but that it is a lifestyle to be continued until a certain predefined time. Thus derives the terminology, "lifestyle abstinence,"[78] that being a lifestyle of abstaining from *all* sexual activity *until* marriage, i.e., selection of lifelong faithful partner, i.e., until sustained mutual monogamy.

"Lifestyle abstinence" as a lifestyle choice will ensure freedom from all sexually transmitted diseases as will sustained mutual monogamy in the case where both partners have abstained until this relationship. Encouraging these health-preserving behaviors is in keeping with most global societal standards. Our patients deserve to understand the health risk that exists with the lifestyle of "serial monogamy," i.e., monogamy for some period of time followed by termination of that relationship followed by monogamy for another period of time with a different individual, and so forth. With each new monogamous relationship, that new partner brings with them a past sexual health history that may not be healthy. If the periods of serial monogamy are each of brief duration then the risk to the health of the individual may not be much improved over networks of concurrent sexual partners. This latter category of sexual lifestyle, whether called concurrency, polygamy, prostitution, sex work, promiscuity, or guised in slang terms of "hooking up," "anonymous partnering," or "friends with benefits" are all highly risky sexual lifestyles for both the individual and for the health of the society (Fig. 13.1).

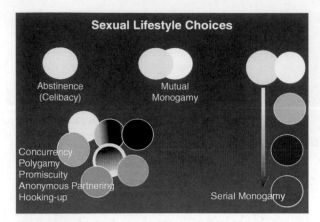

Fig. 13.1 There is no risk of contracting a sexually transmitted disease (STD) in *lifestyle abstinence* or sustained mutual monogamy with an uninfected partner but with each new sexual partner, who may be an asymptomatic STD carrier due to past or current sexual relationships, STD risk occurs and is highest with multiple sexual partners (Adapted from a video by Stephen J. Genuis, courtesy Stephen J. Genuis)

13.10 STD Prevention in the Office: Recommended Guidelines

The medical and scientific practice guidelines clearly recommend counsel regarding behavior change in prevention of STDs and their sequelae. In response to the growing health threats of STDs for our adolescent patients and to assist primary care physicians and other health providers to make preventive services a greater component of their clinical practice, the AMA Guidelines for Adolescent Preventive Services (1997) first recommended that annual "health guidance" regarding responsible sexual behavior include "counseling that abstinence from sexual intercourse is the most effective way to prevent pregnancy and STDs, including HIV infection."[79] The CDCP state in both the 2002 and the 2006 Guidelines for Treatment of STDs that "the most reliable way to avoid transmission of STDs is to abstain from sexual intercourse (i.e., oral, vaginal, or anal sex) or to be in a long-term, mutually monogamous relationship with an uninfected partner."[80,81] The guidelines further state that "counseling that encourages abstinence from sexual intercourse is crucial … for persons who wish to avoid the possible consequences of sexual intercourse (e.g., STD/HIV and unintended pregnancy)."[80,81] A 2005 clinical report from the Committee on Adolescence, American Academy of Pediatrics (AAP), makes as the first, and presumably

primary, recommendation to pediatricians the following: "Encourage adolescents to postpone early sexual activity and encourage parents to educate their children and adolescents about sexual development, responsible sexuality, decision-making, and values."[82]

Nevertheless, adolescents are not routinely being encouraged by physicians to postpone early sexual activity since only 42.8% females and 26.4% males indicated having discussed STD, HIV, or pregnancy prevention at a healthcare visit in the preceding year[83] and counseling in HIV/STD transmission has been reported to occur in only 6.2% of well visits.[84] Barriers to sexual history taking were reported to be difficulties asking sexual history questions, fear of offending patients, and lack of time in more than half of physicians surveyed.[85] Even in the less sensitive realm of counseling young patients in smoking cessation, the perception that counseling is time-consuming and the fear that the parent would be angered were reported as perceived barriers to counseling by over 50% of physicians surveyed.[86]

13.11 STD Prevention in the Office: A Directive Approach

Within my own community private practice of dermatology, I examined the validity of two perceived barriers to abstinence counseling (fear of offending and perception of inadequate time) by observing whether the physician–patient relationship is adversely affected, as assessed by frequency of return for care. I additionally determined whether abstinence counseling is time-consuming by observing its effect on usual scheduling patterns. Due to the broad implications in the area of physician health maintenance counseling, adolescent sexual health, and our role as dermatologists in this realm, I report my findings within this chapter.

My solo private practice is one of four dermatology practices (all of which are open to new patients [NPs]) in Pueblo County, Colorado (population 141,472[87]). The study practice has a payer mix of managed care, preferred provider organizations, private pay, Medicaid, and indigent community clinic patients. Ethnicity was estimated by my observation to be 77% Caucasian, 22% Hispanic, <1% African American, and <1% other. The county served is 57.7% Caucasian, 38% Hispanic, 1.9% African American, and 2.3% other.[87] Ethnicity breakdown and description of payer mix are provided for ease of evaluating applicability of results to other communities and to demonstrate that the practice draws widely from the community. Scheduling allots NPs 20 or 30 min (physician referral) and established patients (FUs) 10 (acne or postoperative) or 15 min. Scheduling is done by the same staff member who has performed in this capacity since 1993.

I undertook to initiate medical guideline recommended abstinence counsel to all youth in my practice and then observe whether return to the office was inhibited by such abstinence counseling beginning on 01 Nov 1998 and continuing to 01 Jan 2001. During this time male and female NPs and FUs, aged 13–19, nonrandomized, regardless of reason for visit, were counseled by me. The NP and FU control groups consisted of the cohorts of male and female patients aged 13–19 not instructed in abstinence in the immediate 10 months prior to the study, January through October of 1998. Analysis showed the control and abstinence-counseled groups to be age and gender matched.

The physician counseling style was concerned, casual, simple, and brief, allowing silence for patient response. After forewarning that an unexpected topic would be initiated, "This has nothing to do with the reason for your visit, but is also important for your health," counseling in the style of asking, informing, and advising began: While handing an abstinence pamphlet[88] I asked, "Have you ever heard of abstinence?" Physician silence followed. Then "lifestyle abstinence"[78] was defined as a lifestyle choice requiring restraint from all forms of sexual intercourse until selection of lifelong partner. Third, the patient was advised that lifestyle abstinence could be initiated despite past or current behavior, thereby preventing disease transmission and ensuring health preservation. Physician silence followed. Throughout, counseling was adapted according to patient response (Fig. 13.2).

If a patient confirmed abstinence/virginity, this was reinforced by physician's affirmation of this behavior as "healthiest," sustained abstinence was encouraged and the patient was enlisted to advise peers and pass the pamphlet on. If a patient declared sexual activity, counseling was modified to risk reduction via an "*informed* condom recommendation," hereby *strictly* defined: First, informing the patient of condom inadequacy in complete protection against all STDs. Second, recommending condom usage as the next best alternative to lifestyle abstinence. Third, advising that

lifestyle abstinence could be resumed, variously termed by peers as renewed-, recycled-, or secondary virginity. Fourth, the option of conversion of the relationship to lifelong monogamy was raised for the patient's consideration.

If there was no verbal response, didactic directive education began with one of the following, "A lot of kids don't realize that … condoms don't fully protect them against diseases,[22,23,78] … one in five people over age 12 already have genital herpes[8] or HPV[89] … dermatologists have to treat STDs … even their skin doctor wants them to stay healthy … that this is a message for boys *and* girls" ending with, "I don't want my patients to say that I never warned them about STDs and how to prevent them. *Now* is the time for you to decide where you will stand in this matter."

The patient and/or parent response to lifestyle abstinence counseling was observed and whether the patient returned for care was determined. A return was recommended only as warranted by the patient's medical condition and the adolescent received medical counsel and treatment regardless of presence or absence of the parent; as per the standard of care for the practice. Counsel in sexual abstinence, specifically, is as recommended by both the CDCP[80,81] and the AAP[82]; it is primary prevention (risk elimination) counsel of universal benefit and therefore no patients were intentionally excluded. Finally, the rate of return to the practice was not calculated for either control or observed cohort until the observation was complete.

Results of in-office adolescent abstinence counsel revealed that 135 new and established patients were counseled. Lifestyle abstinence counseling did not require schedule alteration; hence the observation was not terminated prematurely as had been intended if the physician schedule could not be maintained. In all 51.9% NPs (61.5% females, 42.9% males) not instructed in abstinence returned compared to 69.7% NPs (75.0% females, 64.7% males) who were instructed, ($P=0.151$, $P=0.473$, $P=0.206$); 74.5% FUs (75.9% females, 72.7% males) not instructed in abstinence returned compared to 78.3% FUs (80.6% females, 75.8% males) who were instructed, ($P=0.667$, $P=0.764$, $P=1.00$). Statistical analysis (Fisher's Exact Test, 2-sided) failed to detect a significant difference in population groups, indicating that the abstinence-counseled patients (NPs, FUs, males, females) were at least as likely to return as those who had not been counseled (Fig. 13.3).

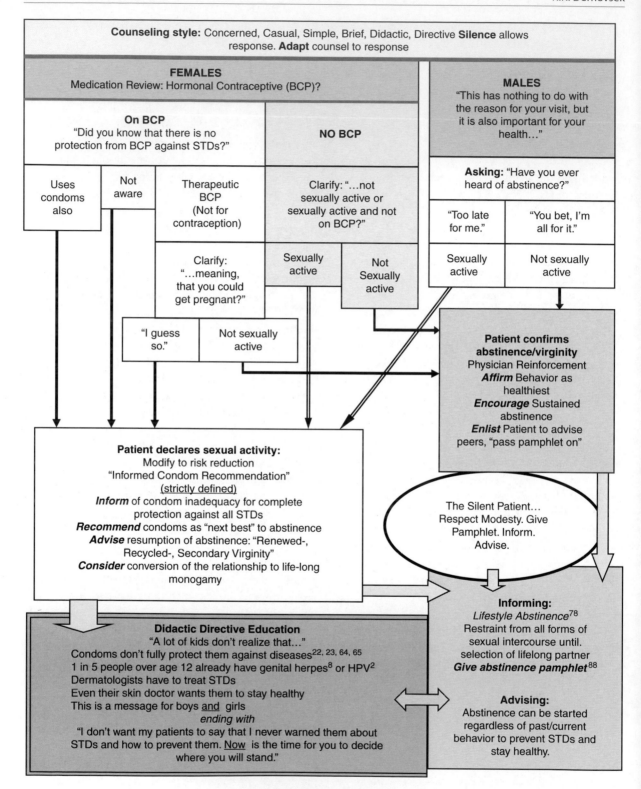

Fig. 13.2 Algorithm for sexual abstinence counsel of the adolescent

Fig. 13.3 The percentage of new (*NP*) and established (*FU*) male and female adolescent patients (aged 13–19) returning for care: comparison of those who received sexual abstinence counseling with those who did not

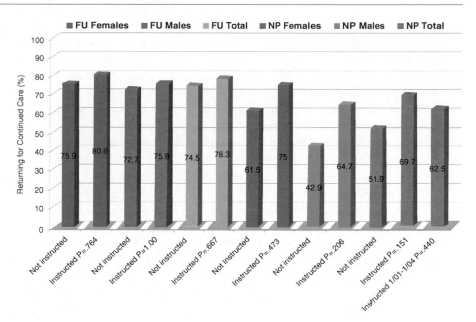

Ninety-seven percent (131/135) of patient responses varied from neutral to positive; 12% (16/135) of patient responses were so positive as to result in role reversal with the patient enumerating reasons for abstinence until marriage with four describing renewed virginity and 12 intending to "stay virgins." Three percent (4/135) of the responses were categorized as negative: All were parents who questioned the "reality" of abstinence.

However, two of four parents were immediately challenged by the adolescent patient who defended abstinence: One countered, "Mom, chastity is cool!" Another muttered, "My mother needs your lessons." Two patients were on oral contraceptives at the next visit: evidence of their commitment to sexual activity, but also evidence that the physician–patient relationship was not adversely affected by the patient's knowledge that the physician recommended sexual abstinence as ideal. A separate patient returned for an STD examination, newly motivated to address health risks of prior sexual activity.

This observation undertaken in a general practice of dermatology shows that new and established patients counseled in lifestyle abstinence were at least as likely as those who had not been counseled to return for care, apparently not inhibited by the abstinence instruction. Furthermore, from 01 Jan 2001 through 01 Jan 2004, since most FUs had already been counseled, this physician continued to counsel NPs ($n=32$, 47% males, average age 15.3 years; 53% females, average age 15.6 years); 62.5% (20/32) returned. Statistical

analysis (Fisher's exact test, 2-sided) of this group compared to the original control group fails to detect a significant difference in population groups ($P=0.440$), again indicating that the abstinence-counseled patients were at least as likely to return as those who had not been counseled (Fig. 13.3). This physician continues counseling in lifestyle abstinence, time-efficiently, with unaltered scheduling to this date.

This in-office observation is limited firstly by failure to enumerate observations; for example, the parental silently mouthed, "thank you" response predominated, yet frequency was not recorded. Secondly, 24 NPs and 22 FUs, i.e., 25% (46/181) of patients in the abstinence-counseled population were not counseled due to severity of illness, psychiatric disorder, mental retardation, current pregnancy, and if already on birth control, received an "informed condom recommendation." Thirdly, other barriers to lifestyle abstinence counseling may exist, including inadequate physician knowledge; the physician is encouraged to review the myriad STDs, their consequences, and the scientific evidence on condom effectiveness (or lack thereof) for STD prevention.[22,23] Finally, no attempt is made to determine whether the patients followed the lifestyle abstinence counsel given; a follow-up survey is under consideration.

This clinical observation of correct counsel of youth in abstinence per guideline recommendations has shown that the physician need not fear offending the patient or disrupting the schedule when providing lifestyle abstinence counseling, even in a dermatology practice, where the advice was somewhat unexpected. Explanation of the relationship between the skin and STDs actually facilitated patient and parent education, since (1) it is no longer commonly known that until 1955, ours was the specialty of *dermatology and syphilology* and (2) patients and their parents were seldom aware that condoms do not fully protect from the skin-to-skin transmission of HSV[90] and HPV.[23] Educating that lifestyle abstinence is "restraint from all forms of sexual intercourse until selection of lifelong partner" is important because disease transmission also occurs with nontraditional forms of sexual intercourse and adolescents who abstain for the longest periods of time will be at least risk. For these reasons, dermatologists and other physicians caring for adolescents can be encouraged to incorporate lifestyle abstinence counseling in health maintenance advice alongside skin cancer prevention instruction.

13.12 STD Prevention: Trends and Expectations

Aligned with the AMA,[79] CDCP,[80,81] and AAP[82] recommendations, 91–95% adults and 92–94% adolescents surveyed annually from 2001 to 2004 agree that it is important for teens to be given "a strong message from society to abstain from sex until they are at least out of high school."[91-95] The community physician likely recognizes the importance of such a message since survey has shown that 49% of people with an STD had gone to a private practice for treatment.[96] Furthermore, sexual abstinence counseling may be most effective if done specifically by the physician since patients who received physician advice on other topics, such as diet and exercise were significantly more likely to engage in risk reduction activities[97] and when physicians provide brief simple advice on smoking cessation there is a small but significant increase in cessation rates.[98] Primary care and pediatrics practices, where health maintenance advice for the adolescent is expected, can be encouraged to include lifestyle abstinence counseling alongside routine counsel against tobacco, drinking, illicit drug use, and promotion of exercise and healthy diet. However, since childhood immunizations are completed at age 12,[99] the primary

care provider may have fewer opportunities to advise the adolescent than the dermatologist.

Ramsay et al. reported in 1986 that both dermatologists and dermatology training program directors overwhelmingly supported an increase in dermatology's role in the treatment of sexually transmitted disease and in public awareness of our interest and ability.[100] More than 20 years later it is expected that dermatologists, who understand skin-to-skin transmission of disease and still regularly treat genital HSV, genital warts and other STDs, are sufficiently motivated to prevent these infections and will assume a leadership role as physicians in educating adolescent patients, of whom they have many. In 1997, a panel addressed the "hidden epidemic" of STDs and called for private sector organizations and for clinicians to assume more leadership in and responsibility for STD prevention especially among adolescents.[1] For example, if dermatology, as a specialty, were to publish a pamphlet for facilitation of youth counsel in abstinence by dermatologists and primary care physicians alike, we might positively impact the sexual health of untold numbers of adolescent patients. This opportunity for prevention is certainly more desirable than the necessity of treatment.

Lowell A. Goldsmith, MD, the Clarence S. Livingood, MD lecturer, said in his address at the national meeting of the American Academy of Dermatology in 2001 that dermatologists should have a goal to think about health promotion every day and to promote the concept to their patients. Aligned with that vision, there is a daily opportunity to reduce morbidity and mortality by encouraging adolescent patients toward the healthiest sexual behavior. Yet, in a 2004 survey of clinicians, 91% of whom agreed that abstinence was a highly effective method for prevention of HPV infection acquisition, only 54% recommended abstinence to their adolescent patients.[101] It appears that we are reluctant to counsel abstinence to our adolescent patients perhaps because we hold little hope that they might choose it. The evidence shows otherwise: the Youth Risk Behavior Surveys showed a *reversal* from 1991 to 2001 in what had been in prior years, elevating trends of teen sexual experience ("ever having had sexual intercourse"),[102] and in both 2007 and 2005, 52–53% of high school students described themselves as not yet having experienced first sexual intercourse.[103,104] Surveys in 2003 of slightly younger adolescents, aged 15–17, revealed 63%[105] and 67%[106] had never had sexual intercourse.

Dermatologists have the expertise in STDs and see adolescents regularly as patients and thus are ideally situated to correctly counsel them. Even if the abstinence counsel were followed only temporarily, postponement of sexual activity would reduce the number of lifetime partners, in turn reducing the risk of STD acquisition. On the other hand, if the lifestyle abstinence counsel were heeded, it would positively impact that patient's health for a lifetime.

13.13 Sexual Behavior Change Yields Health

Is there evidence that people can change sexual behavior with a resultant improvement in health? The answer is found in the story of Uganda. This sub-Saharan African nation reversed what had been the highest rates of HIV/AIDS in the world – and did so without Western world public health direction. Ugandan leadership inspired culturally appropriate sexual behavior change as the means by which to save lives, their culture, and their youth. What followed was a dramatic drop in HIV prevalence rates, as was said in 2003, and still holds true today: "… Uganda has experienced the most significant decline in HIV prevalence of any country in the world …"[107] Without a doubt, what happened in Uganda, at an estimated cost of only $1.80 per adult per year over a 10 year period (1989–1998)[108] is the greatest public health achievement of this millennium. The scientific evidence demonstrating population level risk-avoidance behavior change which in turn resulted in reduced HIV prevalence rates should irrefutably and without delay shift global public health strategy in the fight against AIDS. The Ugandan strategy is a low-cost model with potential for eradicating global AIDS if other countries can implement similar risk-elimination behavior change.

During the years from 1986 to 2001 the dramatic drop in HIV prevalence was observed in Uganda while simultaneously elsewhere in sub-Saharan Africa the HIV prevalence was rising.[109] This remarkable anomaly was first reported in 2002, in a landmark presentation to USAID in which the authors reported that "The most important determinant of the reduction in HIV incidence in Uganda appears to be a decrease in multiple sexual partnerships and networks." They further concluded that "The effect of HIV prevention interventions

in Uganda (particularly partner reduction) during the past decade appears to have had a similar impact as a potential medical vaccine of 80% efficacy."[108]

Most notable was that this strategy was a conceptually simple, financially achievable, culturally appropriate indigenous response incorporating broad-sector community involvement under presidential leadership. The Ugandan president, Yoweri Museveni had entered office in 1986 and found a high percentage of the military infected with HIV. In those tenuous years immediately following the regimes of Idi Amin and Milton Obote, and until about 1995, Uganda was without Western world influences on public health strategy development. President Museveni encouraged Ugandan community leaders in medicine, religion, media, and education to work together toward the goal of preventing AIDS, in order to save Uganda. He and First Lady Janet Museveni (who was to became a key youth motivator via the Uganda Youth Forum) heightened awareness about AIDS, dispelled myths about its cause, and warned people that AIDS caused death, but that AIDS could be stopped. AIDS was a danger to Uganda's survival, so appropriate to African context, they sent out an "alarm" to "call" to all Ugandans that, *by their own sexual behavior of abstaining from sexual activity and being faithful in marriage, they could completely avoid death from AIDS.*[110] This homegrown public health campaign was disseminated widely in schools, from pulpits and taken up by the media and performing arts. It was culturally appropriate and easily understood by an African agrarian population. For example, the idea of sticking only to one partner was called "zero grazing." This concept was easily understood by rural people via communication of a metaphor that made sense to them: "You tether your animal around a tree, and it can only feed where it is tethered."[111] The First Lady encouraged youth to abstain at every opportunity, stating about her efforts, "Young people must be taught the virtues of abstinence, self-control and postponement of pleasure and sometimes sacrifice" and teaching them a different lifestyle "will ensure their survival."[112]

When the Ugandan success was summarized to USAID in 2002, it described the "matter-of-fact," inspirational approach used by President Museveni and thousands of community, religious, and government leaders who encouraged "delayed sexual activity, *a*bstaining, *b*eing faithful, 'zero grazing' and using *c*ondoms (roughly in that order)."[108] As Mrs. Museveni herself has noted, the condom message was targeted to adults who were "already infected with HIV" or were "set in their ways" and unlikely to change their risky behaviors.[110] Uganda's unique strategy had been under scientific scrutiny since the late 1990s by WHO and other organizations and was sometimes "conveniently" abbreviated ABC although "Uganda did in fact emphasize A (abstinence) and B (being faithful) before advising C (condoms)."[113] In other words, the elements of the abbreviation were not equivalent; "their rank order reflects the priority in which they arguably ought to be considered, since it is a basic public health maxim that avoiding a risk is inherently better than reducing a risk."[113]

Others have likewise concluded that the emphasis was on A and B, abstinence and being faithful: "condoms were a minor component of the original strategy."[114] It is reported that prior to 1995 in Uganda there were "few" condoms available in 1987, 15 million in 1989, 12 million in 1991, 10 million in 1992, and 22 million in 1993.[115] Given 4,548,701 men over age 15 in Uganda in 1990[116] it can be calculated that at best, prior to 1995, each Ugandan man had 2–5 condoms in a year that he had any condoms at all.

In fact, condom distribution by the Ministry of Health did not begin until the early to mid-1990s and condom sales did not reach substantial levels until the later 1990s when Population Services International began its more successful condom sales program in 1997.[117] During this time of limited condom availability, the data show that HIV prevalence nationally among pregnant women had peaked in 1991 at 21.1%

and already by 1998 had declined to 9.7% (a decline of 54% apparent in both rural and urban settings) (Fig. 13.4).[114]

It has been concluded that "nearly all of the decline in HIV incidence (and much of the decline in prevalence) had already occurred by 1995" in response to social acceptance of the sexual behavior change messages of abstinence and faithfulness.[117] The role of primary risk avoidance behavior change (reflective of the A, Abstinence) is substantiated by analysis of Ugandan population-based surveys of HIV behavioral risk indicators between 1989 and 1995 which show increase in the age of sexual debut in all youth aged 15–24 except rural females,[114] who traditionally marry young, such that their age of sexual debut remained unchanged (Fig. 13.5). Partner reduction (reflective of the B, Be faithful) is demonstrated by a 60% reduction in persons reporting casual sexual partnerships in the previous year in all population groups studied. (male and female, urban, and rural) (Fig. 13.5). The authors conclude that "HIV reductions in Uganda resulted from public-health interventions that triggered a social process of risk avoidance manifested by radical changes in sexual behavior."[114]

Given the historical and scientific data, it is not surprising that there are Ugandans who reflect that their success would have been more aptly called "AB," write out the abbreviation as ABc while vocalizing, "AB, little c" (personal communications and observations. Dernovsek, KK. Mbarara and Kampala, Uganda, 1–31 Oct 2003), or say it was simply, "AB-Stop!" or "AB-Full

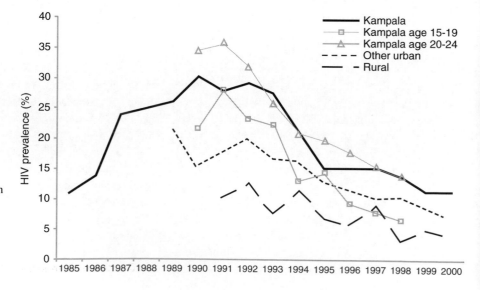

Fig. 13.4 HIV prevalence rates (%) in pregnant women surveyed at antenatal sentinel surveillance sites in Uganda in urban Kampala, other urban sentinel sites, and rural sites from 1985 to 2001 (Adapted from Stoneburner and Low-Beer.[114] Used with permission)

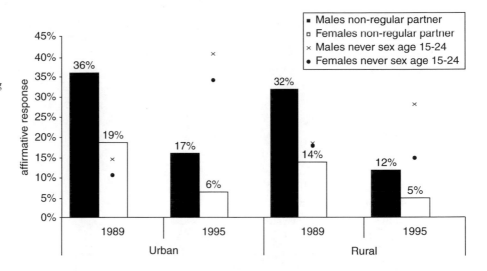

Fig. 13.5 Changes in the proportion of persons reporting sex with a nonregular partner in the previous 12 months and persons aged 15–24 reporting never having had sex in Uganda among adult populations, measured by population-based behavioral surveys performed in 1989 and in 1995, by sex and population characteristics (Adapted from Stoneburner and Low-Beer.[114] Used with permission)

stop!"[118] Indeed, in Washington DC (2003), the Uganda Youth Forum Coordinator wrote out, "*Abstinence and Being faithful are the best Choices.*"[119] In federal testimony, Edward C. Green, PhD, Senior Research Scientist with the Harvard Center for Population and Development Studies, reported concern about a gradual change away from the original endogenously developed Ugandan strategy toward "medical solutions" with less emphasis on sexual behavior. He concluded, "The distinctive Uganda ABC model of the earlier period, the one developed primarily by Ugandans for Ugandans, is the one that seems to have worked best, and is the one that has most to teach the rest of the world."[120] It is no wonder, with increasing condom social marketing[117] to the general population, including youth, that Ugandans should feel frustrated to the point of staging abstinence marches and rallies to "stop abstinence stigma" (personal communication from participant, Oct 2006, Kampala Uganda), finding it counterproductive that the Western world promotes condoms in their country instead of supporting what the evidence showed was successful: their own grassroots AB method of primary behavior change.

13.14 Preventing STDs: The New Global Paradigm

During the last 25 years, a risk-reduction, condom/safe/safer sex public health paradigm has been applied broadly, including to youth, in the United States and

around the globe. The evidence reported herein indicates that both, youth in the United States and the generalized population of Uganda, Africa are capable of risk-avoidance via abstinence, lifetime monogamy (being faithful), and/or motivated toward those lifestyles for personal/social/health reasons. The numbers of STDs, the serious health consequences, the variable effectiveness of existing prevention parameters (condoms, vaccines, microbiocides, treatment) has complicated individual patient management and inevitably will overwhelm an already overburdened healthcare system, especially at the global level.

We stand at a crossroads in public health paradigm that could alter forever the survival of the inhabitants of sub-Saharan Africa, (i.e., the black race), and those human beings in all areas in the world facing the AIDS pandemic. The grim statistics indicate that every 8 s a person is infected with HIV somewhere in the world. This equates to 6,800 new infections per day. Sixty-eight percent of the 33.2 million people with HIV live in Sub-Saharan Africa.[121] It has been a number of years since the HIV prevalence in Uganda reached its low in 2001 at 5% and was reported to the world in 2003. At last survey in 2007, Ugandan HIV prevalence was holding at 5.4%.[122] What role increasing condom social marketing, occurring over the objections of the Ugandans themselves, will have on their success is yet to be observed.

Hearst and Chen have shown graphically that in Cameroon, Kenya, and Botswana, from 1990 to 2001, "urban and rural HIV prevalence have gone up right along with condom sales."[123] Likewise, from 1989 to

2000, South Africa, Botswana and Zimbabwe, had the highest rates of condom availability (seven to ten condoms per year per man) yet had the highest HIV prevalence rates, ranging from 20% to 36%.[124] While causality is unproven, there likewise "is no evidence at the national level in Africa that more condoms have resulted in less AIDS."[124] In 2005, Kajubi et al. reported that gains in condom use by Ugandan men in a condom promotion program seemed to have been offset by increases in the number of sex partners.[125] This phenomenon of "risk compensation" (discussed in Sect. 13.3) refers to the perception of reduced risk being compensated for by a paradoxical increase in risky behavior. In a 2006 commentary published in British Medical Journal, the authors questioned whether vaccines, microbicides, and male circumcision could be *compensated for* by an increase in risky behavior and thus concluded that with regard to HIV prevention, "successful approaches to change behavior must be studied, adapted, and applied with at least the same vigor as the promising host of technological innovations under development."[126]

Time is short as we confront the most serious of all STDs in the global AIDS pandemic. The UNAIDS/WHO 2006 AIDS Epidemic Report challenges all of us who counsel youth: "The future course of the world's HIV epidemics hinges in many respects on the behaviors young people adopt or maintain, and the contextual factors that affect those choices."[127] If we take aim with a goal to prevent all STDs, especially in youth, we need to move quickly and, following the example set by Uganda, align with the same risk avoidance message.

The available scientific evidence supports that the risk-reduction, "safe/safer sex" or "vaccinate, condomize and treat" paradigm was and is not enough. Also established is that the risk-avoidance, Abstinence/Be faithful paradigm is both "realistic" and effective and it is consistent with existing medical guidelines. It is an "umbrella approach," that is best suited to protect vast numbers of people from all STDs whether in-office or around the globe. Subset at-risk populations can be targeted specifically to their risk behavior but always with the goal of moving them toward the healthiest behavior, no different than what a physician would do in the office with an individual patient. The Ugandan model has demonstrated that behavior can be changed, that *sexual* behavior can be changed, that health can be preserved and that lives can be saved.

Dermatologists/venereologists, other physicians, scientists, and leaders, capable of capturing this vision and willing to learn from a developing nation, should be given the lead to establish risk-avoidance strategies worldwide. The Ugandan success model is low cost and simple but requires that community leaders get "on the same page" with a single, clear message that *A*bstinence and *B*eing faithful are the best *C*hoices. That is what the scientific evidence indicates needs to be done for the health of all people around the globe. There is no time to lose.

References

1. Executive summary, committee on prevention and control of sexually transmitted diseases. Institute of medicine. In: Eng TR, Butler WT, eds. *The Hidden Epidemic: Confronting Sexually Transmitted Disease*. Washington, DC: National Academy; 1997:1–17
2. Centers for Disease Control and Prevention. Tracking the hidden epidemics 2000. Available at: http://www.cdc.gov/std/Trends2000/Trends2000.pdf; 2009 Accessed 29.05.09
3. Weinstock H, Berman S, Cates W Jr. Sexually transmitted diseases among American youth: incidence and prevalence estimates, 2000. *Perspect Sex Reprod Health*. 2004; 36(1):6–10
4. Neinstein LS. *Adolescent Health Care: A Practical Guide*. 4th ed. Philadelphia: Lippincott Williams and Wilkins; 2002
5. Kahn JA, Hillard PA. Human papillomavirus and cervical cytology in adolescents. *Adolesc Med Clin*. 2004;15: 301–321
6. Corey L, Handsfield HH. Genital herpes and public health: addressing a global problem. *JAMA*. 2000;283(6):791–794
7. Centers for Disease Control and Prevention. Sexually transmitted diseases treatment guidelines 2006. MMWR 2006:55(No. RR-11):16
8. Fleming DT, McQuillan GM, Johnson RE, Nahmias AJ, Aral SO, Lee FK, St Louis ME. Herpes simplex virus type 2 in the United States, 1976 to 1994. *N Engl J Med*. 1997;337(16): 1105–1111
9. Wald A, Zeh J, Selke S, et al Reactivation of genital herpes simplex virus type 2 infection in asymptomatic seropositive persons. *N Engl J Med*. 2000;342(12):844–850
10. Roberts CM, Pfister JR, Spear SJ. Increasing proportion of herpes simplex virus type 1 as a cause of genital herpes infection in college students. *Sex Transm Dis*. 2003;30 (10): 797–800
11. Tyring SK. Drugs with antiviral activity in clinical dermatology. Dialogues in Dermatology. 1998 Jul;42(4)
12. Xu F, Sternberg MR, Kottiri BJ, et al Trends in herpes simplex virus type 1 and type 2 seroprevalence in the United States. *JAMA*. 2006;296(8):964–973
13. Sonfield A, Gold RB. States' implementation of the Section 510 abstinence education program, FY 1999. *Fam Plann Perspect*. 2001;33(4):166–171

14. Ali L, Scelfo J. Choosing virginity. *Newsweek*. 2002;140(24): 60–64, 66

15. Maw RD, Reitano M, Roy M. An international survey of patients with genital warts: perceptions regarding treatment and impact on lifestyle. *Int J STD AIDS*. 1998;9(10):571–578

16. Reitano M. Counseling patients with genital warts. *Am J Med*. 1997;102(5A):38–43. Review

17. Centers for Disease Control and Prevention. Sexually transmitted diseases treatment guidelines 2006. MMWR 2006; 55[No.RR-11]63. Available at: http://www.cdc.gov/std/treatment/2006/rr5511.pdf; 2009 Accessed 27.05.09

18. Ho GY, Bierman R, Beardsley L, Chang CJ, Burk RD. Natural history of cervicovaginal papillomavirus infection in young women. *N Engl J Med*. 1998;338(7):423–428

19. Winer RL, Lee SK, Hughes JP, Adam DE, Kiviat NB, Koutsky LA. Genital human papillomavirus infection: incidence and risk factors in a cohort of female university students. *Am J Epidemiol*. 2003;157(3):218–226

20. Muñoz N, Bosch FX, de Sanjosé S, Herrero R, Castellsagué X, Shah KV, Snijders PJ, Meijer CJ, International Agency for Research on Cancer Multicenter Cervical Cancer Study Group. Epidemiologic classification of human papillomavirus types associated with cervical cancer. *N Engl J Med*. 2003;348(6):518–527

21. Centers for Disease Control and Prevention. Youth risk behavior surveillance-United States, 2005. MMWR 2006;55 (No.SS–05)

22. National Institute of Allergy and Infectious Diseases, Workshop Summary: Scientific Evidence on Condom Effectiveness for Sexually Transmitted Disease (STD) Prevention, July 20, 2001. Available at: http://www3.niaid.nih.gov/about/organization/dmid/PDF/condomReport.pdf; 2009 Accessed 29.05.09

23. Centers for Disease Control and Prevention, Report to Congress: Prevention of genital human papillomavirus infection. Jan 2004. Available at: http://www.cdc.gov/std/HPV/2004HPV%20Report.pdf; 2009 Accessed 27.05.09

24. Winer RL, et al Condom use and the risk of genital human papillomavirus infection in young women. *N Engl J Med*. 2006;354(25):2645–2654

25. Centers for Disease Control and Prevention, Human Papilloma Virus: HPV information for clinicians. April 2007. Available at: http://www.cdc.gov/std/HPV/hpv-clinicians-brochure.htm; 2009 Accessed 27.05.09

26. Unger ER, Barr E. Human papillomavirus and cervical cancer, conference summary. Emerg Infect Dis 2004 Nov. Available at: http://www.cdc.gov/ncidod/EID/v0110n011/04-0623_09.htm; 2009 Accessed 27.05.09

27. Centers for Disease Control and Prevention, HPV Vaccine Information for Clinicians. June 26, 2008. Available at: http://www.cdc.gov/std/hpv/STDFact-HPV-vaccine-hcp.htm; 2009 Accessed 27.05.09

28. Centers for Disease Control and Prevention, Vaccine information statement (interim) human papillomavirus (HPV) Vaccine. 2007 Feb 2. Available at: http://www.cdc.gov/vaccines/pubs/vis/default.htm#hpv; 2009 Accessed 27.05.09

29. Centers for Disease Control and Prevention, Reports of Health Concerns Following HPV Vaccination. 2009 June 10. Available at: http://www.cdc.gov/print.do?url=http%3A%2F%2Fwww.cdc.gov%2Fvaccinesafety%2Fvaers%2Fgardasil.htm; 2009 Accessed 29.06.09

30. Centers for Disease Control and Prevention, HPV vaccine information for young women. June 26, 2008. Available at: http://www.cdc.gov/std/hpv/STDFact-HPV-vaccine-young-women.htm#hpvvac4; 2009 Accessed 01.06.09

31. Kim JJ, Goldie SJ. Health and Economic Implications of HPV Vaccination in the United States. *N Engl J Med*. 2008; 359(8):821–832

32. Salmon DA, Teret SP, MacIntyre CR, Salisbury D, Burgess MA, Halsey NA. Compulsory vaccination and conscientious or philosophical exemptions: past, present, and future. *Lancet*. 2006;367(9508):436–442

33. Dunne EF, Unger ER, Sternberg M, McQuillan G, Swan DC, Patel SS, Markowitz LE. Prevalence of HPV infection among females in the United States. *JAMA*. 2007;297: 813–819. Erratum JAMA 2007;298(2):178

34. Gostin LO, DeAngelis CD. Mandatory HPV vaccination: public health vs private wealth. *JAMA*. 2007;297(17):1921–1923. Erratum JAMA 2007;298(2):178

35. Sawaya GF, Smith-McCune K. HPV vaccination – more answers, more questions. *N Engl J Med*. 2007;356(19): 1991–1993

36. The FUTURE II Study Group. Quadrivalent vaccine against human papillomavirus to prevent high-grade cervical lesions. *N Engl J Med*. 2007;356:1915–1927

37. Haug CJ. Human papillomavirus vaccination – reasons for caution. *N Engl J Med*. 2008;359(8):861–862

38. Saslow D, Castle PE, Cox JT, et al American Cancer Society guideline for human papillomavirus (HPV) vaccine use to prevent cervical cancer and its precursors. *CA Cancer J Clin*. 2007;57:7–28

39. American Cancer Society. *Cancer Facts and Figures 2009*. Atlanta: American Cancer Society;2009. Available at: http://www.cancer.org/docroot/STT/STT_0.asp; 2009 Accessed 29.05.09

40. Janerich DT, Hadjimichael O, Schwartz PE, et al The screening histories of women with invasive cervical cancer, Connecticut. *Am J Public Health*. 1995;85(6): 791–794

41. Stuart GC, McGregor SE, Duggan MA, Nation JG. Review of the screening history of Alberta women with invasive cervical cancer. *CMAJ*. 1997;157(5):513–519

42. Sung HY, Kearney KA, Miller M, Kinney W, Sawaya GF, Hiatt RA. Papanicolaou smear history and diagnosis of invasive cervical carcinoma among members of a large prepaid health plan. *Cancer*. 2000;88(10):2283–2289

43. Leyden WA, Manos MM, Geiger AM, et al Cervical cancer in women with comprehensive health care access: attributable factors in the screening process. *J Natl Cancer Inst*. 2005;97(9):675–683

44. Parkin DM, Bray F, Ferlay J, Pisani P. Global cancer statistics, 2002. *CA Cancer J Clin*. 2005;55:74–108

45. Department of Health and Human Services. Food and Drug Administration Docket No. 02D-0103. Draft revised compliance policy guide; male condom defects; availability. *Fed Regist*. 2002;67(61):15213–15214

46. Herman BA, Carey RF. Validation of a corona discharge technique to test male latex condoms for pinhole defects. *J Test Eval*. 1999;27(1):3–6

47. World Health Organization. WHO Laboratory Manual for the Examination of Human Semen and Sperm-Cervical Mucus Interaction. 4th ed. Cambridge University Press, UK; New York, NY; 1999:19–21

48. Lytle CD, Routson LB, Seaborn GB, Dixon LG, Bushar HF. Cyr WH. An in vitro evaluation of condoms as barriers to a small virus. *Sex Transm Dis.* 1997;24(3):161–164
49. Modis Y, Trus BL, Harrison SC. Atomic model of the papillomavirus capsid. *EMBO J.* 2002;21(18):4754–4762
50. Carey RF, Lytle CD, Cyr WH. Implications of laboratory tests of condom integrity. *Sex Transm Dis.* 1999;26(4): 216–220
51. Lytle CD, Duff JE, Fleharty B, Bidinger RL, Cyr WH. A sensitive method for evaluating condoms as barriers. *J AOAC Int.* 1997;80(2):319–324
52. Fu H, Darroch JE, Haas T, Ranjit N. Contraceptive failure rates: new estimates from the 1995 National Survey of Family Growth. *Fam Plann Perspect.* 1999;31(2):56–63
53. Morris BA. How safe are safes? Efficacy and effectiveness of condoms in preventing STDs. *Can Fam Physician.* 1993;39:819–822, 827. Review
54. Cates W Jr, Stone KM. Family planning, sexually transmitted diseases and contraceptive choice: a literature update – Part I. *Fam Plann Perspect.* 1992;24(2):75–84. Review
55. Judson FN, Ehret JM, Bodin GF, Levin MJ, Rietmeijer CA. In vitro evaluations of condoms with and without nonoxynol 9 as physical and chemical barriers against Chlamydia trachomatis, herpes simplex virus type 2 and human immunodeficiency virus. *Sex Transm Dis.* 1989;16(2):51–56
56. D'Oro LC, Parazzini F, Naldi L, La Vecchia C. Barrier methods of contraception, spermicides, and sexually transmitted diseases: a review. *Genitourin Med.* 1994;70(6):410–417. Review
57. Grady WR, Tanfer K. Condom breakage and slippage among men in the United States. *Fam Plann Perspect.* 1994;26 (3):107–112
58. Trussel J, Warner DL, Hatcher RA. Condom slippage and breakage rates. *Fam Plann Perspect.* 1992;24(1):20–23
59. Trussel J, Warner DL, Hatcher RA. Condom performance during vaginal intercourse: comparison of Trojan-Enz and Tactylon condoms. *Contraception.* 1992;45(1):11–19
60. Macaluso M, Kelaghan J, Artz L, et al Mechanical failure of the latex condom in a cohort of women at high STD risk. *Sex Transm Dis.* 1999;26(8):450–458
61. Darrow WW. Condom use and use-effectiveness in high-risk populations. *Sex Transm Dis.* 1989;16(3):157–160
62. Warner L, Clay-Warner J, Boles J, Williamson J. Assessing condom use practices. Implications for evaluating method and user effectiveness. *Sex Transm Dis.* 1998;25(6):273–277
63. Rose E, et al The validity of teens' and young adults' self-reported condom use. *Arch Pediatr Adolesc Med.* 2009; 163(1):61–64
64. Crosby RA, DiClemente RJ, Wingood GM, Lang D, Harrington KF. Value of consistent condom use: a study of sexually transmitted disease prevention among African American adolescent females. *Am J Public Health.* 2003;93 (6):901–902
65. Saracco A, et al Man-to-woman sexual transmission of HIV: longitudinal study of 343 steady partners of infected men. *J Acquir Immune Defic Syndr.* 1993;6(5):497–502
66. Anderson JE, Brackbill R, Mosher WD. Condom use for disease prevention among unmarried U.S. women. *Fam Plann Perspect.* 1996;28(1):25–28.
67. Wald A, Langenberg AG, Link K, et al Effect of condoms on reducing the transmission of herpes simplex virus type 2 from men to women. *JAMA.* 2001;285(24):3100–3106
68. Wald A, Langenberg AG, Krantz E, et al The relationship between condom use and herpes simplex virus acquisition. *Ann Intern Med.* 2005;143(10):707–713
69. de Vincenzi I, European Study Group on Heterosexual Transmission of HIV. A longitudinal study of human immunodeficiency virus transmission by heterosexual partners. European Study Group on Heterosexual Transmission of HIV. *N Engl J Med.* 1994;331(6):341–346
70. Fitch JT, Stine C, Hager WD, Mann J, Adam MB, McIlhaney J. Condom effectiveness: factors that influence risk reduction. *Sex Transm Dis.* 2002;29(12):811–817
71. Centers for Disease Control and Prevention. Sexually transmitted diseases treatment guidelines 2006. MMWR 2006; 55(No. RR-11):4
72. Medical Institute of Sexual Health, conference on sexual health in the 21st Century. Fitch JT, oral presentation 2000 Nov; San Antonio TX
73. Department of Health and Human Services. Food and Drug Administration Docket No. 2004N-0556. Designation of special control for condom and condom with spermicidal lubricant; proposed rule. *Fed Regist.* 2005;70(218):69102–69118
74. A series of national surveys of teens about sex:safer sex, condoms and "the pill." 2000 Nov. Menlo Park, CA: Kaiser Family Foundation. Available at: http://www.kff.org/youthhivstds/20001127b-index.cfm; 2009 Accessed 27.05.09
75. National survey of adolescents and young adults: sexual health knowledge, attitudes and experiences 2003 May 19. Kaiser Family Foundation. Available at: http://www.kff.org/youthhivstds/3218-index.cfm; 2009 Accessed 27.05.09
76. Centers for Disease Control and Prevention. Preventing the sexual transmission of HIV, the virus that causes AIDS. Dec 2000. Available at: www.cdc.gov/hiv/resources/factsheets/pdf/oralsex.pdf; 2009 Accessed 27.05.09
77. Dernovsek KK. Sex, Teens and the dermatologist: recognize your role in preventing the spread of STDs. Practical Dermatology. Dec 2004
78. Dernovsek KK. Teens and STDs: a new message for a healthy millennium. School Health Reporter; spring 2003: 1–3. Available at: http://www.thechildrenshospital.org/news/publications/school_health_reporter/2003/std.aspx; 2009 Accessed 27.05.09
79. American Medical Association. Guidelines for Adolescent Preventive Services (GAPS) Recommendations Monograph. Chicago, Il:1997:4. Available at: http://www.ama-assn.org/ama/upload/mm/39/gapsmono.pdf; 2009 Accessed 27.05.09
80. Centers for Disease Control and Prevention. Sexually transmitted diseases treatment guidelines 2002. MMWR 2002; 51(No. RR-6):2. Available at: http://www.cdc.gov/STD/treatment/TOC2002TG.htm; 2009 Accessed 27.05.09
81. Centers for Disease Control and Prevention. Sexually transmitted diseases treatment guidelines 2006. MMWR 2006; 55[No.RR-11]3. Available at: http://www.cdc.gov/std/treatment/2006/rr5511.pdf; 2009 Accessed 27.05.09
82. Klein JD; Committee on Adolescence. Adolescent pregnancy: current trends and issues. *Pediatrics.* 2005;116; 291–286. Available at: http://pediatrics.aappublications.org/cgi/content/full/116/1/281; 2009 Accessed 27.05.09
83. Burstein GP, Lowry R, Klein JD, Santelli JS. Missed opportunities for sexually transmitted diseases, human immunodeficiency virus, and pregnancy prevention services during adolescent health supervision visits. *Pediatrics.* 2003; 111: 996–1001

84. Rand CM, Auinger P, Klein JD, Weitzman M. Preventive counseling at adolescent ambulatory visits. *J Adolesc Health*. 2005;37:87–93

85. Haley N, Maheux B, Rivard M, Gervais A. Sexual health risk assessment and counseling in primary care: how involved are general practitioners and obstetrician-gynecologists? *Am J Public Health*. 1999;89(6):899–902

86. Kaplan CP, Perez-Stable EJ, Feutes-Afflick E, Gildengorin V, Millstein S, Juarez-Reyes M. Smoking cessation counseling with young patients. *Arch Pediatr Adolesc Med*. 2004; 158:83–90

87. U.S. Census Bureau: State and County QuickFacts. Data derived from Population Estimates, 2000 Census of Population and Housing. Available at: http://quickfacts.census.gov/qfd/states/08/08101.html; 2009 Accessed 27.05.09

88. Abstinence because. Austin, Texas: The Medical Institute for Sexual Health

89. Koutsky L. Epidemiology of genital human papillomavirus infection. *Am J Med*. 1997; 102(5A):3–8.

90. Whitley RF, Gnann JW. Herpes simplex virus. In: Tyring S, Yen-Moore A, eds. *Mucocutaneous Manifestations of Viral Diseases*. 1st ed. New York, NY: Marcel Dekker; 2002:103

91. With One Voice: America's adults and teens sound off about teen pregnancy. Washington, DC: National Campaign to Prevent Teen Pregnancy. April 2001. Available at: http://www.teenpregnancy.org/resources/data/pdf/chrtbook.pdf; 2009 Accessed 27.05.09

92. With One Voice: America's adults and teens sound off about teen pregnancy. Washington, DC: National Campaign to Prevent Teen Pregnancy. December 2002. Available at: http://www.teenpregnancy.org/resources/data/pdf/WOV2002_fulltext.pdf; 2009 Accessed 27.05.09

93. With One Voice 2003: America's adults and teens sound off about teen pregnancy. Washington, DC: National Campaign to prevent Teen Pregnancy. December 2003. Available at: http://www.teenpregnancy.org/resources/data/pdf/wov2003.pdf; 2009 Accessed 27.05.09

94. Albert B. With One Voice 2004: America's adults and teens sound off about teen pregnancy. Washington, DC: National Campaign to Prevent Teen Pregnancy. December 2004. Available at: http://www.teenpregnancy.org/resources/data/pdf/WOV2004.pdf; 2009 Accessed 27.05.09

95. Albert B. With One Voice 2007: America's adults and teens sound off about teen pregnancy. Washington, DC: National Campaign to Prevent Teen Pregnancy. February 2007. Available at: http://www.teenpregnancy.org/product/pdf/6_9_2007_15_17_14WOV2007_fulltext.pdf;2009 Accessed 27.05.09

96. Brackbill RM, Sternberg MR, Fishbein M. Where do people go for treatment of sexually transmitted diseases? *Fam Plann Perspect*. 1999;31(1):10–15

97. Center for Disease Control and Prevention. Physician advice and individual behavior about cardiovascular disease risk reduction B seven states and Puerto Rico, 1997. *MMWR*. 1999;48:74–77

98. Lancaster T, Stead LF. Physician advice for smoking cessation. *The Cochrane Database of Systemic Reviews* 2005;3

99. Center for Disease Control and Prevention. Recommended Immunization Schedules for persons aged 0 through 18 years – United States, 2009. MMWR 1–2–09;57(51&52); Q-1-Q-4. Available at: http://www.cdc.gov/mmwR/preview/mmwrhtml/mm5751a5.htm; 2009 Accessed 29.05.09

100. Ramsay DL, Weiss R, Brademas ME. Margolies, R. National survey of dermatologists and residency training program directors on dermatology's role in treating sexually transmitted diseases. *J Am Acad Dermatol*. 1986;14(3):527–531

101. Centers for Disease Control and Prevention. STD-Prevention Counseling Practices and Human Papillomavirus Opinions Among Clinicians with Adolescent Patients – United States, 2004. MMWR 2006;55(41)1117–1120. Available at: http://www.cdc.gov/mmwr/preview/mmwrhtml/mm5541a1.htm; 2009 Accessed 27.05.09

102. Center for Disease Control and Prevention. Trends in Sexual Risk Behaviors Among High School Students – United States, 1991–2001. MMWR 9–27–02/51(38); 856–859. Available at: http://www.cdc.gov/mmwr/preview/mmwrhtml/mm5138a2.htm; 2009 Accessed 27.05.09

103. Center for Disease Control and Prevention. Youth risk behavior surveillance-United States, 2007. MMWR6-6-08/58(SS-4);1. Available at: http://www.cdc.gov/mmwr/PDF/ss/ss5704.pdf Accessed December 5, 2009

104. Center for Disease Control and Prevention. Trends in HIV-related risk behaviors among high school students – United States, 1991–2005. MMWR 8–11–06//55(31); 851–4. Available at: http://www.cdc.gov/mmwr/preview/mmwrhtml/mm5531a4.htm; 2009 Accessed 27.05.09

105. National Survey of Adolescents and Young Adults: Sexual Health Knowledge, Attitudes and Experiences. 2003. Menlo Park, CA: Kaiser Family Foundation. Available at: http://www.kff.org/youthhivstds/3218-index.cfm; 2009 Accessed 27.05.09

106. A Series of National Surveys of Teens About Sex: Virginity and the First Time. Menlo Park, CA: Kaiser Family Foundation. October 2003. Available at: http://www.kff.org/entpartnerships/3368-index.cfm; 2009 Accessed 27.05.09

107. U.S. Agency for International Development. Green EC. Faith-based organizations: contributions to HIV prevention. Sep 2003. Available at: http://www1.usaid.gov/our_work/global_health/aids/TechAreas/community/fbo.pdf; 2009 Accessed 29.05.09

108. U.S. Agency for International Development. Hogle JA, Green E, Nantulya V, Soneburner R, Stover J. What happened in Uganda? Declining HIV prevalence, behavior change, and the national response. Sep 2002. Available at: http://www.usaid.gov/our_work/global_health/aids/Countries/africa/uganda_report.pdf; 2009 Accessed 27.05.09

109. World Health Organization/UNAIDS. HIV/AIDS in sub-Saharan Africa, July 2002. Slide #SSA-5. Available at: www.who.int/hiv/facts/en/Sub-SaharanAfrica.ppt; 2009 Accessed 29.05.09

110. Address by Her Excellency Janet K. Museveni, First Lady of the Republic of Uganda. "Common Ground: A Shared Vision for Health" Conference hosted by Medical Institute for Sexual Health. Washington DC June 17–19 2004. Available at: http://uceglobal.org/pdf/mrsMuseveniAddress.pdf; 2009 Accessed 27.05.09

111. Allen A. "Uganda vs condoms." *The New Republic*. May 27, 2002

112. Address by Her Excellency Janet K. Museveni, First Lady of the Republic of Uganda. Samaritan's Purse "Prescription

for Hope" conference on HIV/AIDS. February 20, 2002 in Washington, D.C Accessed at http://www.usinfo.state.gov/topical/global/hiv/02022710.htm. No longer available

113. Green EC, Herling A. The ABC approach to preventing the sexual transmission of HIV: common questions and answers. Mclean VA: Christian Connections for International Health and Medical Service Corporation International, 2007

114. Stoneburner RL, Low-Beer D. Population-level HIV declines and behavioral risk avoidance in Uganda. *Science.* 2004;304:714–717

115. Success in Uganda: An Overview of Uganda's Campaign to Change Sexual Behaviors and Decrease HIV Prevalence 1986–1995 Douglas Kirby ETR Assoc. 9/2008

116. Available at: http://www.nationmaster.com/red/graph/peo_pop-people-population&date=1990&ob=ws and http://www.nationmaster.com/graph/peo_pop_age_014_of_tot-population-ages-0-14-total&date=1990 and http://www.nationmaster.com/red/graph/peo_pop_fem_of_tot-people-population-female-of-total&date=1990&ob=ws;   2009 Accessed 29.05.09

117. Green EC, Halperin DT, Nantulya V, Hogle JA. Uganda's HIV prevention success: the role of sexual behavior change and the national response. *AIDS Behav.* 2006;10(4): 335–346

118. Ssempa M. Presentation at the International Leadership Conference sponsored by the National Abstinence Clearinghouse. Kansas City KS. Jun 8, 2006

119. Bampata EK. Presentation at "HIV/AIDS Prevention for Young People in Developing Countries," a conference sponsored by USAID Office of HIV/AIDS, Institute for Youth Development, YouthNet/Family Health International. 24 July 2003. Washington DC

120. Green EC. Senior Research Scientist. Harvard Center for Population and Development Studies. Testimony before the African subcommittee U.S. Senate. Available at: foreign.senate.gov/testimony/2003/GreenTestimony030519.pdf; 2008 Accessed 18.05.09

121. Joint United Nations Programme on HIV/AIDS (UNAIDS) and World Health Organization (WHO) AIDS Epidemic update December 2007. Available at: http://data.unaids.org/pub/EPISlides/2007/2007_epiupdate_en.pdf;   2009 Accessed 27.05.09

122. UNAIDS/WHO Epidemiologic Fact Sheet on HIV and AIDS, October 2008 Update, Uganda. Available at: http://who.int/globalatlas/predefinedReports/EFS2008/full/EFS2008_UG.pdf; 2009 Accessed 27.05.09

123. Hearst N, Chen S. Condom promotion for AIDS prevention in the developing world: is it working? *Evidence That Demands Action.* Austin TX: The Medical Institute 2004

124. Green EC. Moving toward evidence-based AIDS prevention. *Evidence That Demands Action.* Austin TX: The Medical Institute 2004

125. Kajubi P, et al Increasing condom use without reducing HIV risk: results of a controlled community trial in Uganda. *J Acq Immune Defic Syndr.* 2005;40(1):77–82

126. Cassell MM, Halperin DT, Shelton JD, Stanton D. Risk compensation: the Achilles' heel of innovations in HIV prevention? *BMJ.* 2006;332:605–607

127. Joint United Nations Programme on HIV/AIDS (UNAIDS) and World Health Organization (WHO) AIDS Epidemic Update. December 2006. Available at: http://data.unaids.org/pub/EpiReport/2006/03-Introduction-2006_EpiUpdate_eng.pdf; 2009 Accessed 27.05.09

Current Vaccinations in Dermatology

Kamaldeep Singh and Robert A. Norman

14

14.1 Introduction

Vaccines have been called medicine's greatest life savers. They have helped eradicate vexing diseases such as smallpox and effectively prevented diseases such as rubella and rubeola. In the present medical landscape vaccinations occupy enormous ground and from first world nations to third world countries they have become part of government policies and legislation to prevent disease. One does not need to study the countless studies and trials that focus on disease reduction from the use of vaccines, but only to go back in history and see the triumph of vaccines over horrific diseases such as polio and tetanus. Edward Jenner would have never envisioned that his use of cowpox to prevent smallpox would have such a paramount impact on medicine. Although the idea behind vaccinating is older than Jenner and records of inoculations can be found as far back as a millennium before Jenner's time, history credits him as being the father of vaccine because his vaccine was safer than inoculation.

Edward Jenner's vaccine was also the first against a disease with cutaneous manifestations and since then many vaccines have been developed including the ones that prevent against diseases with cutaneous components such as measles, mumps, and rubella and more recently diseases caused by varicella zoster virus (VZV) and human papilloma virus. The focus of this chapter is to review the natural history, epidemiology, and diagnosis of VZV and HPV and to emphasize vaccination strategies including the latest CDC guidelines.

K. Singh (✉)
Internal Medicine Resident, Stony Brook University Hospital, Stony Brook, NY, USA
e-mail: drkamaldeep@hotmail.com

14.2 Varicella Zoster Virus

VZV, also known as human herpes 3 (HHV3), is a human neurotropic virus belonging to the family of DNA viruses known as herpesviridae. Its single, linear double-stranded DNA molecule is enclosed within an icosapentahedral capsid making it very similar to herpes simplex virus 1 and 2. The distinguishing factor that is responsible for each virus's unique properties is the lipid envelope consisting of polyamines, lipids, and glycoproteins that encloses this 162 capsomere capsid. More specifically, the glycoproteins are responsible for the distinctive properties of each virus as well as the antigenic capabilities of eliciting an immune response in the host. For example, VZV glycoproteins (gB, gC, gE, gH, gK, gL) correspond with those in the HSV, but HSV gD is not found in the VZV lipid envelope. VZV puts forth a considerable challenge in terms of studying the virus for its biological and pathogenic properties because it only replicates in human cells and tissues for reasons currently unknown.

14.2.1 Epidemiology

Varicella (chickenpox) and herpes zoster (shingles) are both caused by VZV. Chickenpox is a very common childhood illness with peak incidence between 1 and 9 years of age resulting in 90% of the population having positive serology by adolescence and 100% of the population being seropositive by the age of 60. VZV infections are more widespread in winter and spring seasons and have a tendency of epidemics every 2–5 years. The disease is highly contagious and spreads from person to person via direct contact with fluids from vesicles or respiratory inhalation of viral fomites. In immunocompetent persons varicella is a mild-to-moderate illness while immunocompromised persons can suffer from severe complications including death.

Shingles is caused by the reactivation of the latent VZV. It is a disease most commonly of the elderly and immunocompromised and incidence increases with age because of declining immunity. At 60 years of age incidence is reported between 2.5 and 5% and increases to 3–6.8% the age of 70 with lifetime risk of 15–30%. Shingles can also occur in seemingly healthy individuals with incidence of 1.2–3.4%. The disease is worrisome because it poses the potential for severe and debilitating complications such as herpes opthalmicus, postherpetic neuralgia, paresis, myelopathy, myocarditis, depression, and others.

14.2.2 Virus Life Cycle

The VZV life cycle consists of three stages, the primary infection, latent period, and reactivation. The virus gains access to the host's peripheral nervous system via the mucocutaneous surfaces; it replicates, spreads, and causes an immune response resulting in usually self-limiting disease of chickenpox. Thereafter, the virus enters the axonal endings within the mucocutaneous surfaces and travels to the dorsal root ganglia where it remains latent until reactivation. Latency is the presence of viral genome without production of the infective particle. Reactivation occurs in response to stimulus such as immunosuppression, hormonal changes, stress, nerve damage, etc. and causes the virus to once again become active and replicate itself causing shingles. Latency is once again established and potential to reactivate remains.

14.2.3 Varicella (Chickenpox)

Mucocutaneous surfaces most susceptible to VZV are the upper respiratory mucosa and conjunctiva. Upon entering these surfaces VZV replicates in the regional lymph nodes for the next 2–4 days, followed by primary viremia in 4–6 days and then leading to viral replication in the liver, spleen, and other organs. Secondary viremia occurs in 14–16 days leading to the

dissemination of the virus to the skin and vicera and producing the typical vesicular lesions. Prodromal symptoms include fever, malaise, anorexia, and headache. In the United States, universal vaccination policy against varicella was adopted in 1995 and has led to significant reduction in morbidity and mortality associated with VZV (Table 14.1).

14.2.4 Herpes Zoster (Shingles)

Reactivation of the latent VZV causes herpes zoster or shingles. The virus that had remained latent inside the neuronal nucleus maintaining the ability to replicate reverts to its infectious state. It is not clearly known why the reactivation happens but the fact that the disease is more prevalent in the elderly and the immunoincompetent leads to the theory that declining cell-mediated immunity is the culprit. Support for this theory stems from the experimental evidence that, over time, even person with apparent immunity to varicella exhibit T cells with reduced ability to proliferate and produce VZV-specific interferon gamma when exposed to VZV antigen in vitro. Fifty percent of the estimated one million causes of herpes zoster in the United States occur in individuals aged 50 years or older and 50% of individuals 85 or older are expected to develop herpes zoster. Another 300,000 cases occur in the immunocompromised with bone marrow transplant recipients and HIV patients having the highest vulnerability.

In contrast to the primary varicella infection, reactivation tends to occur locally and within dermatomes where the highest viral load was present during the primary infection. Most often these sites are the thorax and the trigeminal distribution of the face. Clear vesicular eruptions appear within a dermatome, becoming turbid and eventually crusting within 5–10 days. Preherpetic neuralgia sometimes precedes shingles and is defined as parasthesias, itching and pain sometimes severe enough to suggest coronary artery ischemia or abdominal conditions. The most common and worrisome complication of the disease is when the pain and itching, usual concomitants of the eruptions, become chronic and lead to the condition known as postherpetic neuralgia. Although self-limiting, postherpetic neuralgia can be debilitating, often difficult to treat, and can leave the patient with poor quality of life leading to social withdrawal and depression.

Table 14.1 Summary of the recommendations of the advisory committee on immunization practices for prevention of varicella United States, 1996, 1999, and 2007

Category	Recommendations		
	1996	1999	2007
Routine childhood schedules	One dose at age 12–18 months	No change	Two doses First at age 12–15 months Second at age 4–6 years
Adults and adolescents aged ≥ 13 years	Two doses, 4–8 weeks apart Recommended for susceptible persons who have close contact with persons at high risk for serious complications Health-care workers Family contacts of immunocompromised persons	Two doses, 4–8 weeks apart No change	Two doses, 4–8 weeks apart Recommended for all adolescents and adults without evidence of immunity
	Should be considered for susceptible persons at high risk for exposure	Recommended for susceptible persons at high risk for expose or transmission	
	Persons who live or work in environments in which transmission of VZV is likely (e.g. teachers of young children, childcare employees, residents and staff in institutional settings)	Persons who live or work in environments in with the transmission of VZV[a] is likely (e.g. teachers of young children, daycare employees, residents and staff in institutional settings)	
	Persons who live and work in environments in which transmission can occur (e.g. college students, inmates and staff of correctional institutions, military personnel)	Persons who live and work in environments in which transmission can occur (e.g. college students, inmates and staff of correctional institutions, military personnel)	
	Nonpregnant women of childbearing age International travelers	Nonpregnant women of childbearing age International travelers Adolescents and adults living in households with children	
	Is desirable for other susceptible adolescents	No change	Second dose recommended for all persons who received one dose previously
Catch-up vaccination	One dose for all susceptible children age 19 months – 12 years (i.e. those with no history of varicella or vaccination)		
HIV[b]-infected persons	Contraindicated	Two doses, 3 months apart Should be considered for asymptomatic or mildly symptomatic HIV-infected children in CDC immunologic and clinical categories N1 or A1 with age-specific CD4+ T-lymphocyte percentages ≥25%	Two doses, 3 months apart Should be considered for HIV-infected children with age-specific CD4+ T-lymphocyte percentages ≥15% May be considered for adolescents and adults with CD4 counts ≥200/mL

(continued)

Table 14.1 (continued)

Category	Recommendations		
	1996	1999	2007
Antenatal screening	None	None	Recommended prenatal assessment and postpartum vaccination
Outbreak control vaccination	None	Should be considered	Recommended two-dose vaccination policy
Postexposure vaccination	None	Recommended within 3–5 days	No change
Vaccination requirements	None	Recommended for children without evidence of immunity attending childcare centers and entering elementary school Should be considered for middle school and junior high school students without other evidence of immunity	Recommended for children attending child-care centers, students in all grade levels, and persons attending college or other postsecondary educational institutions

From Centers for disease control and prevention. Prevention of varicella. Recommendations of the advisory committee on immunization practices (*ACIP*). MMWR 2007;56(RR-4):3
[a]Varicella zoster virus
[b]Human immunodeficiency virus

Various drugs including antivirals and steroids are used to treat and reduce the severity of acute herpes zoster but none can prevent postherpetic neuralgia or other herpes zoster complications. In 2006, the Food and Drug Administration (FDA) approved Zostavax, a live attenuated preparation of VZV. The vaccine has been shown to boost the recipient's immunity to VZV making the reactivation of VZV and development of herpes zoster less likely. The pivotal Shingles Prevention Study, on which basis the FDA approved Zostavax, showed a reduction in the cases of herpes zoster by half and postherpetic neuralgia by two-thirds in a sample of 38,000 older adults.

14.2.5 ACIP Provisional Recommendations

A single dose of herpes zoster vaccine is recommended for adults 60 years of age and older whether or not they report a prior episode of herpes zoster. Persons with chronic medical conditions may be vaccinated unless contraindications or precautions exist for their condition.

Contraindications are:

- A history of anaphylactic/anaphylactoid reaction to gelatin, neomycin, or any other component of the vaccine
- A history of primary acquired immunodeficiency states
- On immunosuppressive therapy
- Women of childbearing age, and is not to be administered to pregnant females

14.3 Human Papilloma Virus

Human papilloma viruses belong to their own family of viruses known as papillomaviridae. These double-stranded DNA viruses are species-specific and infect the skin and mucous membranes of their host. There are more than 100 types of human papilloma viruses that have been identified with each type containing approximately 7,900 base pairs and sharing 90% of DNA base pair homology with other identified types.

Infections with different HPV types result in illness ranging from clinically silent infections, benign skin lesions, and malignant cancers. Certain HPV types associated with squamous intracpithelial lesions and anogential malignancy including cervical, vaginal, and vulvar and anal carcinomas prompt tremendous research effort in order to reduce morbidity and mortality caused by these diseases and to better the treatment and prevention of HPV infections. Types linked to cervical cancer are classified as either high (16, 18), intermediate (31, 33, 35, 39, 45, 51, 52, 58) or low risk (6, 11, 42, 43, 44). Although the high-risk types are linked to 70% of all cases of cervical cancers not all infections with types 16 and 18 lead to cervical cancer. It is the oncogenic potential of different variants of these high-risk types that determine whether a HPV infection has a potential to develop into cervical cancer. HPV infections are also associated with anal cancer and the same high-risk types implicated in cervical cancer have been identified as the culprits for anal cancer. A group of researchers have identified 29 individual HPV types and 10 HPV groups from anal canal of homosexual men.

14.3.1 Virus Life Cycle and Pathogenicity

The pathogenicity of HPV is thought to be caused by proteins E6 and E7 encoded by the HPV DNA. These proteins are part of six early (E) proteins implicated in modifying the cell cycle of infected host cells. Once the HPV virion infects the epithelial tissue through micro abrasions, it gains access to the nucleus of basal epithelial cells via several complex transport mechanisms including alpha integrins, laminins, and several chemical mediators involved in endocytosis within the cell wall and nuclear membrane. Once inside the host keratinocyte the HPV lifecycle follows the keratinocyte's differentiation program. The oncogenes E6 and E7 are thought to modify the function of tumor suppressor gene p53 and retinoblastoma, leaving the keratinocytes cell cycle unchecked. The evidence for oncogenes E6 and E7's role in epithelial cancers is supported by the presence of HPV DNA in tumor biopsies and more specifically the expression of E6 and E7 in tumor material. Additionally, E6 and E7 proteins are required to maintain the malignant phonotype of cervical carcinoma cell lines.

14.3.2 Epidemiology

Currently the bulk of research and emphasis in studying infections caused by human papilloma viruses is placed on genital tract infections that lead to precancerous or cancerous conditions in healthy individuals including cervical intraepithelial neoplasia, cervical cancer, Bowen's disease, and verrucous carcinoma of the penis. Other less severe types lead to mostly benign skin lesions or even clinically silent infections. The prevalence of anogenital tract HPV infection in the United States is quite high with an estimated 20 million infected individuals. The annual incidence is 5.5 million. Incidence is highest among sexually active persons and according to some estimates more than 50% of these individuals are expected to be infected with anogenital HPV infection in their lifetime. With approximately 9,710 cases of cervical cancer and 3,700 deaths annually the cost related to HPV infections are enormous to health care. One study based on a database of cases in Maryland states that the cost of one HPV-related disease alone (the JORRP) costs $57,996 per case with annual cost of between $40 million and $123 million. Combine this with financial burden created by other anogenital diseases caused by HPV infections in both men and women and the dollar figure grows astounding.

14.3.3 Intervention

The CDC states that by age 50, more than 80% of American women will have contracted at least one strain of genital HPV, making them at highest risk of developing HPV-induced cancers, more specifically cervical cancer. Fortunately, development of cervical cancer induced by HPV infection is a slow process requiring many years, giving physicians an opportunity to screen individuals considered to be at risk for HPV-induced cervical cancer.

Papanicolaou (pap) testing is a popular screening test used to detect cervical cytology changes during the developmental phase of HPV-induced cervical cancer. Cells from the cervix are smeared onto a slide and examined under the microscope for presence of precancerous or abnormal cells. The test is 70–80% effective in detection of abnormal cervical cytology caused by HPV. Variations of the test are used to increase the sensitivity including liquid-based cytology known as the thin prep (sensitivity 85–95%), and a pap-HPV DNA test mainly used for women over the age of 30. Adjunct testing including the use of colposcopy and hybrid capture test (the newest FDA-approved method for detecting high risk HPV DNA) may be used if abnormal cytology is suspected. The CDC has several targeted guidelines for routine HPV testing in women to help detect and prevent HPV-induced cervical cancer.

14.3.4 Vaccine

Cervical cancer is the second leading cause of cancer-related deaths in women worldwide and nearly all cases are caused by HPV infections. Although early detection via pap testing has significantly reduced the risk of invasive cervical cancer, there still exists considerable risk. In 2006, a prophylactic HPV vaccine (Gardasil) was approved by the FDA and is currently being marketed by Merck. The vaccine is based upon one of the late proteins of the HPV DNA. The L1 protein is a capsid protein and has the ability to form a virus-like antigenic particle capable of eliciting an immune response and production of high levels of neutralizing antibodies. Gardasil protects against the high-risk type 16 and 18 and types responsible for 90% of genital warts, 6 and 11.

14.3.5 ACIP Recommendations

14.3.5.1 Routine Vaccination of Females Aged 11–12 Years

ACIP recommends routine vaccination of females aged 11–12 years with three doses of quadrivalent HPV vaccine. The vaccination series can be started as young as age 9 years.

14.3.5.2 Catch-Up Vaccination of Females Aged 13–26 Years

Vaccination also is recommended for females aged 13–26 years who have not been previously vaccinated or who have not completed the full series. Ideally, vaccine should be administered before potential exposure to HPV through sexual contact; however, females who might have already been exposed to HPV should be vaccinated. Sexually active females who have not been infected with any of the HPV vaccine types would receive full benefit from vaccination. Vaccination would provide less benefit to females if they have already been infected with one or more of the four vaccine HPV types. However, it is not possible for a clinician to assess the extent to which sexually active persons would benefit from vaccination, and the risk for HPV infection might continue as long as persons are sexually active. Pap testing and screening for HPV DNA or HPV antibody are not needed before vaccination at any age.

Vaccines for melanoma, nonmelanoma skin cancers (NMSCs) such as squamous cell and basal cell cancers, molluscum contagiosum, common warts, and chlamydia have been in trial with mixed results.

14.4 Conclusion

Although many of the cutaneous diseases reviewed in this chapter are self-limiting, they sometimes lead to serious sequelae. While herpes zoster vaccine, Zostavax, prevents shingles and related complications, Gardasil decreases HPV-induced cervical cancer and genital warts. Although yet to be seen, the universal vaccination policy against varicella is further set to decrease the incidence of herpes zoster. The future of medicine is practicing preventative medicine and we only need to study the past starting with Edward Jenner to come to such realization.

Prevention of Skin Infections

15

Dirk M. Elston

15.1 Bacterial Infections

Methicillin-sensitive *Staphylococcus aureus* accounts for most cutaneous infections, including wound infection (Fig. 15.1), folliculitis (Fig. 15.2), and impetigo. Cutaneous injuries commonly become infected. Topical antiseptics can reduce the incidence of infection, but may be contact sensitizers. While topical antibiotics may reduce the overall incidence of infection, they may also cause contact dermatitis. Those with a gram-positive spectrum may increase the likelihood that the infecting organism with be gram negative. Wound care is discussed more thoroughly in the section on prevention of surgical wound infections.

Community-acquired methicillin-resistant *Staphylococcus aureus* (CA-MRSA) has recently emerged as an important skin pathogen. CA-MRSA infections have a high attack rate among wrestlers, football players, weight lifters, and members of amateur and professional sports teams.[1-3] Pre-existing cuts or abrasions and sharing of fomites such as towels and bars of soap are important risk factors for infection. Nasal carriage is associated with sharing of towels and serves as a reservoir for recurrent infection.[4] Carriage also occurs in other moist areas, such as the axillae, groin, and perianal region. Eczematous skin is commonly colonized. CA-MRSA has also been isolated from whirlpools and taping gel.[5]

CA-MRSA strains typically contain the type IV staphylococcal chromosomal cassette that codes for methicillin resistance. Panton-valentine leukocidin (PVL) has been identified as a potent virulence factor.[6] PVL imparts a survival advantage to the organism, and it rapidly replaces other strains of staphylococci. Colonization easily spreads to close contacts. Those who are colonized have a high attack rate of clinical infection.[7,8]

Clinical infection with CA-MRSA generally begins with folliculitis and rapidly evolves into an abscess (Fig. 15.3). Early in the course of disease, pain is often severe and out of proportion to physical findings. Infection commonly begins at sites of minor abrasions such as turf-burns. In weightlifters, abscesses commonly involve the axillae. In women and young children, the thighs and buttocks are often involved. Other common sites of involvement include the neck, back, extremities, nose, and external ear canals.[9]

Prevention of cutaneous CA-MRSA infections requires preventive measures to reduce the incidence of cutaneous injury, elimination of bar soap, policies against sharing of towels, decontamination of mats and

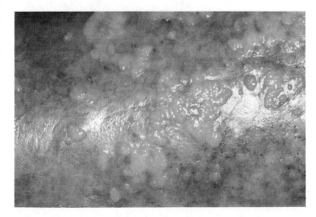

Fig. 15.1 Impetiginized wound

D.M. Elston
Department of Dermatology,
Geisinger Medical Center,
Danville, PA, USA
e-mail: dmelston@geisinger.edu

R.A. Norman (ed.), *Preventive Dermatology in Infectious Diseases*,
DOI 10.1007/978-0-85729-847-8_15, © Springer-Verlag London Limited 2012

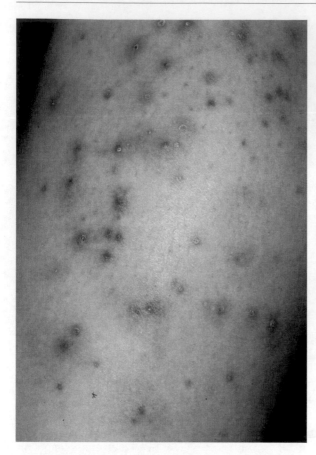

Fig. 15.2 Staphylococcal folliculitis

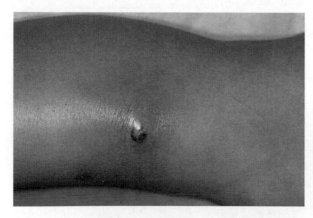

Fig. 15.3 CA-MRSA commonly presents as folliculitis that rapidly evolves to a painful abscess

equipment, as well as treatment of carriers. Cosmetic body shaving is a risk factor for CA-MRSA infection, and should be discouraged.[10]

Sodium hypochlorite (bleach) at a dilution of two tablespoons per bathtub of water can be used to reduce

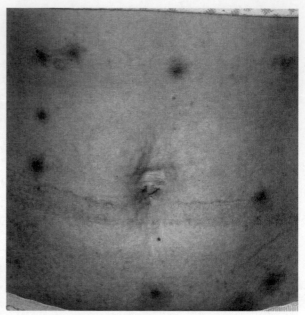

Fig. 15.4 Hot tub folliculitis

colonization of eczematous skin lesions, axillae, and groin regions. Chlorhexidine gluconate washes can also be effective, although resistance is emerging.[11,12]

Seventy percent ethanol is an effective agent for decontamination of mats and equipment.[13] The combination of alcohol and chlorhexidine has also been effective.[14] Triclosan-based hand sterilizers are suitable for use on skin and some equipment. As with chlorhexidine, triclosan resistance is emerging.[15,16] Mupirocin is commonly used for nasal colonization, but resistant strains are now common and eradication may be achieved in fewer than half of those so treated.[17,18] Retapamulin is a newer alternative, but its effectiveness in this setting must be validated in clinical studies.

Group A streptococcal infections complicating cutaneous injuries can result in impetigo, glomerulonephritis, erysipelas, and lymphangitis.[19] Prevention of streptococcal infections is similar to that for staphylococcal infections.

Exposure to fresh or salt water is associated with an increased incidence of skin infection.[20] *Pseudomonas* infections are associated with exposure to water and commonly present as folliculitis restricted to covered or intertriginous areas (hot tub or swimming pool folliculitis). The follicular papules and pustules are typically more pruritic than tender (Fig. 15.4). Warm weather or heated water are risk factors for infection, as free chlorine levels are harder to maintain in the heat. Both chlorine and bromine treated water can be a source of infection, as can contaminated plastic, rubber, or natural loofah sponges.[21,22] The implicated strain is typically type O:11, although types O:1, O:3, O:8, O:10, and O:16 have also been implicated.[23]

Most cases of *Pseudomonas* folliculitis resolve spontaneously, although fluoroquinolone treatment may be required.[24] Prevention involves elimination of standing water and wet sponges, prompt removal of wet bathing suits, and adequate chlorination. Alternative water treatments such as ozone ionization have also been used.

15.2 Viral Infections

Herpes infections (Fig. 15.5) may occur through sexual exposure or by any skin-to-skin contact. Infections are particularly common among wrestlers (herpes gladiatorum), where attack rates are as high as 34%.[25] Ocular involvement can be particularly devastating. Those with genital lesions should refrain from sexual activity during outbreaks and should be aware that asymptomatic shedding occurs. Barrier protection is only partially effective, but oral prophylaxis with acyclovir, valcyclovir, or famciclovir can prevent or reduce the spread of disease. Abrasive shirts create potential portals of entry and are a risk factor for herpes infections among wrestlers.[26] Policies to ban infected individuals from competition and discourage abrasive clothing should be enforced.

Blood-borne pathogens can be spread in the health-care setting, during sexual intercourse, or during competition. Universal precautions should be observed at all times in healthcare settings. Those with open wounds should be barred from competition. Minor wounds may be covered with impermeable adhesive dressings.

15.3 Fungal Infections

Tinea infection is common among military recruits, wrestlers, and swimmers.[27] Asymptomatic carriers are common, and fungal spores are easily recovered from moist surfaces such as the floors around swimming pool.[28,29] There is an inherited susceptibility to *Trichophyton rubrum* infection which may be inherited in an autosomal dominant fashion. Although much of the population is predisposed to infection, it is not inevitable and can certainly be delayed by simple precautions. Those with active tinea should not participate in wrestling matches. Footwear should be worn in locker rooms and other areas with foot traffic and moist floors.

15.4 Prevention of Surgical Wound Infections

The incidence of wound infections following cutaneous surgery is quite low (just over 1%), the benefits of routine antibiotic prophylaxis must be carefully weighed against the cost of treatment, the risks of adverse drug reactions, and the potential for emergence of resistant organisms.[30]

The risk of infection for Mohs surgery is slightly higher (about 2.5%). For any prolonged surgery, the risk of infection can be reduced by avoiding buried suture or allowing the wound to heal by secondary intention. A single preoperative or intraoperative dose of antibiotic can also reduce the risk of infection, but there is no benefit to courses of antibiotic longer than 48 h.[31] Many surgeons favor a single dose of a prophylactic antibiotic before surgery on a site such as the hand where a postoperative infection could be catastrophic. An alternative to prophylaxis with a systemic antibiotic is to add clindamycin to the local anesthetic.[32] This results in a reduction in surgical site infection (to below 1%) with undetectable blood levels and no risk of contributing to the emergence of

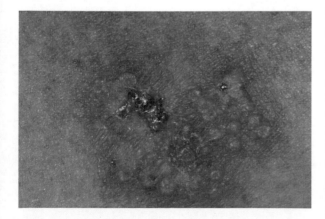

Fig. 15.5 Herpes simplex virus infection

resistant organisms. Clindamycin is also suitable for use in patients with a history of penicillin allergy. The solution is prepared by adding 0.15 mL of clindamycin (150 mg/mL) to 50 mg of lidocaine with 5 mL 8.4% bicarbonate. This results in at concentration of clindamycin of 408 mg/mL.

Elimination of nasopharyngeal staphylococcal colonization with chlorhexidine intranasal ointment and oropharyngeal rinse 4 times daily during the pre-and postoperative periods reduced the incidence of nosocomial infections including respiratory infection, bacteremia, and deep surgical site infections.[33] Data on the use of intranasal mupirocin have generally been disappointing. Studies are needed to determine if newer topical antibiotics such as retapamulin will perform better.

Postoperative use of a topical antibiotic ointment results in a small decrease in the incidence of wound infection at the expense of a significant risk of allergic contact dermatitis. In a randomized, double-blind trial of white petrolatum compared to bacitracin ointment, the infection rate was 1.5% with the former and 0.9% with the latter.[34] Allergic contact dermatitis occurred in 0.9% of those treated with bacitracin. Infections in the bacitracin group were more likely to be gram negative infections, and antibiotics needed to treat them were more expensive. These data make a strong case for the routine use of white petrolatum postoperatively.

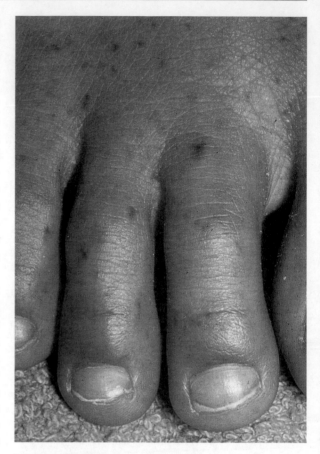

Fig. 15.6 Rocky mountain spotted fever

15.5 Prevention of Arthropod-Borne Infections

Insect bites and stings commonly become infected. Vector-borne illnesses such as leishmaniasis present mainly in the skin. Other diseases such as Rocky Mountain spotted fever (Fig. 15.6) and viral fevers may present with petechial or hemorrhagic skin lesions. Avoidance of infested areas as well as consistent use of repellents and protective clothing can reduce the incidence of infection. Chemoprophylaxis and attention to screening or mosquito netting is important when traveling. At home, public health measures to reduce mosquito and tick populations are important.

In the United States, mosquitoes are vectors for West Nile fever, St. Louis encephalitis, equine encephalitis, dengue, and malaria. North American ticks carry Lyme disease, Rocky Mountain spotted fever, ehrlichiosis, Colorado tick fever, relapsing fever, tularemia, and babesiosis. Homeless patients with ectoparasitic infestation have a high prevalence of infection with *Bartonella quintana*, a cause of endocarditis.[35-37] Fleas transmit plague, bacillary angomatosis, and endemic typhus. Sandflies transmit leishmaniasis. In the United States, *Leishmania mexicana* produces chronic crusted and ulcerative lesions, while *L. donovani* can produce subcutaneous nodules.

Primary prevention of vector-borne disease requires drainage of stagnant water, insecticide spraying programs, use of repellents, and prompt tick removal. Secondary prevention can be accomplished with chemoprophylaxis or early treatment of illness. Anopheline mosquitoes that carry malaria feed mostly at night. Transmission is prevented by staying indoors at night, use of repellents and pyrethroid-impregnated mosquito netting. Mosquitoes that carry dengue tend to bite during the day, and repellents and protective clothing are especially important to prevent transmission.[38,39] Carbon-dioxide–emitting mosquito traps such are helpful. Chemical attractants such as octenol and butanone are often used, although some Culex mosquitoes are repelled by octenol.[40-42]

DEET (*N,N*-diethyl-3-methylbenzamide) is the most commonly used repellent for the prevention of mosquito and sandfly bites. Overall, it has a good safety record, although rare cases of bullous dermatitis, anaphylaxis, and toxic encephalopathy have been reported.[43-46] The American Academy of Pediatrics recommends slow-release products that plateau in efficacy at concentrations of 30%. Many extended duration products formulated for children have concentrations of 10% of less. DEET can be applied to exposed skin and to clothing. The addition of permethrin-treated clothing increases efficacy against a wide range of biting arthropods.[47,48] For those who cannot use DEET, picaridin is a good alternative. A soybean-oil-based product (Bite Blocker for Kids) is suitable for those who wish to avoid chemical repellents. It is not as effective as DEET or picaridin. Citronella has limited efficacy.[49] Neem oil performs better.[50]

Permethrin, applied to clothing, has good efficacy against ticks and chiggers.[47,48] The effect lasts through a number of wash cycles.[51] Permethrin can be applied to clothing, tents, sleeping bags, and mosquito netting. Although southwest Asian camel ticks are attracted by permethrin, this phenomenon has not been reported in North America.[52] Exclusion of deer by means of fencing has been shown to be effective in reducing the number of disease-carrying ticks.[53,54] Feeding stations can be outfitted to deliver topical acaricides to deer.[55-57] Leaf debris should be removed, as ticks are susceptible to dehydration if they do not have access to a layer of leaf debris.[58,59] Ticks are unlikely to transmit disease if they are removed promptly.[60-62] When removing the tick, care should be taken not to squeeze it.[63] The Tick Nipper is an inexpensive plastic device that makes tick removal quite easy.

Fleas can be controlled with lufenuron, a maturation inhibitor that prevents fleas from becoming fertile. It is marketed in oral and injectable formulations for both cats and dogs. Fipronil can be applied to pets to prevent flea and tick infestation.[64] Pet owners should consult a veterinarian for specific recommendations.

References

1. Cohen PR. Cutaneous community-acquired methicillin-resistant *Staphylococcus aureus* infection in participants of athletic activities. *South Med J*. 2005;98(6):596–602
2. Arnold FW, Wojda B. An analysis of a community-acquired pathogen in a Kentucky community: methicillin-resistant *Staphylococcus aureus*. *J Ky Med Assoc*. 2005;103(5): 206–210
3. Centers for Disease Control and Prevention (CDC). Methicillin-resistant *Staphylococcus aureus* infections among competitive sports participants – Colorado, Indiana, Pennsylvania, and Los Angeles County, 2000–2003. *MMWR Morb Mortal Wkly Rep*. 2003;52(33): 793–795
4. Nguyen DM, Mascola L, Brancoft E. Recurring methicillin-resistant *Staphylococcus aureus* infections in a football team. *Emerg Infect Dis*. 2005;11(4):526–532
5. Kazakova SV, Hageman JC, Matava M, et al A clone of methicillin-resistant *Staphylococcus aureus* among professional football players. *N Engl J Med*. 2005;352(5):468–475
6. Carleton HA, Diep BA, Charlebois ED, et al Community-adapted methicillin-resistant *Staphylococcus aureus* (MRSA): population dynamics of an expanding community reservoir of MRSA. *J Infect Dis*. 2004;190(10):1730–1738
7. Calfee DP, Durbin LJ, Germanson TP, et al Spread of methicillin-resistant *Staphylococcus aureus* (MRSA) among household contacts of individuals with nosocomially acquired MRSA. *Infect Control Hosp Epidemiol*. 2003;24(6): 422–426
8. Ellis MW, Hospenthal DR, Dooley DP, et al Natural history of community-acquired methicillin-resistant *Staphylococcus aureus* colonization and infection in soldiers. *Clin Infect Dis*. 2004;39(7):971–979
9. Wang J, Barth S, Richardson M, et al An outbreak of methicillin-resistant *Staphylococcus aureus* cutaneous infection in a saturation diving facility. *Undersea Hyperb Med*. 2003; 30(4):277–284
10. Begier EM, Frenette K, Barrett NL, et al Connecticut bioterrorism field epidemiology response team. A high-morbidity outbreak of methicillin-resistant *Staphylococcus aureus* among players on a college football team, facilitated by cosmetic body shaving and turf burns. *Clin Infect Dis*. 2004;39(10):1446–1453
11. Block C, Robenshtok E, Simhon A, et al Evaluation of chlorhexidine and povidone iodine activity against methicillin-resistant *Staphylococcus aureus* and vancomycin-resistant *Enterococcus faecalis* using a surface test. *J Hosp Infect*. 2000;46(2):147–152
12. Zhang YH, Liu X Y, Zhu LL, et al Study on the resistance of methicillin-resistant *Staphylococcus aureus* to iodophor and chlorhexidine. *Zhonghua Liu Xing Bing Xue Za Zhi*. 2004; 25(3):248–250
13. Suzuki J, Komatsuzawa H, Kozai K, et al In vitro susceptibility of *Staphylococcus aureus* including MRSA to four disinfectants. *ASDC J Dent Child*. 1997;64(4):260–263
14. Kampf G, Jarosch R, Ruden H. Limited effectiveness of chlorhexidine based hand disinfectants against methicillin-resistant *Staphylococcus aureus* (MRSA). *J Hosp Infect*. 1998;38(4):297–303

15. Brenwald NP, Fraise AP. Triclosan resistance in methicillin-resistant *Staphylococcus aureus* (MRSA). *J Hosp Infect.* 2003;55(2):141–144

16. Bamber AI, Neal TJ. An assessment of triclosan susceptibility in methicillin-resistant and methicillin-sensitive *Staphylococcus aureus. J Hosp Infect.* 1999;41(2):107–109

17. Harbarth S, Dharan S, Liassine N, et al Randomized, placebo-controlled, double-blind trial to evaluate the efficacy of mupirocin for eradicating carriage of methicillin-resistant *Staphylococcus aureus. Antimicrob Agents Chemother.* 1999;43(6):1412–1416

18. Mulvey MR, MacDougall L, Cholin B, et al Saskatchewan CA-MRSA Study Group. Community-associated methicillin-resistant *Staphylococcus aureus*, Canada. *Emerg Infect Dis.* 2005;11(6):844–850

19. Falck G. Group A streptococcal infections after indoor association football tournament. *Lancet.* 1996;347:840

20. Shephard RJ. Science and medicine of canoeing and kayaking. *Sports Med.* 1987;4:19

21. Penn C, et al Pseudomonas folliculitis: and outbreak associated with bromine-based disinfectants. *Can Dis Wkly Rep.* 1990;16:31

22. Zichichi L, Asta G, Noto G. Pseudomonas aeruginosa folliculitis after shower/bath exposure. *Int J Dermatol.* 2000; 39:270–273

23. Maniatis AN, et al Pseudomonas aeruginosa folliculitis due to non-O:11 serotypes: acquisition through the use of contaminated synthetic sponges. *Clin Infect Dis.* 1995;21:437

24. Rolston KV, et al Pseudomonas aeruginosa infection in cancer patients. *Cancer Invest.* 1992;10:43

25. Belogna EA, et al An outbreak of herpes gladiatorum at a high school wrestling camp. *N Engl J Med.* 1991;325:906

26. Strauss RH, et al Abrasive shirts may contribute to herpes gladiatorum among wrestlers. *N Engl J Med.* 1989;320:598

27. Adams B. Tinea corporis gladiatorum: a cross-sectional study. *J Am Acad Dermatol.* 2000;43:1039–1041

28. Bolanos B. Dermatophyte feet infection among students enrolled in swimming pool courses at a university pool. *Bull Assoc Med Puerto Rico.* 1991;83:181

29. Auger P, et al Epidemiology of tinea pedis in marathon runners: prevalence of occult athlete's foot. *Mycoses.* 1993;36:35

30. Whitaker DC, Grande DJ, Johnson SS. Wound infection rate in dermatologic surgery. *J Dermatol Surg Oncol.* 1988;14: 525–528

31. Griego RD, Zitelli JA. Intra-incisional prophylactic antibiotics for dermatologic surgery. *Arch Dermatol.* 1998;134:688–692

32. Huether MJ, Griego RD, Brodland DG, Zitelli JA. Clindamycin for intraincisional antibiotic prophylaxis in dermatologic surgery. *Arch Dermatol.* 2002;138:1145–1148

33. Segers P, Speekenbrink RG, Ubbink DT, et al Prevention of nosocomial infection in cardiac surgery by decontamination of the nasopharynx and oropharynx with chlorhexidine gluconate: a randomized controlled trial. *JAMA.* 2006;296(20): 2460–2466

34. Smack DP, Harrington AC, Dunn C, et al Infection and allergy incidence in ambulatory surgery patients using white petrolatum vs bacitracin ointment. A randomized controlled trial. *JAMA.* 1996;276:972–977

35. Guibal F, de La Salmoniere P, Rybojad M, et al High seroprevalence to Bartonella Quintana in homeless patients with cutaneous parasitic infestations in downtown Paris. *J Am Acad Dermatol.* 2001;44:219–223

36. Foucault C, Barrau K, Brouqui P, Raoult D. Bartonella quintana bacteremia among homeless People. *Clin Infect Dis.* 2002;35(6):684–689

37. Raoult D, Foucault C, Brouqui P. Infections in the homeless. *Lancet Infect Dis.* 2001;1(2):77–84

38. Coosemans M, Van Gompel A. The principal arthropod vectors of disease. What are the risks of travellers' to be bitten? To be infected? *Bull Soc Pathol Exotique.* 1998;91:467–473

39. Carnevale P. Protection of travelers against biting arthropod vectors. *Bull Soc Pathol Exotique.* 1998;91:474–485

40. Rueda LM, Harrison BA, Brown JS, et al Evaluation of 1-octen-3-ol, carbon dioxide, and light as attractants for mosquitoes associated with two distinct habitats in North Carolina. *J Am Mosq Control Assoc.* 2001;17(1):61–66

41. Kline DL. Comparison of two American biophysics mosquito traps: the professional and a new counterflow geometry trap. *J Am Mosq Control Assoc.* 1999;15(3):276–282

42. Kline DL, Mann MO. Evaluation of butanone, carbon dioxide, and 1-octen-3-OL as attractants for mosquitoes associated with north central Florida bay and cypress swamps. *J Am Mosq Control Assoc.* 1998;14(3):289–297

43. Brown M, Hebert AA. Insect repellents: an overview. *J Am Acad Dermatol.* 1997;36:243–249

44. Fradin MS. Mosquitoes and mosquito repellents: a clinician's guide. *Ann Intern Med.* 1998;128:931–940

45. McKinlay JR, Ross V, Barrett TL. Vesiculobullous reaction to diethyltoluamide revisted. *Cutis.* 1998;62:44

46. Miller JD. Anaphylaxis associated with insect repellent. *N Engl J Med.* 1982;307:1341–1342

47. Young GD, Evans S. Safety and efficacy of DEET and permethrin in the prevention of arthropod attack. *Mil Med.* 1998;163:324–330

48. Gupta RK, Sweeny AW, Rutledge LC. Effectiveness of controlled-release personal use arthropod repellent and permethrin-treated clothing in the field. *J Mosq Contr Assoc.* 1987;3:556–560

49. Lindsay LR, Surgeoner GA, Heal JD, Gallivan GJ. Evaluation of the efficacy of 3% citronella candles and 5% citronella incense for protection against field populations of Aedes mosquitoes. *J Am Mosq Contr Assoc.* 1996;12: 293–294

50. Caraballo AJ. Mosquito repellent action of Neemos. *J Am Mosq Contr Assoc.* 2000;16:45–46

51. Schreck CE, Mount GA, Carlson DA. Wear and wash persistence of permethrin used as a clothing treatment for personal protection against the lone star tick (Acari: Ixodidae). *J Med Entomol.* 1982;19:143–146

52. Fryauff DJ, Shoukry MA, Schreck CE. Stimulation of attachment in the camel tick, Hyalomma dromedarii (Acari: Ixodidae): the unintended result of sublethal exposure to permethrin-impregnated fabric. *J Med Entomol.* 1994;31:23–29

53. Stafford KC 3 rd. Reduced abundance of Ixodes scapularis (Acari: Ixodidae) with exclusion of deer by electric fencing. *J Med Entomol.* 1993;30(6):986–996

54. Daniels TJ, Fish D, Schwartz I. Reduced abundance of Ixodes scapularis (Acari: Ixodidae) and Lyme disease risk by deer exclusion. *J Med Entomol.* 1993;30(6):1043–1049

55. Mount GA, Haile DG, Daniels E. Simulation of management strategies for the blacklegged tick (Acari: Ixodidae)

and the Lyme disease spirochete, Borrelia burgdorferi. *J Med Entomol.* 1997;34(6):672–683

56. Pound JM, Miller JA, George JE. Efficacy of amitraz applied to white-tailed deer by the '4-poster' topical treatment device in controlling free-living lone star ticks (Acari: Ixodidae). *J Med Entomol.* 2000;37(6):878–884

57. Solberg VB, Miller JA, Hadfield T, et al Control of Ixodes scapularis (Acari: Ixodidae) with topical self-application of permethrin by white-tailed deer inhabiting NASA, Beltsville, Maryland. *J Vector Ecol.* 2003;28(1):117–134

58. Strey OF, Teel PD, Longnecker MT, Needham GR. Survival and water-balance characteristics of unfed Amblyomma cajennense (Acari: Ixodidae). *J Med Entomol.* 1996;33: 63–73

59. Slowik TJ, Lane RS. Nymphs of the western black-legged tick (Ixodes pacificus) collected from tree trunks in woodland-grass habitat. *J Vector Ecol.* 2001;26(2):165–171

60. Katavolos P, Armstrong PM, Dawson JE, Telford SR 3rd. Duration of tick attachment required for transmission of granulocytic ehrlichiosis. *J Infect Dis.* 1998; 177(5):1422–1425

61. Berger BW, Johnson RC, Kodner C, Coleman L. Cultivation of Borrelia burgdorferi from human tick bite sites: a guide to the risk of infection. *J Am Acad Dermatol.* 1995;32(2 Pt 1): 184–187

62. Piesman J, Mather TN, Sinsky RJ, Spielman A. Duration of tick attachment and Borrelia burgdorferi transmission. *J Clin Microbiol.* 1987;25(3):557–558

63. Piesman J, Dolan MC. Protection against lyme disease spirochete transmission provided by prompt removal of nymphal Ixodes scapularis (Acari: Ixodidae). *Med Entomol.* 2002;39(3):509–512

64. Young DR, Arther RG, Davis WL. Evaluation of K9 Advantix vs. Frontline Plus topical treatments to repel brown dog ticks (Rhipicephalus sanguineus) on dogs. *Parasitol Res.* 2003;90(Suppl 3):S116–S118

Index

MIX
Papier aus verantwortungsvollen Quellen
Paper from responsible sources
FSC® C105338

FSC
www.fsc.org

Printed by Books on Demand, Germany